W9-BZN-921

ATOMIC DOCTORS

Atomic Doctors

Conscience and Complicity at the Dawn of the Nuclear Age

JAMES L. NOLAN, JR.

THE BELKNAP PRESS OF
HARVARD UNIVERSITY PRESS
Cambridge, Massachusetts
London, England
2020

Printed in the United States of America

Second printing

Library of Congress Cataloging-in-Publication Data is available from loc.gov
ISBN: 978-0-674-24863-2 (cloth)

To *Póvi Tsáy*

Contents

ATOMIC DOCTORS

Introduction

On the morning of June 17, 1945, Captain James F. Nolan, MD, boarded a plane in Albuquerque, New Mexico. In his briefcase was a highly sensitive report prepared by Nolan, along with other Manhattan Project physicians and two physicists, that expressed concerns about potential radioactive fallout from what would be the first nuclear bomb ever exploded. The plutonium bomb, or Gadget, as it was called, was scheduled for detonation in the Alamogordo bombing range of New Mexico in less than a month. Nolan and his colleagues hoped to persuade General Leslie Groves, military head of the Manhattan Project, to approve safety and evacuation procedures for the so-called Trinity test. After a flight delay, a missed connection, and a long train ride from Cincinnati to Knoxville, Nolan finally arrived at the Oak Ridge Site of the Manhattan District at six thirty the next morning. At Oak Ridge, about twenty-five miles outside Knoxville, Nolan eventually met with the large and imposing Groves, who was not at all pleased to receive the report.

Groves made Nolan sit outside his office while he read the document and discussed it with his aides. When he finished, Groves called Nolan in and addressed him dismissively: "What are you, some kind of Hearst propagandist?" The comment—with its reference to William Randolph Hearst, known for his sensationalist journalism—was indicative of Groves's overriding concerns with security and secrecy. He feared that if the proposed plan were implemented, information about the top-secret Manhattan Project might leak out to people living near the Alamogordo bombing range. Such a response from Groves was not unexpected. In Nolan's view, the military was concerned only with making a bomb for the purposes of warfare; worries about radiation hazards "were entirely secondary." Groves, in Nolan's words, "had rifle-barrel vision," which "made him a great soldier" but limited him to "thinking only of the security aspect."[1] As it turned out, the Manhattan Project physicians were right to be worried about fallout from the Trinity test. Groves eventually approved some of the safety measures, but concerns about the long-term effects of radiation on the region around the test site persist to this day.

Although the Manhattan Project doctors warned the military about dangerous fallout from the Trinity test, they also participated in downplaying the harmful effects of radiation following the test. The doctors' complicated role in this instance is emblematic of what happened a number of times at the dawn of the nuclear age. Manhattan Project doctors would offer warnings, particularly with respect to the dangers of radiation exposure. Military leaders would not take the warnings seriously, giving greater weight to military and scientific concerns. Doctors would then be put in a position of helping the military to hide or minimize the negative consequences of radiation exposure, often out of fear of litigation.

Atomic Doctors focuses on the physicians who were involved in the Manhattan Project, paying particular attention to Nolan, as well as his colleagues Louis Hempelmann and Stafford Warren—all of whom were part of the project from its earliest days and then played important roles in the unfolding drama of the atomic age. All three doctors had training in radiology and thus knew more than most about radiation—the critical and defining, yet mysterious, feature of the new weapon. How they gained and managed their knowledge about radiation, and how they treated (or didn't treat) those who were affected by it, is a central theme of this book. It's a theme that intersects with the continuing debate about the necessity and morality of detonating, and then continuing to develop and stockpile, atomic weapons. We will see how the doctors were used, with or without their cooperation, either to support or to refute competing historical narratives about the atom bomb.

James F. Nolan was my grandfather. I first became aware of the nature and scope of his contribution to the Manhattan Project when my mother visited me several months after my dad had passed away. She brought with her a box of materials that no one else in the family even knew existed. When I opened the box and began sorting through its contents, I was astonished by what I found. The box contained a treasure trove of data about my grandfather and his role in the Manhattan Project. I discovered photographs of the Trinity test, the USS *Indianapolis,* Tinian Island, Bikini Island, and Hiroshima and Nagasaki (taken just weeks after the bombs were dropped on the two cities). Also inside were my grandfather's military papers, travel itineraries, artifacts, souvenirs, weather maps, newspaper clippings, written accounts of his experience, and correspondence, including with Robert Oppenheimer, the scientific head of the Manhattan Project.

Discovery of this material marked the beginning of my own journey through the early nuclear age, with my grandfather acting as my guide. In a sense, Nolan served as my Virgil, taking me through a divine comedy of sorts. He introduced me to fascinating people, including those who had visions of a technophilic new paradise. He also showed me a horrifying inferno—the image conveyed by the Japanese doctors with whom Nolan interacted in Hiroshima and Nagasaki immediately after the war. The contents of my grandfather's secret box of materials led me on exploratory trips to a number of archives across the United States, to Los Alamos and Oak Ridge, to the San Ildefonso Pueblo, to a reunion in Indiana with the still-living survivors of the USS *Indianapolis,* and to Hiroshima and Nagasaki. The more I explored, the more interesting and troubling the story became. The Virgil image also works in the sense that the story is not so much about Nolan—though he is clearly a central figure—as it is about the dramatic and utterly transformative historical period he lived through.

My grandfather participated in many of the crucial events of this period. He was involved in some way with the first eight nuclear bombs ever detonated. He was there at Los Alamos—indeed, he was one of the first recruits. He helped plan the safety and evacuation measures for the Trinity test. He was one of two men tasked with escorting Little Boy, the bomb that would be dropped on Hiroshima, from Los Alamos to the Pacific Islands. He was one of the first Americans to visit Japan and investigate the bomb sites after the war. He was present for the subsequent atomic tests on the Bikini and Enewetak Atolls in the Marshall Islands. And, at the very end of his life, he joined about one hundred others to attend the fortieth reunion of the start of the Manhattan Project in Los Alamos, an event that provided the scientists who built the bomb an opportunity for tortured reflection on all that had become of their invention. This book follows Nolan through these episodes and considers the ethical and medical issues faced by the doctors working on the project.

My interest in my grandfather's journey is more than personal and more than historical. As a sociologist with a long-standing interest in the role of technology in modern society, I find that Nolan's story provides insights into our fraught relations with technology. Discovery of the bomb generated a host of nuclear technologies—in the military, in energy, and in medicine—along with a variety of related technologies that continue to shape our lives. Lessons from the early atomic age help us deepen our understanding of how humans engage not only with nuclear and nuclear-engendered technologies but also with such emerging technologies as genetic engineering, robotics, and nanotechnology. The forceful impact of technology, nuclear and otherwise, on human life is one of the multiple meanings of "delivering little boy" that will be explored as we follow Nolan's passage through the early atomic age.

1

Life at Los Alamos

It was the best of times, it was the worst of times . . . it was the spring of hope, it was the winter of despair, we had everything before us, we had nothing before us, we were all going direct to Heaven, we were all going direct the other way.

—Charles Dickens, *Tale of Two Cities*

The youngest of three brothers, James Findley Nolan was born in Chicago on September 5, 1915, to Joseph and Bernice Nolan. When he was five years old, the family moved to St. Louis, where he would reside until leaving for college in 1931. For high school, my grandfather attended the John Burroughs School, where he met his future wife, my grandmother, Ann Lawry. Nolan spent his undergraduate years at the University of Missouri, from which he graduated in 1935, and attended the Washington School of Medicine in St. Louis, where he completed his MD in 1938. His parents, who were not wealthy, dedicated what resources they had to helping their youngest son complete medical school. Nolan's two older brothers, Joe Jr. and Eugene, would instead enter the military.

James Nolan married Ann Lawry in August 1936. Two years later and just a couple of months after Nolan graduated from medical school, they welcomed a son, my father, James Lawry Nolan, into the world. Following medical school, Dr. Nolan completed a one-year internship in surgery, followed by three years of residency and assistantships in obstetrics and gynecology, all in St. Louis–area hospitals. In 1942, Nolan moved with his young family to New York City to take up a fellowship at Memorial Hospital for more specialized training in physics and radiation therapy for the purposes of treating gynecologic cancer. This particular specialty had been a growing interest of Nolan's since encountering the reputable radiology department at Washington University.[1]

Nolan's fellowship at Memorial Hospital was cut short in February 1943 when he received a life-changing phone call from Louis Hempelmann, a good friend and medical school classmate. Hempelmann, who graduated the same year as did Nolan, had spent six months at Berkeley in 1941 on a Commonwealth Fellowship, during which time he met Robert Oppenheimer. A few weeks before calling Nolan, Hempelmann had met with Oppenheimer in Chicago. The new scientific director of the Manhattan Project very candidly briefed Hempelmann on the purpose of the project and invited him to lead the Health Group at Los Alamos. "He was very open about it," Hempelmann recollected. "He said they were going to try to make an atomic bomb."[2] Hempelmann, however, wasn't Oppenheimer's first choice. Oppenheimer had originally invited John Lawrence, brother of Berkeley physicist Ernest Lawrence, to head up the "medical and health aspects" of the work in Los Alamos. When John declined because of other commitments, Oppenheimer asked him to suggest someone else. He recommended his friend and squash partner, Louis Hempelmann.[3]

Nolan also wasn't Oppenheimer's first choice. He had initially invited Hannah Peters, a close friend and the wife of Bernard Peters, one of Oppenheimer's doctoral students at Berkeley, "to take care of the health of the community." It's not entirely clear why the Peters ultimately did not go to Los Alamos. "They were coming out there," said Hempelmann. "Then they didn't, or couldn't or something. I don't know the exact story there."[4] Hempelmann probably knew more than he was willing to admit in this instance, as it's likely the Peters didn't go to Los Alamos because of their communist affiliations and their failure to pass the security clearance.[5]

When things didn't work out with Hannah Peters, Hempelmann recommended Nolan instead, an outcome Hempelmann regarded as very fortunate. "And I say fortunately, because I met her [Peters], when I moved to Rochester in 1950. She had the laboratory next to me. And she was the nicest person in the world and very bright. She could no more handle the surgery and the obstetrics here than I could. And I know that I would have had to do all of this and I am not very good at this sort of thing. So, fortunately, when she dropped out, Oppie asked me if I knew of anybody."[6] At this point he turned to Nolan. "My friend Nolan," explained Hempelmann, "had been trained as a surgeon, as an obstetrician, and he had also been involved in using radium to treat cancer patients. He was a very down-to-earth, practical, person and an excellent doctor."[7]

After accepting the offer to join the nascent Manhattan Project in late February 1943, Nolan, as he recounted, was taken "on a strange secret mission to Washington to meet Dr. Oppenheimer and General Groves, where I was filled in on the idea of the Manhattan District and was, of course, briefed on secrecy."[8] It's significant and telling that secrecy was the memorable idea communicated to Nolan in this very first meeting with Groves and Oppenheimer, as secrecy would be an oft-repeated theme that would define and have serious consequences for the Manhattan Project and for Nolan's participation on it.

At this initial meeting, Oppenheimer asked Nolan to recruit several nurses to join him in working at the hospital to be built on the mesa. Oppie, as he was commonly called, thought that having medical facilities in place would aid his efforts in recruiting top physicists to the project. "I think that it will be reassuring to the people who come in," Oppenheimer wrote to Nolan in early March, "that we have a doctor and a nurse or two available."[9] A few days later, Nolan confirmed with Oppenheimer the good news that he had successfully recruited two "willing and able" nurses from St. Louis—Harriet "Petey" Peterson and Sara Dawson. St. Louis would serve as the primary recruiting place for most of the medical staff who worked at the Los Alamos Hospital during the war.[10] Nolan was pleased not only that Peterson and Dawson were prepared to relocate quickly but also that both had training in pediatrics, an expertise, as would soon become clear, that would prove invaluable for work in the remote military hospital.[11]

In late March, Nolan and Hempelmann joined Oppenheimer in Los Alamos to survey the mesa at the base of the Jemez Mountains in New Mexico.[12] At the time, though construction was already under way, no one was living at the site except one soldier whose quarters were furnished with little more than a sleeping bag. The only functional buildings on the property were from the former Los Alamos Ranch School, an institution that had been in operation since 1917 but that had just been forced off the mesa by the military in order to build the secret wartime lab. The members of the school's 1943 graduating class were made to accelerate their studies in order to participate in a late January graduation ceremony.

After the survey trip in March, it was decided that Hempelmann would remain a civilian and work in the Technical Area, or Tech Area, as it was known, monitoring radiation hazards, while Nolan would enter the military and serve as post surgeon for the new hospital, providing for the general medical needs of the community. This particular division of labor was never strictly observed, as the two friends aided each other in their respective assignments. Particularly during the first year in Los Alamos, when radiation issues were less pressing in the lab, Hempelmann would help out at the hospital.[13]

Likewise, Nolan was never too far from the health and safety concerns of the lab. Even in Oppenheimer's first letter to Nolan, he discussed not only matters related to setting up a hospital but also the need for medical personnel to help with blood counts. Oppenheimer wrote to Nolan, "Our whole radiological program will depend on having these counts made early in the game before there are any radiation hazards."[14] Oppenheimer thus conveyed both that he expected Nolan would be involved in some aspects of radiation safety and that he was keenly aware of the hazards to which workers would soon be exposed once the processed uranium and plutonium began to arrive at the lab. It was initially understood that the medical staff would serve a small community of several hundred people. However, the population at Los Alamos grew steadily and eventually surpassed, by a considerable margin, original estimates. Indeed, by the end of the war the population at Los Alamos exceeded 6,500 civilian and military personnel.

Also recruited to the Manhattan Project at this time was Stafford Warren, a 1922 graduate of the University of California Medical School, who had, since 1926, been on the faculty of the University of Rochester in the Department of Radiology. The older and more experienced Warren was recruited directly by Groves to serve as the chief medical officer for the Manhattan District. However, the forty-six-year-old Warren would be stationed not in Los Alamos but at Oak Ridge, Tennessee, which had become the new official headquarters for the Manhattan Engineer District. At approximately the same time that Nolan and Hempelmann were visiting Los Alamos in March 1943, Warren and Hymer Friedell, another early medical recruit to the Manhattan Project, were surveying an expanse of land twenty-five miles outside Knoxville, Tennessee, which would become the home of Site X. Here, too, major construction was under way for the development of the enormous Clinton Engineer Works, which would ultimately produce the purified uranium (U-235) for the Little Boy bomb to be dropped on Hiroshima.

It was determined that Warren, like Nolan, should enter the military. Warren insisted that he be given the rank of colonel. Unlike Nolan, who was never really comfortable with military life, Warren relished his role as an army officer. According to one account, he showed up on his first day of work "in combat boots with a .45 revolver strapped to his waist."[15] Of these three primary Manhattan Project doctors—Nolan, Hempelmann, and Warren—the last identified most closely with the military character of the operation. As journalist Eileen Welsome observes, though "Warren was also a scientist . . . he clearly saw himself as a military officer whose loyalty belonged to General Groves."[16]

This particular allegiance resulted in a bit of tension between Warren and some of the other doctors, including Robert Stone, who had become the head of the Health Division of the Metallurgical Lab, or Met Lab, in Chicago, though still in a civilian capacity. Friedell, who became Warren's deputy at Oak Ridge, recalled that almost immediately after Warren became the chief medical officer of the Manhattan District, as an army colonel, "there was polarization between the army and the University of Chicago, particularly Dr. Stone."[17] The division, as such, was rooted in the essential differences between a scientific and a military perspective, a clash, as we will see, that was evident in a broader sense at Los Alamos as well.[18]

In keeping with Groves's emphasis on compartmentalization—that is, that one should only be concerned with, and know about, one's particular assignment—Warren was not, at first, allowed to visit Los Alamos. During the first year of the project, he did not even know about Los Alamos.[19] Hempelmann acknowledged that "in the early days of the Manhattan Project, Staff Warren was not allowed to come out here. And the reason is known only to General Groves."[20] After encountering Warren at a meeting (likely in Chicago), Hempelmann determined that it would be useful for Warren to visit Los Alamos. He and Nolan then successfully appealed to Oppenheimer to make this happen. As Nolan recalled, "We convinced Oppie to get SW [Stafford Warren] to come here so we could get things done!"[21] Because Warren reported directly to Groves, the Los Alamos doctors thought that, with Warren more directly involved, they would have more of a voice with the general. Thereafter, the chief medical officer of the project would visit Site Y with some frequency.[22] During these trips, Warren typically stopped by Oppenheimer's office, chatted with his secretary, Priscilla Green, and sometimes had a cup of coffee with the director, though on these occasions he "was always accompanied by either

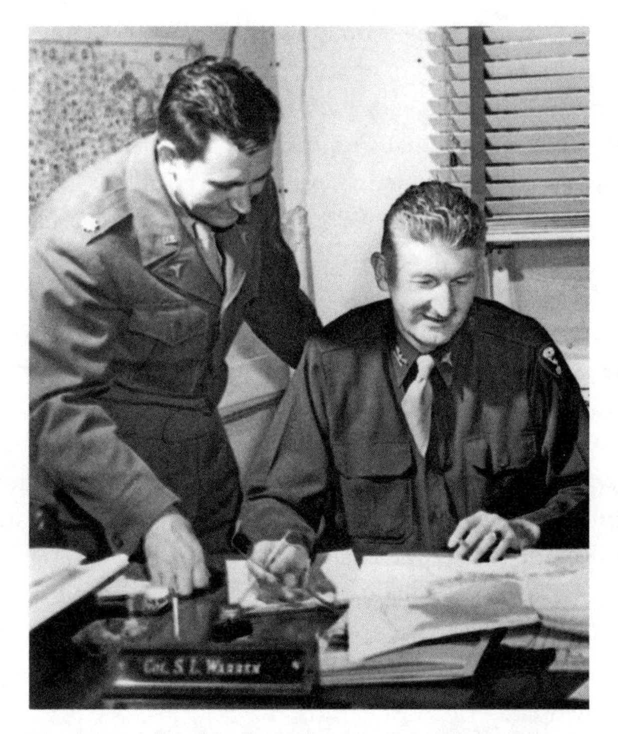

Hymer Friedell and Stafford Warren at Oak Ridge, 1945.

Nolan or Hempelmann," with whom he spent most of his time while visiting Los Alamos.[23]

Competing Paradigms

Present on the Manhattan Project, beginning in 1943, then, were three unique professional communities, which emphasized distinct, and sometimes conflicting, vocational characteristics: the academics, the military, and the much smaller community of medical doctors. The academics were primarily concerned with scientific discovery. Was it possible to harness the energy of an atom into a nuclear explosion? The Manhattan Project scientists, including eight Nobel Prize winners, were from the country's (and the world's) leading universities.[24] They were accustomed to the open exchange of ideas through seminar-style discussions and colloquia. The military, on the other hand, wanted a bomb for combat purposes. It emphasized secrecy, security, and a strict hierarchy of authority. Instead of the open sharing of ideas, it wanted an operational structure with clearly defined compartmentalization of tasks.

Much has been written about the tension between the military and the scientists on the Manhattan Project. The academics chafed against the military culture, and the military cared little for the scientists.[25] Groves referred disparagingly to the academics at Los Alamos as "the children," "long hairs," the "greatest bunch of prima donnas ever assembled in one place," or, even more unflatteringly, "the largest collection of crackpots ever seen."[26] The unfavorable feelings were rather mutual, as many in the scientific community disliked Groves and the regimented and security-conscious ways of the military, whom they referred to as fascists.

As Jane Wilson, wife of the Princeton physicist Robert Wilson put it, "Security was almost always inconsistent, often high-handed, and sometimes unjust. As a group, we civilians disliked the security office."[27] Or as the physicist Joseph Hirschfelder characterized the relationship between Groves and the scientific community, "He [Groves] never understood the scientists and they thoroughly hated him."[28] Such an attitude led to many complaints and frequent roasts of the military, and of Groves in particular. "We poked fun at security and censorship," Eleanor Jette, wife of the metallurgist Eric Jette, remembered, "and barbecued Our General to a lush, crisp brown at regular intervals. We garnished him with the things we lacked and flamed him with rum before we served him."[29]

The medical doctors were marginally part of both communities but not fully members of either. At least in theory, they were principally focused on matters of health and safety, on preserving and protecting life. This was not a top priority for either the military or the scientific community, and the doctors sometimes had difficulty getting members of these other groups to take their concerns seriously, particularly as they related to the dangers of nuclear radiation. As Nolan recalled in a 1957 letter to the author Richard Newcomb, "The radiation phase and possible hazards were not too important in those days. There was a war going on, and the engineers [that is, the military] were interested in having a usable bomb and protecting security. The physicists were anxious to know whether the bomb worked or not and whether their efforts had been successful. . . . The bomb was designed as a weapon of warfare primarily utilizing blast and heat for destructive forces, and radiation hazards were entirely secondary."[30] Thus, the doctors were placed in a unique and difficult position, one that "linked the arts of healing and war in ways that had little precedent."[31] The salience of scientific and military commitments—and the unusual combination of both—pressed in on the doctors in ways that clearly challenged the core of their medical callings. How were they to manage these pressures? What compromises were they willing to make?

Adding to the difficulties of their unprecedented roles in the context of the Manhattan Project, the physicians did not always feel entirely respected by the scientists. Henry Barnett, a pediatrician and a later recruit to the Los Alamos Hospital, noticed this attitude when he arrived with his wife, Shirley, in July 1943. Barnett, who had also been a classmate of both Hempelmann's and Nolan's at Washington University, had always regarded medicine as a rather prestigious profession. Thus, he was a bit taken aback by the attitude of some of the physicists when he began work at Los Alamos. "I had thought being a doctor was pretty far up on the pole, but not there," Barnett remembered. "The physicists, many of them, sort of looked down on doctors," in part because the hospital doctors were technically part of the military.[32] Warren likewise noted the difficulties faced by the Los Alamos doctors working with the world-renowned scientists at Site Y. Even though "Dr. Nolan and his crew were top flight," Warren recounted, "those PhDs would go to the library and ask for books and look up symptoms and make their own diagnosis half the time," thus causing "quite a problem to the doctors there."[33]

In one instance, a worker with a broken leg was taken to the Los Alamos Hospital. While Nolan sometimes directed more serious injuries to Bruns Hospital in Santa Fe, in this case he determined that he and his staff could handle the patient's medical needs. The worker's scientific supervisor from the lab, however, questioned Nolan's assessment and advised that the patient be sent to Bruns Hospital. Nolan turned the tables on this "amateur doctor" in order to push back on the unwelcome and not entirely atypical interference. "Tell me, how is the work going in your department?" Nolan asked the supervisor. "I mean, are you getting the work done? You know I'm very interested in this because I think it's important to the whole Project. Do you need any help in your department? Perhaps I could come in for a few minutes and set a few things right. You know, I've often thought that a new and uninformed point of view could do wonders in these scientific things."[34] The group leader stammered in response, "Well, I hardly think . . ." Nolan continued, "Oh, that's all right. But if you need advice on anything, just call me. Be glad to help." According to Shirley Barnett, who overheard this conversation, Nolan's humorous repartee "solved the problem"; he had "found a perfect solution for avoiding acrimonious discussions on medical subjects with such amateurs."[35]

In the context of the competing vocational paradigms, it appears as though the three doctors—Warren, Hempelmann, and Nolan—in keeping with their particular institutional assignments, handled the pressures placed on the medical community differently, representing, one might argue, three ideal-typical orientations: the military, the scientific, and the medical. Of the three, Hempelmann, who reported directly to Oppenheimer, was the one most oriented toward the scientific paradigm. Nolan said of Hempelmann that "he never treated people . . . he was a 'theoreticer' rather than a practitioner"; he was more "the archetype of the . . . pure scientist."[36] Hempelmann, as head of the Health Group in Los Alamos, was very close to Oppenheimer and, after a stint doing research at Rochester University after the war, returned to Los Alamos to work at the lab. He never really worked as a doctor.

Nor, for that matter, did Warren. As Nolan put it, Warren was "supposed to be a radiologist, but really wasn't."[37] After the war, Warren continued to work in more administrative capacities, including as dean of the new University of California, Los Angeles, Medical School, and, as noted earlier, was, of the three doctors, the one most comfortable with the military character of the project. Nolan, on the other hand, as his son Lawry put it, saw himself "first and foremost [as] a physician whose No. 1 concern was the welfare of his patients."[38] His assignment as the post's hospital doctor, therefore, was in line with, and helped to foster, this primary vocational understanding. Unlike either Warren or Hempelmann, after the war, Nolan was keen to return to his role as a doctor, a medical practitioner.

The three doctors, nevertheless, worked closely together during the war years and beyond, and they shared similar concerns about how best to protect people from the hazards of nuclear radiation, about which little was known at the time. While they seem to have worked well together, there were also, evidently, some tensions between the three doctors. Hempelmann and Nolan were and remained close friends; and while they respected Warren in many ways, they also regarded him as something of a politician, self-promoter, and storyteller who was prone to exaggeration. Nolan remarked of Warren that he was "a complete politician"; he was a "great salesman," good at what he did, but also "full of it."[39] Hempelmann said that Warren was "very flamboyant . . . a teller of tales." Because of this, it was difficult "to believe anything he [said]."[40]

More recent assessments of Warren's character and leadership style echo Nolan's and Hempelmann's accounts. Eileen Welsome, for example, describes Warren as "garrulous and full of bravado . . . an extraordinary blend of contradictions: flamboyant and cautious, amiable and shrewd, a storyteller who kept secrets."[41] Similarly, the author and lawyer Jonathan Weisgall depicts Warren as "an energetic scientist, always amiable and polite. A dynamic speaker, he was also flamboyant and given to histrionics."[42]

These characterizations of this larger-than-life military doctor are borne out in the introduction to Warren's lengthy oral history project with the revealing title *An Exceptional Man for Exceptional Challenges,* put out by the Regents of the University of California. In the laudatory introduction to the publication, Warren's friend and colleague Paul Dodd acknowledges that Warren had his critics, who regarded him as "too much of a 'builder,' too much of a 'one man' man of action."[43] The interviews for the oral history project were conducted in 1966 and 1967, though the edited version was not published until 1983. The long delay was mainly a result of difficulties the editing staff faced in corroborating the details of many of Warren's stories. Publication, in other words, was hampered because of Warren's exaggerations and chronic (and evidently well-known) inability to accurately recall people and places.[44]

Warren's specific Manhattan Project assignment, as a military doctor reporting directly to Groves, placed him in a difficult position. His personality and storytelling proclivities may have afforded him the dexterity to traverse the distinctive parameters of the medical and military paradigms, but one also senses that, at least at times, he was quite troubled by the nearly impossible task of balancing these not always congruent vocational commitments. That is, he was, at the same time, meant to oversee the health and safety of thousands of military and civilian personnel—working in unprecedented conditions with hazardous materials about which there was little understanding—while also obeying the directives of a demanding and difficult military boss, one described by his immediate deputy as "the biggest son of a bitch I have ever worked for."[45] The difficulties of this particular balancing act would only intensify over time, and not always in ways that benefited those in need of medical care.

Shangri-La

After Nolan and Hempelmann's exploratory visit to Los Alamos in March 1943, Nolan returned east to retrieve his family. By early April he was back in New Mexico with his wife, Ann, who was five months pregnant at the time, and their five-year-old son, Lawry.[46] Nolan received an early lesson on the military's obsessive preoccupation with security and secrecy when, upon arrival in April, he was asked to destroy the pass issued to him during the March visit. He was required to write and sign a statement testifying that the pass "was destroyed by burning."[47] Dorothy McKibbin—the project's friendly and resourceful gatekeeper, who with indefatigable alacrity greeted new arrivals at her headquarters at 109 East Palace Street in the center of Santa Fe—arranged for the young family to stay in temporary housing below the mesa until their apartment building on "the Hill," as it was commonly called, was completed.

Sometime in late April, the Nolans moved into one of the hastily constructed four-unit Sundt apartment buildings, named after the contracting company that built the charmless, army-issued, olive-colored structures. Occupying the rooms directly above the Nolans was the family of physicist Dana Mitchell. Lawry Nolan would often play with the Mitchells' son DD, who had an electric train set extending the length of his room and circling up three levels, as well as a chemistry set, which included solutions for making disappearing ink. In their building's other two apartments were the families of photographer Julian Mack and physicist Sam Allison (who would two years later give the audible countdown for the Trinity test). The Nolans' four-room dwelling (Apt. A of Building T-135) was, like the other Sundt units, fully equipped with a large and unwieldy wood-burning stove. Ann Nolan was afraid of the bulky stove, referred to on the Hill as a "Black Beauty," and preferred instead to cook on an electric hot plate, which, because of multiple complaints about the wood stoves, were eventually issued to families living in the Sundt apartments.

Among the four families in the Sundt unit next door to T-135 were the Tellers. The prickly Hungarian physicist Edward Teller, an advocate of the super, or hydrogen, bomb, kept unusual hours, sometimes playing his Steinway grand piano late into the night, which, because of the apartments' thin walls, could be heard by his neighbors. Adjacent to the Sundt Apartments was Bathtub Row, so named because these were the only homes on the Hill with bathtubs. The houses on Bathtub Row, previously occupied

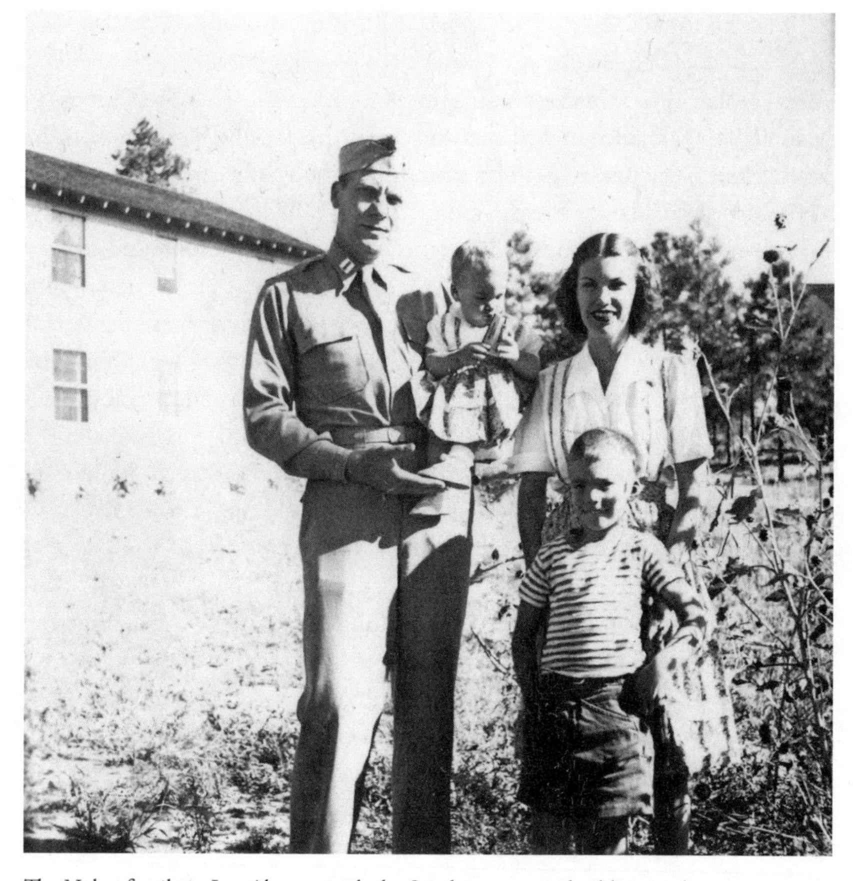

The Nolan family in Los Alamos, with the Sundt apartment building in the background, 1944.

by the administrative and teaching staff at the Ranch School, were the homes of the upper echelon of project personnel, including the Oppenheimers and the families of physicist Kenneth Bainbridge and navy captain William "Deak" Parsons.

Particularly during the first year in Los Alamos, when the community was smaller and when the pressure to complete the bomb was less intense, it was an exciting and exhilarating place to live. Situated atop the Pajarito Plateau between the Sangre de Cristo Mountains to the east and the Jemez Mountains to the west, the isolated mesa was stunningly beautiful. Oppenheimer, who played a role in selecting the location, had, for a long time, been in love with the region, which he regularly visited in the years before the war. He and his brother, Frank, owned a small ranch house in the nearby Pecos Valley, called Perro Caliente, which was about a forty-mile horse ride from Los Alamos. Oppenheimer wrote to a friend in 1929, "My two great loves are New Mexico and physics. Too bad they cannot be combined."[48] With Los Alamos these two affections were united, though years later, when Oppenheimer had come to regret much of what had become of the scientists' revolutionary invention, he lamented, "I am responsible for ruining a beautiful place."[49]

In the early months on the Hill, residents worked hard and played hard. On Sundays, which Oppenheimer insisted be a day off, residents explored the region, taking long hikes and horse rides, visiting the ancient ruins of Bandelier National Monument, or picnicking in the surrounding countryside. Kitty Oppenheimer, among others, was an avid and accomplished horse rider, and the stables from the former Ranch School were used for boarding the animals. During the winter, residents skied and ice-skated.

Not only did Nolan and Hempelmann work together on the Hill, their families were close during their time in Los Alamos. When Nolan's daughter, Lynne, was born, the first baby to be born at Site Y, Hempelmann and his new bride, Elinor, were asked to be her godparents. Two months before Lynne's birth, Hempelmann had briefly left Los Alamos and returned to St. Louis in order to marry Elinor Pulitzer, daughter of Joseph Pulitzer II, the editor and publisher of the *St. Louis Post-Dispatch,* and granddaughter of Joseph Pulitzer, the founder of the Pulitzer Prize.

Adjusting to life on the Hill was not entirely easy for the lovely and high-society Elinor Hempelmann, who continued, in spite of her new, nearly camp-like surroundings, to dress impeccably and in keeping with the more refined social world to which she was accustomed. Though generally a good sport and able to make fun of her altered circumstances, she once commented in exasperation to Shirley Barnett, "I'm just so sick of looking at all the ugly people in the Commissary!"[50] The Hempelmanns, who never had children of their own, were also the godparents of Robert and Kitty Oppenheimer's children, Peter and Toni. The Hempelmanns remained close to the Oppenheimers after the war. In fact, Peter and Toni stayed with the Hempelmanns during Oppenheimer's disastrous tribunal in 1954, and Peter Oppenheimer and his young family lived for a season with the Hempelmanns outside Santa Fe. Lynne remembers her godparents as "very charming people."[51]

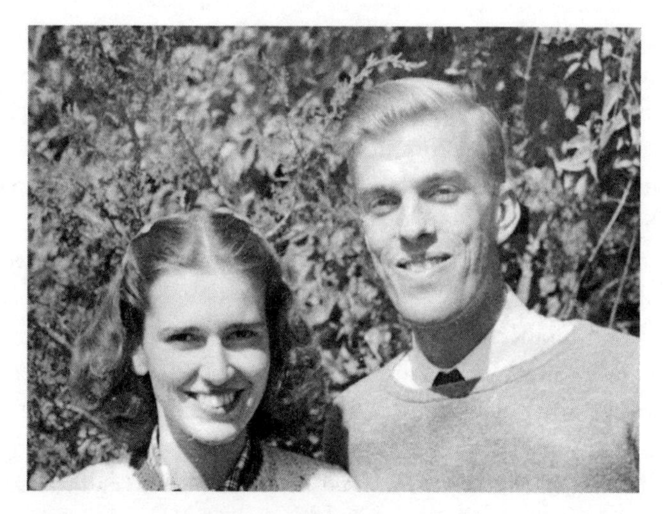

Elinor and Louis Hempelmann in 1944.

With a relatively young population living on the Hill, the place was renowned for its spirited parties. Shirley Barnett recalled that "the parties were naturally pretty wild" and all "drank like fish."[52] At an elevation of 7,400 feet above sea level, the alcohol was all the more potent. Elsie McMillan, wife of future Nobel Prize–winning physicist Ed McMillan, remembered drinking more at the Los Alamos parties than she ever had before. She viewed it as almost a necessity, given the immense pressure placed on the scientists; it was a way "to let off steam, you had to let off this feeling eating your soul, oh God are we doing right?"[53]

Among the many parties thrown on the Hill was a costume party sponsored by the Nolans and the Hempelmanns at the PX (post exchange) with the provocative theme, "Come as your suppressed desire." Oppenheimer dressed as a waiter, wearing an ordinary suit with a napkin over his arm. Dorothy McKibbin, making the thirty-five-mile drive from Santa Fe for the event, wore a leopard-skin outfit with a long coat draped over her shoulders. The overworked medical staff came in their pajamas, with pillows strapped to the back of their heads, expressing their wish for an uninterrupted night's sleep. Hempelmann sheepishly admitted that, while in pajamas and a robe, he also wore a sign that read, "I am Rita Hayworth." Alice Helmholtz, wife of physicist Lindsey Helmholtz, conveying her desire to escape the confines of the isolated military post, came dressed in city clothes, with gloves and a suitcase. As Hempelmann remembered, "She wanted to get the hell out of there as fast as she could." Others dressed up as celebrities, starlets, or historical figures. Someone came wearing roller skates and made circles around the PX during the evening. "That was a very gay party," Hempelmann reminisced.[54]

Another memorable party was the one Kitty Oppenheimer threw to celebrate her husband's fortieth birthday on April 22, 1944. During the celebration, Oppenheimer made his famous martinis, and the alcohol flowed rather freely. "Everybody, even the most sober people like [Isidor] Rabi, were feeling no pain at all," recalled Hempelmann. "Everyone was dancing, and we all had a marvelous time."[55] Some of Oppenheimer's former Berkeley colleagues put together a mock yearbook to commemorate the event. Using the mug-shot-like pictures from the site's security passes, the publication was organized in the style of a high school yearbook, with Oppenheimer as class president, Dorothy McKibbin as the "Welcoming Committee," and Hempelmann, Nolan, and Barnett, along with six nurses, as "The 4-H Club," likely an allusion to the fact that the medical staff sometimes engaged in veterinarian services on the Hill.[56]

The British Mission sponsored one of the last big parties on the Hill just after the war ended. A group of some twenty members of the British Mission, led by the prominent British physicist Sir James Chadwick, had arrived beginning in December 1943 to join the effort at Los Alamos. In addition to Chadwick, members of the delegation included British physicist William Penny, with whom Nolan would later travel to Japan, and the German-born Klaus Fuchs, who would eventually be tried and found guilty in a British court for passing valuable nuclear secrets to the Russians. Perhaps the most famous member of the British Mission was the beloved Danish physicist Niels Bohr, who went by the code name Nicholas Baker or, as he was affectionately called by most in Los Alamos, Uncle Nick.

The British Mission party was held at Fuller Lodge, a handsome and sturdy log building left over from the Ranch School days and mostly used for dining during the war years. Entertainment at the big event featured British physicist Ernest Titterson on the piano and a comical English pantomime mocking the Trinity test, security, and other aspects of life on the Hill. The climax of the evening, Dorothy McKibbin recalled, was "when everyone rose to their feet, brandishing their paper cups, and drank to the King's health with sparkling Burgundy."[57]

In addition to the parties, other recreational activities included twice-weekly fifteen-cent movies at the Post Theater, square dances, choral and

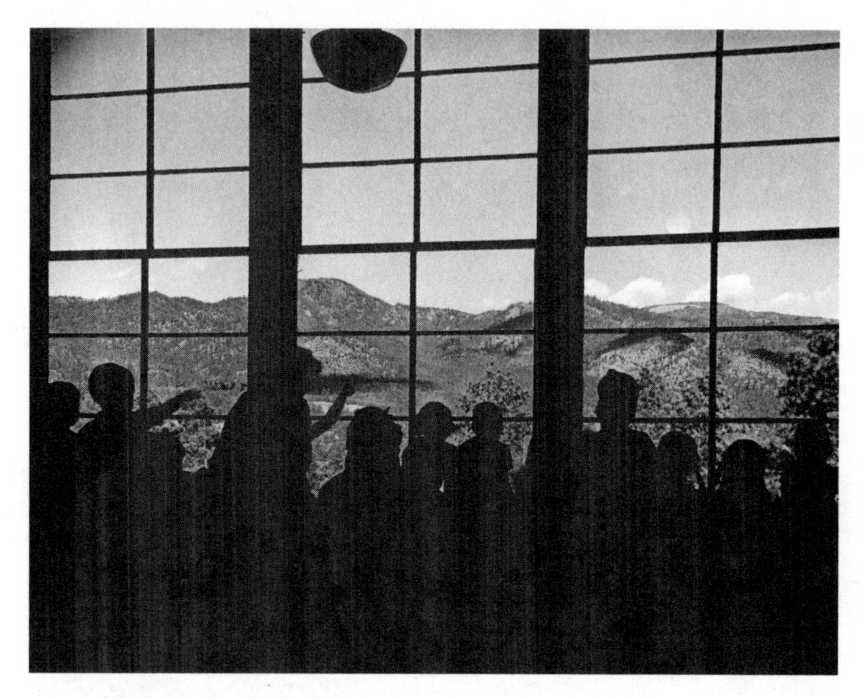

Views of the Jemez Mountains from the Los Alamos school building.

theater groups, chess club, and Spanish classes. Residents also formed a PTA, participated in a basketball league, and played softball, tennis, and even golf. Protestant and Catholic church services were offered in the Post Theater on Sunday mornings, often requiring considerable cleanup from the party or dance held in the same building on the previous evening. Residents would occasionally escape the confines of the fenced-in military compound for trips to Santa Fe, where they would eat and drink at La Fonda, a favorite drinking hole in the center of Santa Fe, or gather for small parties, and even a number of weddings, at Dorothy McKibbin's house.

After their arrival, Lawry Nolan was soon enrolled in kindergarten, which, before the new school building was completed, at first met in an apartment across the street from their unit. Lawry's first teacher, Mrs. Tinsley, would ring a bell to announce the start of the school day. The new school building, when it was completed, offered breathtaking views of the Jemez Mountains through large paned windows.[58] Lawry found life on the Hill enchanting and the families of the famous physicists fascinating. He enjoyed the games and adventures the children created on the site and in the surrounding hills.

In addition to his work at the hospital, Dr. Nolan was elected to the town council established by the civilians at Los Alamos. He also helped to equip the new nursery school, while his wife, Ann, played a role, along with Elinor Hempelmann, in setting up a laundry facility that was used by both military and civilian personnel and established, in part, with the goal of easing the tensions between the two communities.

Though there was much to enjoy among the various activities initiated by the creative and ingenious people living at Shangri-La, as it was sometimes called, residents also had to endure considerable hardships and inconveniences, not the least of which was the intense surveillance to which the scientists and their families were relentlessly subjected. Mail was censored and telephone calls were monitored and sometimes recorded. Security even followed some of the scientists when they traveled off the Hill. Because of his early years as an admitted fellow traveler of communist causes, Oppenheimer was among the most scrutinized of the scientific community. His surreptitious visit in June 1943 to the home of his former mistress, Jean Tatlock, who was still living in Berkeley, did not help matters. Tatlock's communist ties were well known, and Oppenheimer's visit was carefully observed by security.

Peer de Silva, head of security at Los Alamos, was so suspicious of Oppenheimer that, a few months after Oppenheimer's clandestine visit to Tatlock's Berkeley home, he offered to his superiors his opinion that Oppenheimer was "playing a key part in the attempts of the Soviet Union to secure, by espionage, highly secret information which is vital to the security of the United States."[59] Oppenheimer was largely shielded from the repercussions of such warnings because of Groves's interventions and protection. In one of the most improbable partnerships imaginable, the radically different Groves and Oppenheimer worked well together. Groves saw Oppenheimer as essential to the project and, as such, was willing to overlook his communist-leaning past.

However, Groves's support did not stop ongoing surveillance of the project's scientific director. According to Robert Wilson, Oppenheimer "complained constantly that his telephone calls were monitored."[60] The director was not the only member of the community who grumbled about, and deeply resented, military oversight and surveillance. Wilson's wife, Jane, found the military scrutiny to be oppressive, unreasonable, and excessive. "I couldn't write a letter without seeing a censor pouring [*sic*] over it," she wrote. "I couldn't go to Santa Fe without being aware of hidden eyes upon me, watching, waiting to pounce on that inevitable misstep. It wasn't a pleasant feeling." In short, she said, "living at Los Alamos was something like living in jail."[61]

One day, Ann Nolan was preparing to go to the PX to pick up a few items for her family and for the Hempelmanns, because Elinor was at home with a head cold. The two friends reviewed their respective shopping lists over the phone. As Ann stepped out of her Sundt apartment, standing at her door were two military police officers. Two others were at the Hempelmanns' apartment. Ann and Elinor spent an hour and a half explaining themselves and asserting their innocence. Evidently, they had inadvertently used the secret password for the day during their phone conversation, which happened to be "peanut butter." The experience "intimidated the hell out of them," Lynne Handy remembers. "It was paranoia city up there. Really it was."[62]

In addition to the resentment toward heavy-handed military surveillance, residents also struggled with the difficulties of living in crowded and cheaply built housing. The Sundt apartments were among the nicer housing options at Site Y. Smaller and more shoddy units—which included squatty hutments, government trailer units, and large and utilitarian barracks for the Women's Army Corps and enlisted men—were quickly built to accommodate the ever-increasing number of people living and working in Los Alamos. With limited comforts and the almost slum-like conditions of these sprawling housing units, it's no wonder the comparatively more commodious four-family Sundt unit complex was sometimes referred to as "Snob Hollow." Though the military town continued to expand, the roads remained unpaved, resulting in dusty summer months and frustratingly muddy conditions in the late winter and early spring, in which cars sometimes got stuck. Water on the mesa was also an ongoing problem, causing the doctors no little anxiety. Warnings about water rationing were a regular item in the community's *Daily Bulletin.* With all the hazardous materials and explosive testing on the site, the doctors constantly worried about potential fires. They feared that, in case of a fire, they "just didn't have enough water to save the buildings."[63]

Nolan and the Los Alamos Hospital

With the interesting people and the varied extracurricular activities atop the gorgeous mesa—the military oversight and other trying conditions

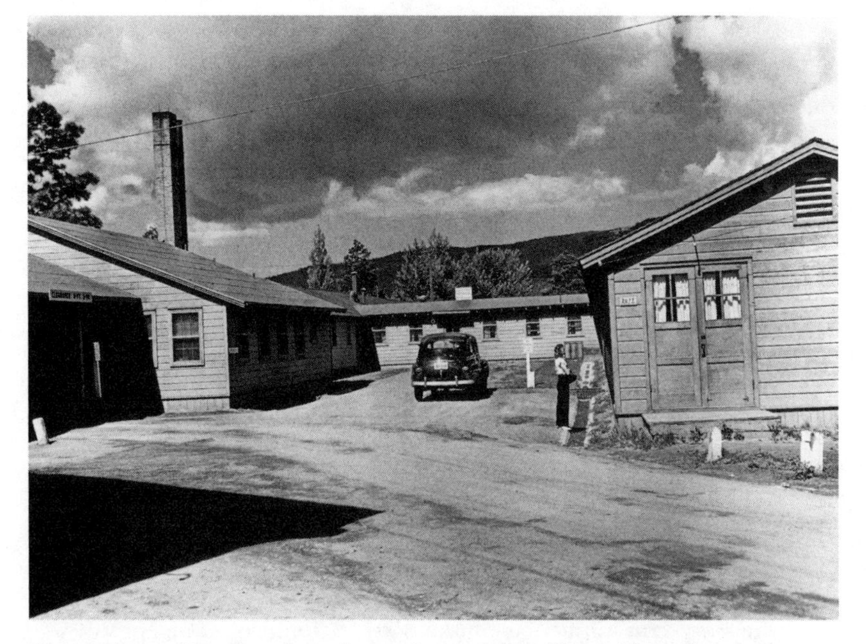

Visitor talking with patient through a window at the Los Alamos Hospital.

notwithstanding—it was a unique and exciting time. Nolan's principal preoccupation, however, was with his work at the new hospital. With Henry Barnett's arrival in July 1943, the hospital staff comprised Nolan, Barnett, and three nurses. The staff also included a secretary and two boys from a nearby pueblo serving as hospital orderlies.[64] At this time, the hospital had only six beds and an operating room, with a few additional small rooms that served as offices, conference rooms, and a pharmacy. The facility was so small that visitors had to stand outside the building, sometimes on crates or packing boxes, in order to visit patients through the window. When the operating room was in use, those waiting for appointments were also made to stand outside.

The hospital, which was situated across from the Tech Area on the opposite side of Ashley Pond, was in the center of the growing town. The lights in the operating room were bright enough that everyone at Site Y knew when the doctors were operating at night. One evening, Ann Nolan and Shirley Barnett were waiting for their husbands outside the hospital building. At the time, Ann was only weeks away from giving birth to her daughter Lynne, and the community was anxiously looking forward to the first newborn on the Hill. As the two women waited in the dark, the driver of a passing car, noticing the lights on in the hospital, slowed down to ask Shirley whether Ann was in the delivery/operating room. In answer to this inquiry, Ann stepped out of the dark shadows to reveal her still very pregnant condition. The experience made the shy and somewhat reserved Ann hope that she would give birth during the more inconspicuous daytime hours.[65]

Ann's wish was not realized, as her daughter was born on the evening of August 16, 1943. Given that her husband was the only ob-gyn in town, and Hempelmann was evidently queasy at the sight of blood (it was rumored that he actually passed out during one attempt at a delivery), Nolan was made to deliver his own child.[66] Hempelmann was originally meant to deliver Lynne, but at the last minute, Nolan decided he didn't trust his friend with the job and instead assigned Hempelmann the role of anesthetist. Hempelmann acknowledged that this was a wise choice: "Jim, as I said, was a first-rate obstetrician, a very good doctor. He worked well with his hands."[67]

In the small community, as Shirley Barnett recalled, Lynne's birth was regarded as "a major event and a matter of loud huzzah."[68] The local San Ildefonso Pueblo community celebrated the occasion by giving Lynne the Tewa name Póvi Ts'áy, which means "yellow flower," presumably because of her blond curls, an unusual sight on the mesa. A day of dancing in the plaza of the nearby pueblo was offered in commemoration of Lynne's birth—likely the Corn Dance, which is performed in the late summer or early fall. Fittingly, the purpose of the Corn Dance is for "the fertility of all things, the crops, the beasts, and man himself."[69]

Lynne's birth may have been the first on the Hill, but it was hardly the last. With the average age of residents at twenty-five, starting and growing families was a popular activity. Because medical care was free, the hospital was nicknamed RFD for "rural free delivery."[70] In the first year alone, eighty babies were born, which kept Nolan and Barnett very busy. Sometimes when a delivery occurred late at night, army sergeant Myron Weigle would drive to Nolan's home, enter his bedroom, awaken him, and then escort the doctor to the hospital in the ambulance. He would return Nolan to his apartment in the same manner after the delivery. The most celebrated birth on the Hill was that of Toni Oppenheimer, Robert and Kitty's second child, who was delivered by Nolan on December 7, 1944. Demand to see the director's baby daughter was so high that the doctors suspended normal visiting hours and posted a hand-written sign over the baby's crib that read

OPPENHEIMER, so that the long line of curious well-wishers knew where to look for the boss's new baby.[71]

The high fertility rate became a matter of some concern to Groves, so much so that he complained to Oppenheimer and asked him to do something about it. His worries did little to curtail the fecundity of the place, as the high birth rate continued unabated. By the end of the war, more than two hundred babies had been born on the Hill.[72] An oft-quoted jingle was written ribbing Groves over the matter:

> The general's in a stew
> He trusted you and you.
> He thought you'd be scientific
> Instead you're just prolific
> And what is he to do?[73]

When the commissary perpetually ran low on diapers and baby formula, young mothers suspected it was a conspiracy to discourage further births.[74] Because of the top-secret nature of the Manhattan Project, the birth certificates of all babies born at the secret military site read, "P.O. Box 1663, Santa Fe, New Mexico." Los Alamos residents joked about the overcrowded nature of this PO box.

Nolan was highly commended for his work as post surgeon. Hempelmann said of Nolan that he was "a very competent person" and a "most fortunate choice" for the job.[75] Testimonies from others make clear that this was not simply the affectionate overstatement of a close friend. Reflecting the views of many, Ruth Marshak, whose husband, Robert, was deputy head of the Theoretical Physics Division, remarked that, though people complained about many aspects of life on the Hill, "there were few criticisms of the hospital. The doctors were competent and popular."[76]

One example of such competence occurred in mid-June 1943, just a couple of months after Nolan arrived in Los Alamos, when Will Harrison and his wife brought their sick daughter, Linda, to the small hospital. After examining the infant, Nolan discerned that the baby had a serious case of pneumonia. Utilizing a makeshift apparatus, he attempted to administer oxygen. The child failed to respond properly, and by midnight her condition had worsened. Not satisfied with the limited facilities at Los Alamos, Nolan ordered an ambulance and accompanied the child, with her mother and a nurse, to Bruns Hospital in Santa Fe. Five days later the child was released, having fully recovered. So grateful were the parents for Nolan's efforts that they wrote a letter to the post's commanding officer, Lieutenant Colonel Whitney Ashbridge, lauding his work. "We believe," they wrote, "Nolan's decisiveness in handling the case is largely responsible for our baby being with us today, and consider ourselves, and all in the Los Alamos civilian area, as fortunate in having available the service of this able physician."[77]

In addition to his capable medical skills, Nolan was also known to have a dry and sardonic wit, evident, as noted earlier, in the manner in which he handled the meddling "amateur doctors." According to Beverly Agnew, whose baby Nolan delivered, when someone with athlete's feet would ask Nolan what he or she should do about it, Nolan would say something like, "Well, if I were you, I would itch." While acknowledging that he "was a very good doctor," Agnew remembered that he made similarly wry comments to the pregnant women under his care.[78] When the expecting Rose Frisch, for example, went to the hospital for an appointment with Nolan, she asked whether she could use the restroom, to which Nolan reportedly replied, "Oh no you don't, I've lost too many babies down the toilet."[79] Another patient, Elsie McMillan, spent considerable time in the hospital after suffering a skull fracture from a car accident on the winding road up to Los Alamos. She was once in the hospital with her cocker spaniel named Borrego Mac. Perusing his medical charts, Nolan wondered aloud why Elsie's "chart read 'thinner and thinner,' while Borrego Mac was getting fatter and fatter."[80] Nolan was also known to offer such advice as, "Why sit down when you have the energy to lie down?"

Nolan once made a house call to see an ailing Eleanor Jette. After a preliminary examination, he was concerned that her condition might be something serious and had her taken by ambulance to the Los Alamos Hospital. At the hospital, Nolan and Paul Hageman, another later recruit to the Hill, did a more thorough examination. Hageman, a specialist in internal medicine, was hired in January 1944 and, like the other Los Alamos doctors, was from St. Louis, though he graduated from medical school four years earlier than did Nolan, Hempelmann, and Barnett. After consulting with Hageman, Nolan returned to Jette's hospital bed with good news, though offered, as Jette recalled, in notably colloquial terms: "You lucky girl, this is a mechanical thing. A piece of your female plumbing slipped its moorings and was being pinched by an attack of acute indigestion. It's a wonder more people don't get their innards knocked loose on the rough roads in the valley. Exercises will take care of the slipped plumbing, but what did you have for dinner last night?"[81]

Jette explained that, after saving her ration tickets, she had purchased and eaten steak. Feigning a shocked look, Nolan replied, "My heart isn't in good enough condition after the scare you gave me. . . . Don't eat any more steak. Meat rationing shrinks the stomach. You can't digest rich things like steak. For my sake, please stick to hamburger!" In concluding her telling of this anecdote, Jette recalled of Nolan, "He was a grand guy." The only trouble with Nolan and the other doctors, she added, imagining the benefits of more of the same, was that "each of them should have been triplets."[82]

The Expanding Community and Growing Pressures

Accounts of life in Los Alamos often make note of the differences between the first year and the years that followed. As pressure to complete the bomb intensified and as more and more people moved to the Hill to work at the site, the already overtaxed resources became seriously strained, at times almost to the breaking point. While the lively social life continued, more cliques developed and some had the impression that the early arrivals were somehow part of a special and more exclusive in-group. Among other concerns, rumors circulated that a prostitution ring was being run out of one of the Women's Army Corps dormitories.[83] Hempelmann's recollections are emblematic of what many remembered of the changing nature of the community: "At first, it was lots of fun, but then as things wore on and everybody got tired, tense, and irritable, it was not so good."[84]

The growing population placed considerable pressures on the hospital staff. It became increasingly clear that the limited facilities and the small medical staff were simply not adequate to handle the growing number of patients. On June 9, 1944, Nolan sent an urgent memo to the commanding officer of the post pleading for more resources. "There are now available in extremely crowded conditions, only 24 beds," wrote Nolan, which he viewed as dangerously inadequate. Instead, he argued "that approximately 55–60 beds will be required to handle the present population with any degree of safety." Not surprisingly, with the large number of births on the Hill, the lack of necessary resources was especially pronounced in the areas of obstetric and pediatric care. "There are three beds now assigned to obstetrical cases and at the present time there are five obstetrical patients hospitalized," wrote Nolan. "There are ten pediatrics beds and on the basis of use, sixteen would be required to meet the demand."[85]

Stafford Warren, who was by this time working more closely with Nolan and Hempelmann, followed up two weeks later requesting from Groves an expansion of hospital facilities and staff to a level that would accommodate fifty to sixty "sick patient" beds. Not long after these pleas, the hospital was enlarged and more medical staff were hired. In addition to Barnett and Hageman—who were added in July 1943 and January 1944, respectively—two more St. Louis doctors were procured in the second half of 1944: Jack Brookes, a nose and throat specialist, and Alfred Large, a general surgeon. The hospital continued to expand thereafter, though in a rather piecemeal fashion. By the summer of 1945, there were more than one hundred staff members working at the Los Alamos Hospital.

Health and safety measures were similarly becoming more of a challenge in the lab. Hempelmann recalled a clear difference between the first year in Los Alamos, when "the project was small and the health and safety needs were few," and the months that followed, when "problems became more complex and numerous."[86] Beginning in February 1944, microscopic amounts of plutonium began arriving in Los Alamos. As the processing plants at Oak Ridge, Tennessee, and Hanford, Washington, became more productive, larger quantities of processed uranium and plutonium were delivered to Site Y. With the presence of more toxic materials and the growing pressure to make progress on the bomb, Hempelmann struggled to maintain and manage necessary levels of safety in the Tech Area.

In light of these challenging circumstances, the Health Group wanted to better understand the biological effects of radiation exposure, a deeper knowledge of which would aid them in more accurately explaining the risks to workers and in providing more appropriate and adequate safety measures. With these concerns in mind, Hempelmann and representatives from the Met Lab and from Oak Ridge took a trip to visit the Luminous Paint Company on the East Coast. In the 1920s, women factory workers in the northeast would detail the dials of luminous watches with paint containing small amounts of radium. The workers would use their lips to point the paintbrushes in a method called tipping, thus ingesting some of the radium remaining on their brushes. A number of these workers, as a result, contracted bone cancer, especially in their jaws, and eventually died. The subsequent safety measures that were implemented at the watch factories served as a model for setting up similar procedures in Los Alamos.

"We patterned our whole operation on the basis of what they'd learned," Hempelmann explained. "We tried to use their operation as a model."[87] However, what was happening in Los Alamos was much more complicated than what took place in the watch factories. Though a related radioactive element, plutonium had different effects on the human body, effects that were not very well understood at the time. "We were working with kilograms of plutonium," Hempelmann said. "Their operation was very simple, but ours were very complex: some of them being chemical engineering and metallurgical operations. It was many orders of magnitude more difficult here."[88]

Thus, more scientific data and more Health Group personnel were required. Such concerns became all the more pronounced when, in the summer of 1944, an accident occurred in which a worker ingested traces of plutonium. As a consequence, there was growing dissatisfaction among workers in the lab and in the Health Group regarding issues of safety, particularly given the doctors' and the physicists' limited knowledge about the biological effects of exposure to these new toxic elements. Just as Nolan had requested more resources for the hospital, Hempelmann asked for more help in the lab. Subsequently, another physician, Harry O. Whipple, was assigned to help with medical examinations, and Richard Watts, an expert on radiation-monitoring instrumentation, was given permission to devote three-quarters of his time to the Health Group, an assignment that would eventually become full time.[89]

At the same time, Hempelmann was increasingly concerned about the vulnerability of the project to legal challenges. In fact, Hempelmann viewed "protecting . . . the legal interests" of the project as one of the important functions of the Health Group.[90] As the size of the lab grew, the Health Group could not keep up with maintaining an accurate and complete hematology record (that is, taking blood counts), enforcing safety procedures, and even determining the actual levels of risk to which workers were being exposed. Hempelmann had to rely on the cooperation of various group leaders in the lab for obtaining records, and, much to his frustration, not all "cooperate[d] to the fullest extent."[91]

"The group leaders were mainly academic people," Hempelmann explained, "who were used to operating on their own. They didn't like to be regimented like that. They were pretty casual."[92] In fact, "the more scholarly and inquisitive the person, the greater the tendency to ignore the recommended procedures."[93] Or as Nolan put it, "We were looked upon as cops."[94]

The lack of proper records, Hempelmann worried, made the project vulnerable to potential legal claims. Fear of legal repercussions would remain a concern of Hempelmann's and other Manhattan Project doctors at other stages in the first years of the atomic age; and the efforts by the doctors to cover themselves against anticipated legal actions—even, in some instances, to the detriment of actually protecting the health of individuals—would become a common preoccupation.

As the size of the community continued to expand and as pressure from Groves to complete the bomb intensified at the beginning of 1945, "a serious effort was made to obtain adequate personnel for the Health Group."[95] In February 1945, several more members were added to Hempelmann's team, including Wright Langham, Joe Hoffman, and J. H. Allen. Additionally, Nolan was asked to assume the role of alternate group leader for the Health Group and thus moved away from his primary role as the hospital's post surgeon. Barnett replaced Nolan as the head physician at the hospital.[96] In this new capacity, however, most of Nolan's time was dedicated not to work in the lab but to health and safety measures related to the testing of the first atomic bomb to be exploded in human history, the so-called Trinity test, scheduled for detonation in the Alamogordo bombing range in July 1945.

2

The Trinity Test

> What went down at Trinity that Monday morning must go down as one of the most significant events in the last thousand years.
>
> —Ferenc Szasz, *The Day the Sun Rose Twice*

Early in 1945, everything at Los Alamos began to speed up. Two types of bombs were being built, one using processed uranium (U-235) and the other a plutonium isotope (P-239) as the core explosive material. The former was being produced at Oak Ridge and the latter at the facility in Hanford, Washington. The two substances required different designs to generate a nuclear explosion. The scientists determined that it was not necessary to test Little Boy, the uranium-based bomb. For one, producing U-235 proved more difficult than producing P-239, and in the late spring of 1945 there only existed enough processed uranium for a single weapon. Second, scientists had more confidence in the success of the rifle-shot design of Little Boy, which involved firing one piece of subcritical U-235 into another. The plutonium bomb, on the other hand, was based on the more complicated implosion model. For the implosion design, a core sphere of plutonium was surrounded by explosives, which, when detonated simultaneously, would compress the sphere inwardly, forcing criticality and a nuclear blast.

It was this second model that would be tested in the New Mexico desert in July 1945 and then, less than a month later, dropped on Nagasaki. As the scientific community was preparing for this test, important developments were unfolding far from the remote mesa in New Mexico. Beginning in the fall of 1943, Leslie Groves had launched a project to investigate how close the Germans were to developing an atomic bomb. The espionage project, called Alsos (the Greek word for *grove*), included on its team an army officer named Robert Furman, a Princeton grad who had worked with Groves on building the Pentagon and would soon accompany James F.

Nolan in the delivery of Little Boy to Tinian Island. Members of the Alsos team followed close behind Allied troops as they advanced across France in the latter part of 1944.

By the end of the year, members of the mission had uncovered a nuclear lab hidden in the wing of a hospital in Strasbourg, which contained revealing and decisive information about Germany's nuclear project. The Alsos team found that Germany was not remotely close to building a bomb. "The conclusions were unmistakable," said Samuel Goudsmit, one of the Alsos physicists on the secret mission. "The evidence at hand proved definitely that Germany had no atom bomb and was not likely to have one in any reasonable time."[1] Not long after their time in Strasbourg, and excited about the mission's discoveries, Goudsmit declared to Furman, "Isn't it wonderful that the Germans have no atom bomb? Now we won't have to use ours." Furman countered, "Of course you understand, Sam, if we have such a weapon, we are going to use it."[2] Though surprised by Furman's response, Goudsmit realized that he was "utterly correct."[3] Robert Oppenheimer seemed to agree that what had been set in motion would necessarily be carried to completion. As he put it, "The decision [to use the bomb] was implicit in the project."[4]

For many of the scientists, the race to beat the Germans in building a nuclear weapon was the raison d'être for the Manhattan Project. A number of the scientists had escaped Nazi-controlled regions of Europe and feared that Hitler would produce an atomic bomb before the Allies would. However, after receiving the intelligence that the Nazis had no bomb—and even after Germany's defeat and surrender about five months later—the Los Alamos scientists continued to work on the bomb. By many accounts, they worked with greater intensity and fervor than ever before. Why did they carry on without more reflection and reconsideration? In the years after the war, some of the physicists looked back and asked themselves just this question.

Robert Wilson, for example, who had a Quaker background and had been a pacifist before the war, in retrospect wished that he had thought and acted differently. "I would like to think now that at the time of the German defeat that I would have stopped, taken stock, thought it all over very carefully, and that I would have walked away from Los Alamos at that time." Based on his long-held outlook and values, this is what Wilson would have expected of himself. "And in terms of everything that I believe . . . I cannot understand why I did not take and make that act." Grasping for an explanation, he remembered that such an idea "simply was not in the air . . . Our lives were directed to do one thing. It was as though we were programmed to do that and as automatons were doing that."[5]

The physicist Frank Oppenheimer, Robert Oppenheimer's brother, who moved from Oak Ridge to Los Alamos in 1945 and worked closely with Kenneth Bainbridge on preparations for the Trinity test, likewise recalled that the scientists, even after Germany's surrender, were carried forward as though directed by a force outside themselves. "It's amazing," he remembered, "how the technology tools trap one. They are so powerful." He acknowledged that the original impetus for building the bomb came from the "anti-fascist fervor against Germany." Yet "when VE Day came along no one slowed down a bit. We all kept working. . . . The machinery had caught us in its trap and we were anxious to get this thing to go."[6] In other words, a sort of "technological momentum," to borrow Thomas Hughes's term, compelled the scientists forward, despite their latent reservations.[7]

Not all, however, carried on without any reflection. At the Met Lab in Chicago, which was institutionally less directly accountable to military oversight, a group of physicists, led by James Franck, issued the so-called Franck Report on June 11, which argued against an unannounced attack on a Japanese city and recommended instead a demonstration bomb dropped on an uninhabited area. Then, in early July, Leo Szilard, the same Hungarian physicist who had originally urged Albert Einstein to approach Franklin D. Roosevelt about starting a nuclear program back in 1939, circulated a petition warning against a military attack on Japan. The petition, signed by seventy Manhattan Project scientists, noted that with the defeat of Germany, the object of their original fears had been averted. The petition also advocated for a careful and serious consideration of the moral responsibilities involved in any use of the weapon.

At least one scientist did walk away from the project, demonstrating that the technological momentum at play was not entirely irresistible. When Joseph Rotblat, a Polish physicist who was part of the British Mission, learned in late 1944 that "the Germans had abandoned their bomb project," he realized that his "whole purpose for being in Los Alamos ceased to be." Therefore, he "asked for permission to leave and return to Britain," and just before Christmas in 1944 he departed from Los Alamos. Even before learning of Germany's negligible nuclear capacities, he came to understand that the American military was already thinking about Russia. In the course of a dinner one evening at James Chadwick's house in Los Alamos, Rotblat was shocked to hear Groves assert that "the real purpose of the bomb was to subdue the Soviets."[8] As with the discovery of Germany's moribund nuclear program, this information confirmed for Rotblat that his reasons for being part of the project had vanished.

Rotblat asked himself why other scientists did not choose to leave after learning of Germany's defeat. This was a question he explored with his colleagues both before and after the war. "The most frequent reason" offered to Rotblat by his Los Alamos colleagues was that of "pure and simple scientific curiosity—the strong urge to find out whether the theoretical calculations and predictions would come true." Operating within the investigative mentality of the scientific paradigm, the physicists were thinking not so much about the wartime use of a weapon as they were about the final outcome of their intensive research, experimentation, and theoretical predictions. "Only after the test at Alamogordo," Rotblat's colleagues told him, would "they enter into the debate about the use of the bomb."[9] This was certainly Robert Oppenheimer's understanding of the process: "When you see something that is technically sweet, you go ahead and do it and you argue about what to do about it only after you have had your technical success. That is the way it was with the atomic bomb."[10]

As the scientists approached the test at Alamogordo in the early months of 1945, compelled as they were by the quest for scientific discovery, the machinations of international diplomacy added further pressure to the almost frantic pace of their work in New Mexico. Officials in Washington wanted to know whether a bomb would soon be available for use in Japan. Harry S. Truman was preparing for his upcoming meeting with Winston Churchill and Joseph Stalin in Potsdam, Germany. Knowledge of a potentially war-ending super weapon would give the new American president strength in negotiating with Russia. Though an ally during the war, US officials were already anticipating a competitive and adversarial postwar relationship with Russia, as illustrated in Groves's statement to Chadwick.[11] Therefore, Oppenheimer and the other scientists were pressing hard to test the Gadget, the successful results of which would strengthen Truman's hand in Potsdam.

Pressure on the Doctors

These factors—both the international developments and the concomitant technological momentum that was "in the air" at Los Alamos—had a singular and direct impact on the work of the doctors on the project. As noted in Chapter 1, the delivery of more plutonium to the Hill, and the speed with which workers were made to labor, caused Louis Hempelmann and others in the Health Group serious trepidation. As the Trinity test approached, there would be similar concerns in Alamogordo. As a result of these developments, Nolan, by his own account, "became detached from the Hospital in order to help out in the setting up of safety measures at the Alamogordo testing ground."[12] The Alamogordo bombing range—the site for the upcoming Trinity test—was located in the Jornada del Muerto (Journey of Death) desert located about two hundred miles south of Los Alamos. Hempelmann remained mostly at Los Alamos, at least until the days immediately before the Trinity test, in order to manage the growing plutonium hazards in the Tech Area.

Thus, though both doctors were now working in the Health Group, a division of labor remained between the two friends. "Jim Nolan was in charge of . . . the health and safety and monitoring" at the Trinity Site, Hempelmann explained. "He gave up his job as head of the hospital and moved over with us. And he is a very competent person and did an excellent job of planning. . . . He did all the planning. I didn't have anything to do with it until shortly before the test."[13] A unique health concern for the Trinity test was the possibility of radiation fallout from the explosion. Neither military nor scientific personnel worried much about radiation. As Rotblat also observed, the scientists were primarily motivated by, and focused on, discovering whether their innovation would work; and the military wanted a bomb for combat purposes. Again, in Nolan's words, "the radiation hazards were entirely secondary."[14]

It is commonly understood that the curious name for the test, Trinity, was given by Oppenheimer in reference to a John Donne poem. When Kenneth Bainbridge, the physicist assigned to direct the Trinity test, asked Oppenheimer to provide a name for the experiment, Oppie had been reading Donne's *Holy Sonnets.* Lines from Sonnet XIV read,

> Batter my heart, three-personed God; for you
> As yet but knock, breathe, shine, and seek to knock
> That I may rise and stand, o'erthrow me, and bend
> Your force, to break, blow, burn, and make me new.[15]

To be sure, the physicists were developing a destructive technology that would break, blow, and burn with an unimaginable force, a weapon that would bring about something fundamentally new for humankind, though not quite in the sense conveyed by Donne.

Indeed, where the seventeenth-century poem pleads for a profound humility, the quest of the twentieth-century physicists could contrastingly be characterized as a sort of scientific hubris. Princeton physicist Freeman Dyson, reflecting on the work of the Manhattan Project scientists, noted "the technological arrogance that overwhelms people when they see what they can do with their minds."[16] This poetic reference to the Trinity of Christian theology would not be the last time religious imagery would be invoked to make conceptual sense of this powerful new weapon.

In keeping with the language of the Donne poem, the scientists were primarily concerned with understanding the blast and heat effects of the bomb. As historian Sean Malloy puts it, "The handling of the Trinity test was characteristic of the entire approach at Los Alamos, which aimed at speedy development of a weapon whose effects were primarily understood to be those of a large blast bomb."[17] Few of those working at Los Alamos, except the doctors, were worried about potential radiological fallout from the bomb, a situation that frustrated the doctors. "Everybody was too busy with getting the bomb fabricated to worry about what happened afterwards," Stafford Warren recollected. When the doctors tried to raise concerns, they would get "brushed off."[18] The physicists "were interested only up to time zero and when the bomb went off," Warren continued. "I was the only one," he added, "with Hempelmann and Nolan to do any worrying about [what would happen] afterwards."[19] More succinctly, Hymer Friedell recalled, "The idea was to explode the damn thing"; people were not "terribly concerned with the radiation."[20]

Though a general lack of concern about radiological fallout prevailed among military and scientific personnel, Manhattan Project physicist Joseph Hirschfelder and physical chemist John Magee were two notable exceptions. According to Warren, after long conversations and arguments with some of the scientists, the doctors "were finally able to get the ear of Joseph O. Hirschfelder."[21] He was, according to Warren, "the only one of the physicists who was interested in what Hempelmann and Nolan were saying and asking."[22] In March 1945, then, Hirschfelder joined Hempelmann and a few others for two ad hoc meetings in Los Alamos in which "initial plans for protection of personnel" at the Trinity test were discussed, including matters related to radiation fallout.[23]

Following these meetings, both Hempelmann and Hirschfelder made preliminary calculations in an effort to get some sense of how radiation would be deposited in the area following the detonation. Hirschfelder succeeded in convincing his friend and colleague Magee that they should investigate these matters further. Magee distinctly remembered the day in April when Hirschfelder burst into his office and shouted, "What about radioactivity?"[24] Magee immediately recognized the importance of his friend's concerns and began working with Hirschfelder and the doctors to better understand and raise awareness about potential radiological fallout from the upcoming test bomb. Hempelmann gave much credit to Hirschfelder and Magee for alerting (or at least for trying to alert) the community about the dangers of radiological fallout.[25]

On April 25, 1945, Hirschfelder sent a memo to Oppenheimer confirming earlier calculations made by Hempelmann and asserting that in the case of an induced thunderstorm, "the radiation effects might cause considerable damage in addition to the blast damage." Hirschfelder even warned that though the blast damage would only extend to less than a mile, under these conditions, the "radiation from the active material and fission products would be sufficient to render an area of from one to one-hundred square kilometers uninhabitable."[26] Hirschfelder calculated a radiation level of 720 roentgens in an area of one square kilometer one day after the explosion.[27]

Around this time, the meteorologist Jack Hubbard was brought into the mix.[28] He had been hired by Groves to study weather patterns and make recommendations about the ideal meteorological conditions for conducting the test. Among the first people he met upon his arrival to Los Alamos in mid-April were Warren and Hirschfelder. Hubbard was taken with Warren, whom he described as a "tremendous man" who "chain smoked and used a waste paper basket, pulled in front of him, for an ashtray."[29] Warren right away told Hubbard that he "was most concerned about the radioactive fallout." Hirschfelder, whom Hubbard found more "unassuming in appearance," likewise communicated his interest "in the carry of radioactive products."[30]

Hubbard offered useful input to Hirschfelder, Magee, and the doctors on how temperature, humidity, wind speed and direction, and rain might affect potential fallout. Hubbard endured serious bullying from Groves, who famously threatened to personally hang Hubbard should his weather predictions for the morning of the Trinity test prove inaccurate, and this after Groves moved forward with a test date that Hubbard had not recommended.[31] In fact, Hubbard had specifically recommended against July 16, "because of anticipated thunderstorms."[32] When Hubbard learned that the date for the Trinity test had been fixed for July 16, he recorded in his diary, "Right in the middle of a period of thunderstorm. . . . What son-of-a-bitch could have done this?" He was told that "it had something to do with a conference in Potsdam."[33]

The TNT Pretest

An opportunity to further investigate radiation hazards from the bomb presented itself when it was determined that there would be a pretest to the Trinity test. In military parlance, these two tests would be coded TR1 and TR2. Based on Hubbard's forecast regarding ideal weather conditions, the pretest, TR1, was scheduled for May 7, 1945—the same day, as it would turn out, as Germany's formal surrender—and would involve the detonation of a one-hundred-ton pile of TNT stacked on a twenty-foot platform. A sample of plutonium was procured from Hanford, Washington, and the pile was spiked with fission material in order to investigate how radioactivity might be distributed following the explosion.

As noted earlier, scientific and military personnel were mainly concerned about the blast and heat effects of the bomb, as they would be with any conventional weapon. While the doctors were pressing for greater attention to the possibility of radiation fallout, they also helped with some of the measurements of the blast effects of the bomb at TR1. Toward this end, the doctors attached live rats to wires using battery clips at distances of one thousand, two thousand, and three thousand feet from the one-hundred-ton pile. Because they set up this experiment late on the night before the detonation, which was scheduled for early dawn, Oppenheimer was critical of their efforts, fearing they might trip over cables or electrical wires. Evidently, the experiment proved largely fruitless. When the doctors collected the rats after the blast, they found that, not surprisingly, the closest ones had all died. At further distances, some were torn loose by the blast, some had died, and some "simply twirled around the wires a bit." The last, according to Nolan, were "a bit dizzy but were not badly hurt." When Wright Langham suggested that such twirling could be prevented through the assembly and use of a special rack, the proposed invention was dubbed "Wright's Micerack."[34]

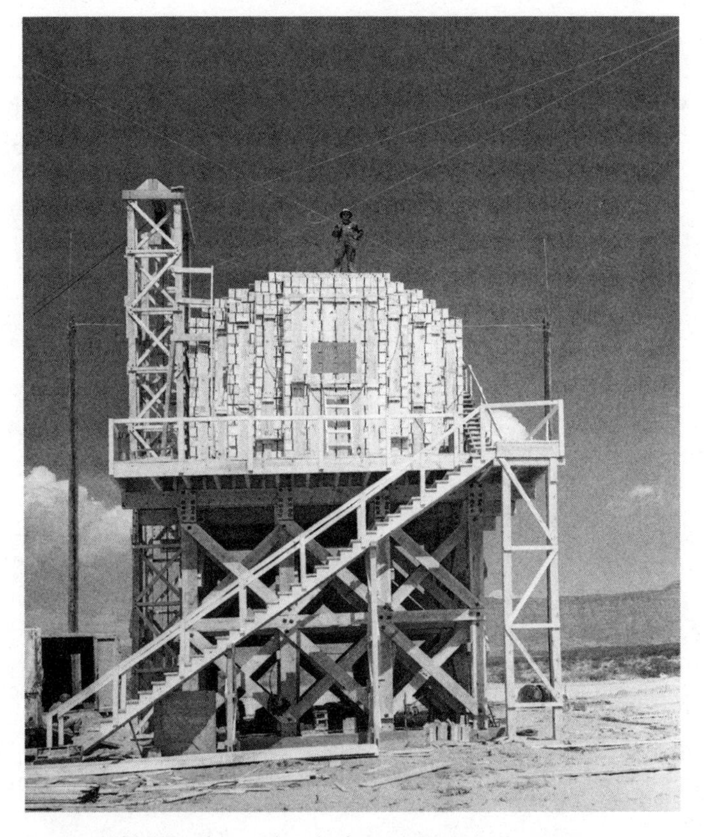

Preparing for TR1, the one-hundred-ton pretest.

More significantly, the doctors observed the movement of the cloud following the blast. With the sympathetic scientists, they used findings from TR1 to calculate anticipated levels of radiological fallout from the upcoming explosion of the Gadget. What they estimated caused them considerable concern. On June 15, Hubbard had run into both Bainbridge and Nolan and could tell that both were seriously troubled about something. "Bainbridge was very worried," Hubbard reported in his diary. "Captain Nolan was also worried. Something is going on to worry these people. . . . I can't put my finger on it."[35] The likely source of their apprehensions would become clear the next day.

Based on input from the meteorologist about weather—and projections based on the results of the one-hundred-ton test—Hirschfelder and Magee issued an alarming report on June 16 that was sent to Bainbridge and circulated to Warren, Hempelmann, and Nolan, among others. "There is a definite danger," they wrote, "of dust containing active material and fission products falling on towns near Trinity and necessitating their evacuation." The two scientists were primarily focused on radioactive dust raised up from the ground into the mushroom cloud and then distributed over the surrounding area.[36]

The June 16 memo was not well received by the scientific community. Hirschfelder was decidedly frustrated that, in spite of all their calculations and warnings, "very few people believed us when we predicted radiation fallout from the atom bomb."[37] He perceived that "the dangers represented by fallout[,] . . . on the basis of his calculations, were simply not taken seriously enough" and that "the government acted very cavalierly toward the danger."[38] Hempelmann concurred, "They were awfully cavalier." Then, as if checking his unguarded response during this particular interview, he added, "I shouldn't be saying all of this sort of thing."[39]

The day after Hirschfelder and Magee issued their memo, an uneasy Nolan departed from Los Alamos to meet with Groves in Oak Ridge. Nolan traveled with a briefcase containing his secret report and carried with him a government-issued .45-caliber revolver. He disliked guns and sought permission from Peer de Silva, head of security at Los Alamos, to put the revolver in his briefcase and the ammo clip in his pocket. Nolan's aversion toward, and lack of knowledge about, weaponry would soon take a rather comical turn.

His early-morning flight from Albuquerque on June 17 was delayed, which resulted in a missed connection in Cincinnati. Instead, Nolan boarded an overnight train to Knoxville, which departed from Cincinnati at eleven o'clock on the night of June 17. He did not finally arrive at Site X until six thirty the next morning.[40] At the time of his visit, the massive Y-12 facility at Oak Ridge had 1,152 operational calutrons (the brainchild of Berkeley physicist Ernest Lawrence) producing enriched uranium.[41] More than twenty-two thousand employees were now working on the sixty-thousand-acre site, which had been acquired by the government in 1942. From Y-12 would come the majority of the U-235 used in the Little Boy bomb.

Nolan and Groves in Oak Ridge

Once at Oak Ridge, the travel-weary Nolan personally handed his report to Kenneth Nichols, Groves's deputy in charge of the Oak Ridge Site, and

John Lansdale, a top counterintelligence and security officer. Nolan was made to sit outside Groves's office "for hours" while "Groves 'held court' with his aides."[42] Nolan's report spelled out the medical group's monitoring and evacuation plans for the Trinity test, the purpose of which was "to anticipate possible dangers to the health of scientific personnel, residents of nearby towns and casuals; to provide means of detection of these dangers; and to notify proper authorities when such dangers exist." If necessary, the doctors proposed that the "evacuation of towns or inhabited places will be carried out."[43] The document included an organizational chart detailing the responsibilities of nineteen personnel leading the operation, including Hempelmann as "Chief of Medical Group," Nolan as his "Deputy at TR," and Warren and Friedell as "Consultants." The use of protective clothing (including booties, gas masks, and gloves), radiation-measuring instruments, vehicles for evacuation purposes, and the identification of specific monitoring locations were all addressed in the document.[44]

The end of the report included an "additional measure" of sending film badges to post offices in the region. "We sent films in envelopes," Hempelmann explained, "we mailed them to various little post offices and then asked them to return them to us sometime after the shot."[45] When the packages were returned to Los Alamos, film from the post offices in the towns of Bingham and Cedarvale indicated measurable levels of radiological contamination, while most came back blank. Though Hempelmann thought that the "one-man man of action" Warren took too much credit for the planning and execution of their Trinity efforts, he conceded approvingly that the strategy for sending the film was Warren's idea.

After considering the document with his aides, Groves invited Nolan into his office and offered his now famous response, "What are you, some kind of Hearst propagandist?"[46] Nolan understood this reaction to reflect Groves's single-minded preoccupation with security and secrecy. Executing the plans detailed in the report, Groves feared, would risk alerting people in the surrounding areas to the secret military operation. The general was loath to support movements that would "send a lot of MPs [military police officers] and trucks into these towns for evacuation. . . . Security might be compromised and news of the test might reach the newspapers." Nolan perceived that Groves was "genuinely sore at [him] for bringing up the prospects of radioactive contamination."[47]

Nolan's confrontation with Groves is poignantly captured in *Doctor Atomic*, an opera about the Trinity test composed by John Adams with a libretto by Peter Sellars. Sellars's rendition of the encounter has Nolan challenging Groves further about his hyperactive security concerns. In the opera, Nolan responds to Groves's worries about secrecy and security by retorting, "With respect, sir, anyone with two good eyes could have found Los Alamos just by following the beer cans from Santa Fe." In this instance, Sellars was taking poetic license, just as he was in placing the Nolan-Groves encounter at the Trinity Site rather than at Oak Ridge, where it actually took place. Though Nolan certainly could have said something like this, in this instance, he was not the source. Rather, the statement was offered by Louis Jacot, a member of the Special Engineer Detachment on Nolan's evacuation team, in an interview with Lansing Lamont for his book *Day of Trinity*.[48]

As recorded by Lamont, Jacot stated, "Talk about security precautions—anyone with two good eyes could have found where Los Alamos was, just by following the beer bottles from Santa Fe."[49] The statement speaks not only to the partying ways of Los Alamos personnel but also to the perception among the scientists that security practices were often misdirected and not entirely rational. Heavy-handed measures were coupled with apparent carelessness in completely missing more obvious, egregious, and consequential security breaches. One need only consider the high level of surveillance concentrated on Oppenheimer, while at the same time physicists Klaus Fuchs and Ted Hall and machinist David Greenglass were passing classified materials to the Russians wholly undetected.[50]

In any case, Nolan found Groves uninterested in the doctors' concerns and his response indicative not only of the general's "rifle-barrel" focus on security but also of his lack of regard for medical doctors more generally. "Groves didn't believe in Medical Corpsman," Nolan observed, "and spit on them." In reflecting on this unpleasant encounter in Oak Ridge, Nolan remembered how, when Groves visited Los Alamos, he would typically inspect the mess hall and menus. The general apparently disapproved of fatty foods. Nolan found this ironic in that the overweight Groves was hardly the model of health and fitness. Nolan and others were well aware of Groves's habit of always keeping "a Hershey bar in his safe" in his office, which he consumed and replenished with frequency. Though Groves seemed unyielding following this encounter at Oak Ridge, the doctors did not give up.[51]

Warren later flew to Washington in early July in another effort to get Groves's ear on the matter. According to Nolan, Warren, who also served as Groves's personal physician, was "the only one who could get the General

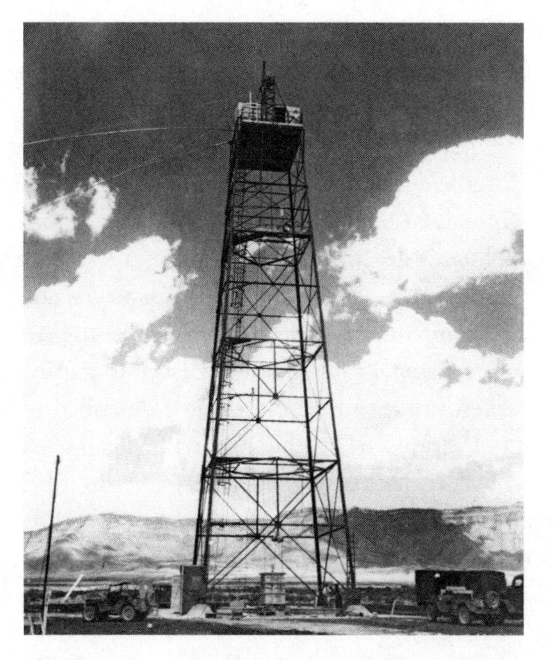

The Trinity test tower with the Gadget at ground zero.

to listen to anything medical."[52] With help from Hirschfelder, Warren put together a letter with a diagram illustrating a possible fallout pattern. After inspecting the document in his office, Groves entered the anteroom where Warren was sitting. "Well, you sure play hob with everything," Groves said.[53] Though not enthusiastic, Groves allowed the doctors to move forward with their plan, but committed limited resources to the effort.[54] Groves did, however, contact the governor of New Mexico, informing him of the possibility of imposing martial law should an evacuation prove necessary.

Preparing for Trinity

What happened back in New Mexico after Nolan's encounter with Groves is not easy to interpret. On June 22, 1945, the day after Nolan returned to Los Alamos from Oak Ridge, he and Hempelmann submitted a memo to Bainbridge, responding to Hirschfelder and Magee's June 16 memo. In the short two-page report, the two doctors sought to determine what might be "the actual danger to personnel in the contaminated area" based on the scientists' earlier calculations. They found that the distribution of fission products would result in an "integrated amount" of sixty-eight roentgens of "external radiation" in the first fourteen days, which, while not insignificant, "would certainly not result in permanent injury to a person with no previous exposure to radiation."[55]

The doctors argued that "even if dust falls from the cloud in the manner described by Hirschfelder and Magee, there is little likelihood of serious damage to individuals in neighboring towns unless the contamination is 2–3 times that which is described."[56] This seems a rather significant reassessment of, perhaps even a retreat from, earlier concerns raised by the doctors and the two sympathetic scientists. However, the next line in the memo offers an important, though somewhat ambiguous, caveat: "This should not be taken to mean that the hazards described by Hirschfelder and Magee are not serious and to be avoided if possible. All precautions should be taken for evacuation of the countryside should the contamination be worse than described."[57]

How does one make sense of this statement, and the document more generally? Historian Sean Malloy concludes, in direct reference to this memo, that "those in charge of safety for the test . . . were largely dismissive" about the dangers of fallout.[58] This is an implausible conclusion, and somewhat surprising, given the careful and insightful quality of the rest of Malloy's analysis. In light of the doctors' comprehensive monitoring and evacuation plans, Nolan's exceptional trip to Oak Ridge, Warren's follow-up trip to Washington, and the doctors' numerous statements about their worries regarding radiation exposure, both during and after the early summer of 1945, it's difficult to conclude that they were "largely dismissive" about the dangers of fallout—far from it.

Indeed, the historian Ferenc Szasz, in his estimable book on the Trinity test, comes to a very different conclusion about the doctors' efforts at Trinity. Szasz commends the "elaborate preparations . . . the physicians made to ensure the safety of the area" and adds that the "health physics arrangements by the medical group were the most sophisticated that the world had ever seen."[59] Nevertheless, it is understandable how one might interpret the June 22 memo as an effort to downplay the effects of fallout. Did Groves's dismissive reaction to their plan just a couple of days earlier in Oak Ridge, and the broader technological momentum of the larger project, cause the doctors to adjust their previously articulated apprehensions?

A further blow to alerting the community about the dangers of radiation fallout came two weeks later—and just ten days before the scheduled Trinity test—when Hirschfelder and Magee sent a revised assessment of their earlier calculations to Bainbridge, which was again cc'd to Hempelmann, Nolan, and Warren, among others. In this July 6 report, Hirschfelder and Magee argued that "the amount of active material sedimenting onto a nearby town may be less by a factor of from 2 to 10 than the amount estimated in our previous memorandum."[60] This was also a notable modification. As Hempelmann recalled, "Hirschfelder and Magee corrected their calculations and they came up with radiation levels which were high, but they weren't as bad as they had been before."[61] These "further calculations and estimations . . . got it down to be borderline or just marginally safe," enough, anyway, to justify going forward with the shot.[62] Was this recalculation simply the natural progression of normal science, offering an ostensibly more objective and accurate presentation of scientific truth, or did certain social factors enjoin the physicists to adjust their original findings?

Suggesting that it may have been at least partly the latter, Hempelmann recollected that there were considerable efforts in the lab to challenge Hirschfelder and Magee's original calculations. It was Hempelmann's distinct impression that, after the June 16 memo was circulated, "much of the effort of the laboratory was directed at trying to disprove them." A falsification of the scientists' conclusions was important, according to Hempelmann, because had Hirschfelder and Magee's earlier estimations been correct, "we really shouldn't have done the test."[63] Moreover, Hempelmann remembered the palpable pressure placed on the community at the time to keep moving forward. The clear message and the overwhelming climate of the place and time was that "the work has to go on. Truman is going to meet with Stalin on the 16th and we have to have not only bombs, but we have to have it tested by then."[64]

As a consequence of this pressure, both at Alamogordo and in the lab, significant dangers were being ignored or downplayed. In the lab, workers were "excreting high levels" of plutonium; in fact, Hempelmann "thought they were probably lethal levels." In more normal circumstances they "would have been pulled off their jobs."[65] But these were far from normal circumstances. In a 1986 interview, Hempelmann was asked directly whether "the Trinity test would have been held up" had Hirschfelder and Magee's calculations "shown there was a danger." He answered, with little equivocation, "No." That is, the international pressures and the technological momentum were such that, regardless of the scientists' final calculations, they would have gone forward with the test. In another interview Hempelmann elaborated, "We couldn't have stopped it in any possible way."[66]

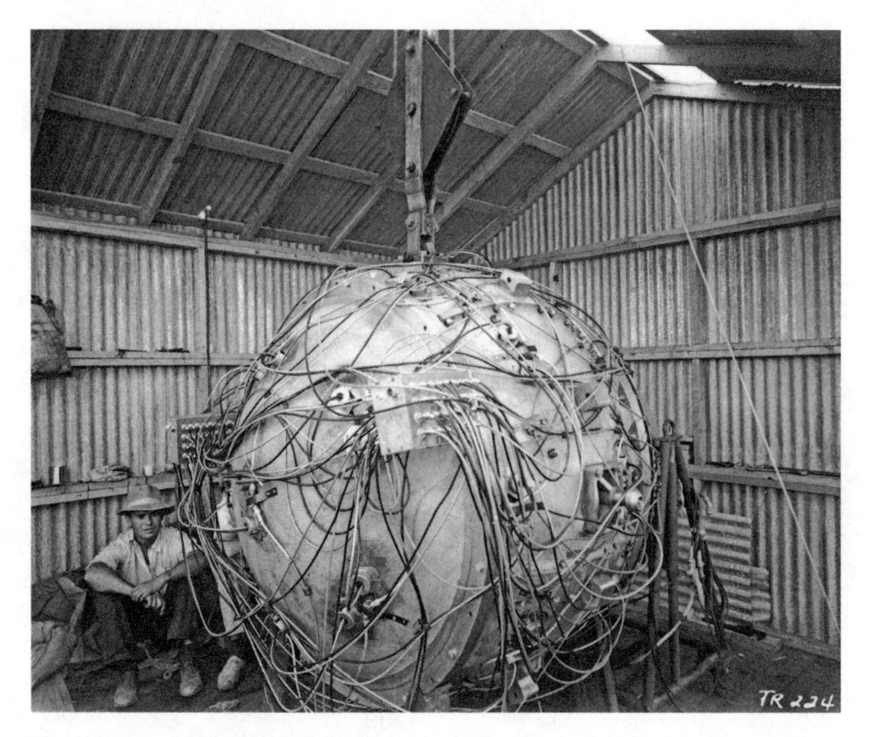

The Gadget in the one-hundred-foot tower.

Why would they go forward despite the expected dangers? Because "there was great excitement just as the time of the test approached," Hempelmann explained. "Truman wanted the results by the time of the Potsdam conference and they would have shot in the middle of the rainstorm if it were necessary to get the results."[67] A rainstorm would be the least favorable of conditions, as Hubbard and others clearly understood, because the rain would push higher levels of radioactivity to the earth's surface and would complicate efforts to photograph and measure various aspects of the explosion. In the end, much of what Hirschfelder and Magee predicted in their original June 16 memo was realized. As Szasz concludes, "The initial calculations of Hirschfelder and Magee proved basically correct."[68]

Regarding Hempelmann and Nolan's June 22 memo, a case could be made that their assessment, rather than constituting a retreat, sought something of a middle ground. That is, as with Hirschfelder and Magee's revised calculations, the doctors provided enough information to justify moving forward with the test, thus appeasing their forceful military boss—and acquiescing to the force of the project's forward momentum—while they also more or less maintained their previous warnings. In other words, though they downplayed the likelihood of significant radiation damage, they asserted, with qualification, that precautions should be observed and that the hazards described by Hirschfelder and Magee should still be taken seriously. Such a middle ground would arguably protect (or at least was aimed at protecting) the doctors and the project from possible legal challenges, should the hazards prove as harmful as originally anticipated.

In support of this interpretation of their memo, there is considerable evidence to suggest that the doctors were ever mindful of potential legal consequences and careful to take precautions to protect themselves and the military from future litigation.

Medicolegal Concerns

Indeed, the first ad hoc meetings about fallout between Hempelmann, Hirschfelder, and others in March 1945 focused on three main topics, the second of which was "the medico-legal aspects of these hazards."[69] A month later, Hempelmann was still concerned that "the medical legal complications of the shot have not been considered thoroughly as yet."[70] When Groves visited Los Alamos in April, the very first question he asked during a meeting was about legal matters associated with the Trinity test. On April 18, following the meeting, Groves told Bainbridge that he was going "to get additional legal talent to consider and act on the legal aspect of the TR tests."[71]

Among other procedures, this additional legal talent encouraged radiation monitors to "get permanent records of the measurements in the shelters as well as in the towns for future reference."[72] The "permanent records," as such, would equip the military with the necessary legal documentation to challenge future legal claims. Instructions from military lawyers about proper documentation were detailed and obsessive. Following a July 7, 1945, meeting with Nolan, Hempelmann, and Lieutenant John Davies, the Trinity project's claims officer, for example, monitors were given the following guidelines: "Keep as complete notes as possible in your own handwriting to be signed and filed away by you for future reference. These notes can be written up more fully at a later date but in any court proceedings it is necessary to present your original data."[73] Monitors were instructed further to keep all their records, as these would be "used as evidence in future legal proceedings. You will be the chief witness for off-site contamination."[74]

To ensure the legal validity of such records, a member of Davies's team would accompany each monitor. The presence of military personnel would "permit an affidavit to be made as to the time, place, and nature of the radiation measurement."[75] These detailed instructions make clear that the military was fully cognizant of the possibility of future litigation and aimed to direct and manage the doctors and radiation monitors accordingly.

Recollections from both Warren and Hempelmann provide further evidence as to the pressures the doctors were facing in this regard, as well as the continuing concerns they had about radiation. As mentioned earlier, while Nolan was the point person for setting up the safety and evacuation procedures at Trinity, Hempelmann remained at the lab, where he continued to worry about the levels of radiation to which the workers were being exposed. About a week before the Trinity test, Nolan was asked to escort Little Boy to Tinian, and thus would depart two days before the actual test. At this point, Oppenheimer frantically called Hempelmann and instructed him to get to the Trinity Site as quickly as possible. "What are you doing up there?" Oppie said. "Get the hell down here."[76]

When Hempelmann arrived at the Trinity Site around July 11 or 12, he was bothered by what he saw. For one, he perceived that aspects of the operation were set up not because of valid health and safety concerns but in order to protect the army from legal claims. Hempelmann recollected, "I think it was all set up this way on the books, so that if something happened, the army wouldn't be blamed."[77] When Hempelmann learned from Hubbard and others about plans to go forward with the test despite the less than ideal weather conditions in the forecast, he was "horrified." Perhaps a bit ironically, his first impulse was likewise to establish a legal record whereby the doctors would not receive the blame. "I spent most of my time writing memos saying we can't take responsibility for shots conducted under these conditions." Given the way in which the military ignored previous warnings from the doctors, the response to his memos was not surprising. "Of course I got no response," Hempelmann said. "All my memos were put in the wastebasket."[78]

Warren also perceived that the army's instructions regarding the documentation of monitoring measurements and the like were more about legal protection than ensuring health and safety. "Everyone wanted to get the test over with," Warren said. "The Army and Government lawyers were scared of legal complications. They wanted to put it all out of sight and mind as quickly as possible."[79]

Maximum Tolerance Dose

In setting up safety measures at Trinity, the doctors were put in the unusual position of having to determine what constituted an acceptable or tolerable dose of radiation. Both U-235 and P-239 were new elements, and understandings of their radiological effects were incomplete at best, though they were clearly known to be dangerous. How were the doctors, then, able to determine what was an acceptable level of exposure? Recall that in Hempelmann and Nolan's perplexing June 22 memo, they suggested that sixty-eight roentgens, though high, would not cause serious damage, at least not to anyone who had no previous exposure. A roentgen, named after Wilhelm Conrad Röntgen, who discovered the x-ray in 1895, constitutes a unit of radiation exposure—that is, a unit measuring the ionization of air. In 1934, the US Advisory Committee on X-Ray and Radium Protection recommended 0.1 roentgen as an acceptable tolerance dose.[80]

The doctors, of course, were aware of this standard. As Nolan recalled, "The standard limit or tolerance dose then was 1/10 of a roentgen." However, he added, "no one knew really how much radiation a human could stand." In fact, the scientists on the project, some of whom had been working with radioactive materials for years in places like the Radiation Lab, or Rad Lab, in Berkeley and the Met Lab in Chicago, thought that they could handle much more, as much as "25 or even 50 roentgens," and would ask Nolan, "How much radiation are you going to let me take?" Nolan, no doubt with some irony, would turn the question back on the scientists: "How much do you want?" They finally settled on 5 roentgens as the "maximum dose," which was, in fact, the level identified in the evacuation plan Nolan gave to Groves at Oak Ridge.[81] But even this higher level was not taken entirely seriously. One week before the test, Warren proposed that he would only worry if the dose peaked at a level of 10 roentgens. In his view, an integrated dose of 60 to 100 roentgens over a two-week period would "not be harmful provided there would be no further exposure to radiation." Evacuation, he suggested, should only be considered if contamination reached these levels.[82]

The one-time dose of exposure (5 roentgens), which was formally agreed on in a seemingly arbitrary fashion, was fifty times higher than the official standard at the time. Warren's revised level (10 roentgens as the maximum permissible dose) was one hundred times higher than the official standard. Not long after, even the standard of the mid-1940s would be regarded as far too high. During his 1965 interview with Lansing Lamont, Nolan acknowledged that by the 1960s the "maximum safe dose" had been lowered to "6 miliroentgens (or 6 one-thousandths of a roentgen)."[83] In other words, the agreed-on level of "safe" exposure during the Trinity test was more than eight hundred times higher than what would be viewed as acceptable only two decades later. Currently, the standard is even lower. "Today," Eileen Welsome observes, "most scientists generally agree that any amount of radiation, no matter how small, has the potential of causing harm."[84]

Hempelmann admitted that what they determined to be an acceptable level of radiation exposure at the time of the Trinity test was "just arbitrary . . . these things were awfully arbitrary." When asked by Barton Hacker in a 1980 interview how the working standard at the time was determined, Hempelmann again answered, "I don't know. It was just arbitrary." He acknowledged further, "We didn't know what the hell we were doing. . . . Nobody had had any experience like this before . . . and we were just hoping that the situation wouldn't get terribly sticky."[85]

Nolan's Departure and Warren's Letter

Matters did become sticky for Hempelmann when, about a week before the test, Nolan was informed by Peer de Silva that he would leave New Mexico as one of two escorts who would carry the uranium bomb from Los Alamos to Tinian Island. Nolan was not sure why he was selected for this role. "I do not remember specifically how the decision was made to have a scientific courier accompany the material in addition to the security courier, who was Major Robert Furman." He knew, though, that Oppenheimer, Warren, Hempelmann, and de Silva had been involved in making the decision. "The main idea," Nolan remembered, regarding his unusual assignment, "was that one of our medical group should accompany the material during transport, and remain at the laboratory at the Island of Tinian for the problems associated with the assembly of the bomb, take-off, etc."[86] In keeping with his generally contemptuous attitude toward medical corpsmen, Groves told Admiral William Purnell, the navy liaison to the Manhattan Project, that "the Medical Officer will merely go along to hold someone's hand if they get excited."[87]

Nolan's departure complicated matters at the Trinity Site. Hempelmann recounted, with some disappointment, that, "just before the Trinity Test, Dr. Nolan, who had been in charge of . . . the health and safety at the Trinity

Test site, he was ordered overseas to accompany one of the atomic bombs going by ship to Tinian." He regarded Nolan's departure as "a severe blow to us" and was not sure how they would make up for his absence.[88] That said, because the safety, monitoring, and evacuation procedures had been carefully laid out, there wasn't much else to do but follow what had been put in place. In other words, as Hempelmann put it, because "the whole thing had been planned out, everybody knew what they were going to do."[89]

Thus, Nolan departed on July 14, two days before the Trinity test. He would not actually learn about the success of the test until after he reached Tinian Island. Almost a week after the test, Warren wrote a letter to Nolan explaining the results of the test and providing information that he viewed as relevant for the delivery of the bombs to Japan. In this remarkable handwritten letter, Warren made a number of revealing statements about the test and his perception that a major deathly catastrophe had been narrowly averted.

The letter included some personal information to Nolan, such as, "Your wife got off ok. Everybody wishes you luck—they all miss you." Following her husband's departure, Ann Nolan had left Los Alamos with their two children to live with her sister, Jane Reynolds, and her family in Los Angeles during the time Nolan was overseas. The main thrust of the letter, though, was about the Gadget and its effects. First, Warren communicated that, while the basic monitoring and evacuation plan had worked, the blast was more powerful than anticipated: "The organization worked fine except that: the energy released was 3–5x greater than expected. The cloud went up 50–70,000 ft.," though it had been expected to rise to about twelve thousand feet. In the letter, he described the three different directions in which the cloud dispersed and how after three hours, "it then disintegrated in thin sheets." Significantly, he noted that the radiation monitors found radiation at levels as high as thirty to forty roentgens "near a lot of houses" and, in "one hot canyon" northeast of Bingham, radiation "totaling 230r."[90]

While these were high levels—even higher than the "safe" levels agreed on through the doctors' negotiations with the scientists—no one in these areas was evacuated. Even more significantly, Warren admitted that it could have been much worse. "Boy what a narrow escape. If we had laid it down in a steady wind as planned when you left we would have had a *high mortality!!* It was terrific" (emphasis in original).[91] This is, of course, a major concession as to the dangers of the radioactive fallout from the bomb. Had the levels of radioactivity detected in the canyon near Bingham been deposited on more-populated areas surrounding ground zero, there would have been, according to Warren, a high number of casualties.

It seems that one reason there were less concentrated deposits of radioactivity, in spite of the higher-than-expected potency of the bomb, was the extended elevation of the cloud.[92] Because of this, radioactive material was dispersed more widely and thus more diffusely. Had fallout been distributed in populated areas closer to ground zero in a more concentrated manner, the consequences could have been devastating, or rather, one might argue, more immediately and visibly devastating. Near the end of the letter, Warren presciently added, "You missed a show but you will live longer! as a result. Nobody was hurt but it was a close shave."[93]

Hempelmann agreed with this basic assessment—that is, that it was a "close shave" and could have been much worse. "We were terribly lucky, just unbelievably lucky because there could have been really serious fallout." He admitted that "parts of New Mexico were fairly heavily exposed, but there weren't very many people there."[94] Again, Hempelmann asserted, "We were just awfully damn lucky."[95]

On the day before writing his letter to Nolan, Warren had constructed a memo to Groves. Absent in this communication was the more alarmist and colorful language found in the letter to his fellow physician. For example, in his memo to Groves, Warren made no mention of potentially "*high mortality!!*" or of the 230 roentgens discovered in the radiated canyon. However, Warren did communicate to Groves his understanding that "the dust outfall from the various portions of the cloud was potentially a very serious hazard over a band almost 30 miles wide extending almost 90 miles northeast of the site." He also offered his recommendation that any future tests should take place not in Alamogordo but in a region "with a radius of at least 150 miles without population." He also acknowledged that, at the time of his memo (five days after the test), there was "still a tremendous amount of radioactive dust floating in the air."[96]

Trinity and Its Aftermath

Much has been written about Trinity and the profound effect it had on the Manhattan Project scientists. The explosion itself was stunning and breathtaking and, as noted in Warren's letter, much more powerful than had been expected. The blast of the explosion was estimated to have yielded a force of twenty kilotons. William L. Laurence, the *New York Times* journalist who was hand-picked by Groves to observe, and ultimately report on, the Trinity explosion, described the spectacular display of the detonation in religious-like terms: "And just at that instant there rose from the bowels of the earth a light not of this world, the light of many suns in one. . . . One felt as though one were present at the moment of creation when God said: 'Let there be light.'" About one hundred seconds after the visual spectacle there came a thundering boom, which Laurence described as "the first cry of a newborn world."[97]

Laurence was not alone in invoking such language. Hubbard, for example, recalled that the "unlocking of nuclear energy had been seen by some of us as the birth of a beautiful child." Having "achieved a victory over ignorance," he added, "some of us felt that we had been permitted to play on the harps of God."[98] As the atomic age unfolded, Laurence would continue to divinize nuclear power, reflecting what some have termed nuclearism. It was as though only religious imagery was evocative enough to appropriately depict the power of the bomb. Conceiving of the bomb in such ethereal terms, arguably, is also indicative of a broader enthusiasm with which modern humans perceive and then embrace the ostensible benefits of technological innovations more generally. Not all, however, were unambiguously celebratory in their reaction to the Trinity test.

Many, after initially reveling in the success of their colossal effort, became soberly awakened to the frightening reality of what they had created. Oppenheimer remembered, while at first feeling relieved that the bomb had worked, calling to mind lines from the Bhagavad Gita: "I am become death, the destroyer of worlds." Kenneth Bainbridge, the director of the Trinity test, walked over to Oppenheimer, shook his hand, and said, "Well, now we're all sons of bitches." An assistant to photographer Julian Mack, Nolan's Sundt apartment neighbor, declared, "My God, it's beautiful," to which Mack replied, "No, it's terrible."[99] The recollections of Victor Weisskopf, head of the Theoretical Physics Division, represent a nice summation of the conflicting and evolving emotions experienced by the scientists: "Our first feeling was one of elation, then we realized we were tired, and then we were worried."[100]

For the doctors and the radiation monitors, in certain respects, their work had just begun. In all, about forty monitors were involved in collecting radiation data. One of them was the pediatrician Henry Barnett, who was stationed at N-10,000—that is, at the observation station that was ten thousand yards north of ground zero. Less than thirty minutes after the

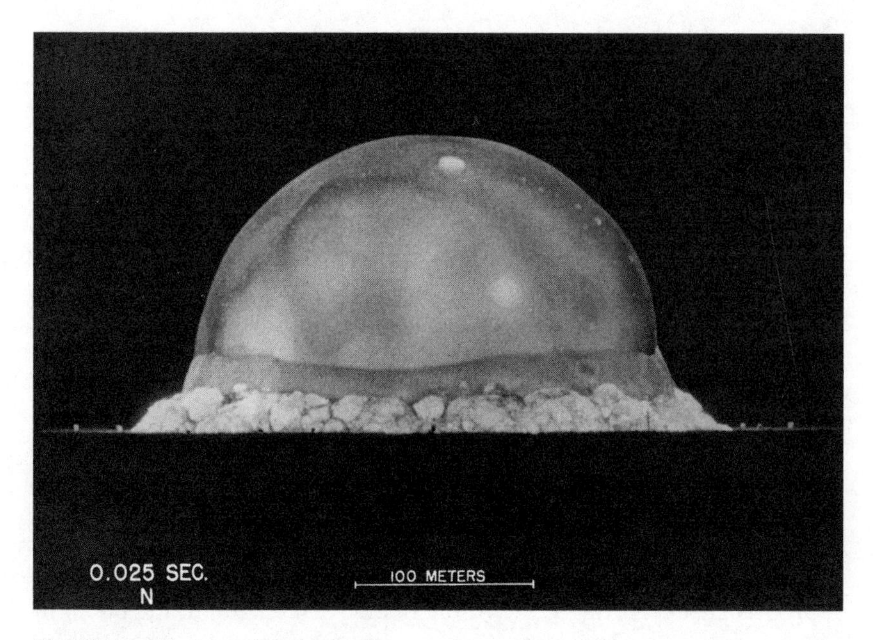

The Trinity explosion at 0.025 seconds.

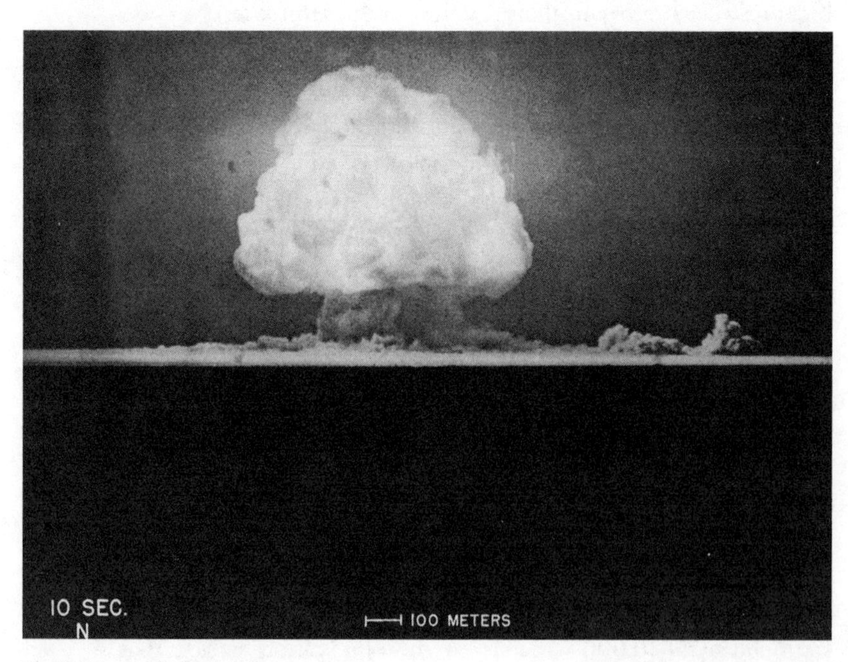

The Trinity explosion at 10 seconds.

detonation, Barnett's monitoring meters began indicating levels of radiation between ten and thirty-five roentgens. Physicist Robert Wilson and others at N-10,000 then noticed a red-and-brown-colored cloud with "stuff" descending toward them. Wilson ordered an evacuation, and the men piled into cars and headed for base camp.[101]

As noted in Warren's letter to Nolan, high levels of radiation were also found in a canyon near Bingham, about twenty miles north of ground zero. This "Hot Canyon," as it came to be called, was first discovered by John Magee. Magee's measuring instrument indicated a level of 20 roentgens. When he radioed the information to Hempelmann at base camp, he was instructed to take another measurement. Magee remeasured, checked his reading with Joe Hoffman, and again reported a level of radioactivity at 20 roentgens. Shortly after this second reading, their communication with base camp was unexpectedly cut off. Magee viewed the situation as a disaster and thought the canyon should be evacuated. Years later, he still remembered his discovery of the Hot Canyon as one of the most dramatic events that had ever happened to him. After returning to base camp, he showered but didn't have the nerve to test himself, though the film badge he was wearing registered 5.5 roentgens.[102]

The next day, July 17, Friedell and Hempelmann returned to the Hot Canyon and were alarmed to discover that two families of ranchers, the Raitliffes and the Wilsons, were living within a mile of where Magee had made his measurements. These families had not been identified when Manhattan Project personnel surveyed the area before the Trinity test. After discovering the ranchers, Friedell contacted Lieutenant Davies and inquired about potential legal issues. Davies, in turn, contacted Groves. As Davies's communication was recorded in Groves's diary, "Friedell's boys had made some further observations and are concerned about one family to the extent that they want to get in touch with that family to see how they feel. They called me [Davies] to ask about the legal end—told them there was nothing I could do about it."[103]

Thus, even in a case in which there was an acknowledged high level of radiation exposure, the military, and the complicit doctors, were evidently more concerned about legal outcomes than with the health of the individuals who had clearly been exposed. The ranchers in the Hot Canyon were never evacuated, nor were they told about the Trinity bomb or the reasons for the doctors' return visits to check on them. In early August, Hempelmann and Warren went back to the area and chatted with the Raitliffes and others in the areas and took additional measurements. Warren continued to worry about this region for years after the war.

About ten miles beyond Bingham and more than thirty miles from ground zero, along the Chupadera Mesa, more evidence of radioactivity was discovered. On the mesa, with its average elevation of about seven thousand feet, cattle showed evidence of beta burns on their skin. When fur from the radiated skin grew back, it came in gray or white in color. Some cows were speckled with white spots, while others looked as if they had been covered with a dusting of snow. The ranchers who owned the cattle had difficulty selling the contaminated cows. In October, a lawsuit against the government was filed. Hempelmann visited the area in November and eventually the government purchased four cows, determined that the burns were indeed a consequence of radiation fallout, and eventually paid full market value for dozens more. Seventeen cows were taken to Los Alamos for further testing and the rest were shipped to Oak Ridge.[104]

Given these discoveries, the doctors wanted to investigate radiation issues further, but they were discouraged from doing so, even though they knew there was significant radiological fallout and that people had been exposed. Hempelmann admitted later that a few people in the region of the Trinity test "were probably overexposed, but they couldn't prove it and we couldn't prove it. So we just assumed that we got away with it."[105] Warren agreed that there was not much interest in honestly investigating the extent of radiation exposure in the area. And he perceived that this lack of concern was motivated, at least in part, by a fear of legal consequences. "No one really wanted to pursue the radiation possibilities for fear of getting involved in litigation."[106]

As a consequence, efforts to understand and document the full extent of radiation fallout in the months immediately after the Trinity test never occurred, though it's clear that there was extensive fallout. Concerns about the long-term health effects from this fallout have persisted for decades. Residents in the towns surrounding ground zero complain that higher-than-average rates of cancer and other radiation-related sicknesses have plagued their communities for years. Among the many stories is that of Barbara Kent and a group of eleven other girls who, at the time of the test, were at a summer camp in the mountains of Ruidoso, situated about fifty miles from ground zero.

In the early morning of July 16, Kent remembers hearing a large explosion, the force of which knocked some of the campers off the top bunks in their cabin. Fearing that the camp's water boiler had exploded, the girls' counselor urged the campers to run outside. Within about five minutes "everything went bright," Kent remembers. "It went from dark to bright."[107] Later in the afternoon, the campers noticed white material floating down from the sky. The girls asked for and were given permission to go down to the river and play in the "snow." As they frolicked in the water, the young campers ran around catching the descending white ash, rubbing some of it on their faces. Unlike snow, however, the white material felt warm to the touch.

According to Kent's brother, Bob Keller, only two of the twelve girls lived past thirty. "The rest died of cancer."[108] The counselor and her step-daughter, who helped at the camp, also died from cancer. Not long after playing in the fallout material, a streak of Kent's blond hair turned and remained white, the same sort of discoloration that occurred with the contaminated cows collected by Manhattan Project officials. Kent is the only camper from the group still alive, though she too has suffered from various forms of cancer over the years, including endometrial cancer and skin cancer, and has had her gall bladder removed.[109]

In recent years, under the leadership of Tina Cordova, the Tularosa Basin Downwinders Consortium has been working to achieve some sort of recognition and remuneration for the suffering of Trinity test downwinders.[110] "We were unknowing, unwilling, and uncompensated guinea pigs in the world's largest science experiment," Cordova argues.[111] She and others in the consortium have been lobbying Congress to include the Trinity downwinders in the Radiation Exposure Compensation Act, a federal law passed in 1990 that is aimed at compensating mostly those who suffered radiation exposure from the Nevada testing grounds in the years after the war. The bill was amended in 2000 and then again in 2002, but to date Trinity test downwinders have not been included in the compensation legislation.

Truman Learns of Little Boy's Big Brother

News of the successful test was communicated to Truman in Potsdam via two secret cablegrams. The first arrived at seven thirty in the evening Berlin time on July 17 and was sent to Secretary of War Henry Stimson from his assistant and advisor, George Harrison. Curiously, the message was coded using medical nomenclature: "Operated on this morning. Diagnosis not complete but results seem satisfactory and already exceed expectations."

Given his attitude toward the medical officers on the Manhattan Project, it may seem ironic that the attending physician here was "Dr. Groves," who was "pleased" with the outcome of his operation and on his way home to Washington.[112] The next coded cable, again sent from Harrison to Stimson, arrived early the next morning and offered more details on the results of the test. "Doctor has just returned most enthusiastic and confident that the Little Boy is as husky as his big brother. The light in his eyes discernible from here to Highhold and I could have heard his screams from here to my farm."[113] The substance of the decoded message was that "Dr. Groves" had returned to Washington and was confident that the Little Boy bomb, now traveling across the Pacific Ocean, would be as formidable as the Gadget. The Trinity bomb was so powerful that light from the explosion could be seen as far away as 250 miles, the distance between Washington and Stimson's Highhold estate on Long Island, and could be heard as far away as 50 miles, the distance from Washington to Harrison's farm in Upperville, Virginia.

It's hard to reconcile how such seemingly innocuous images as a successful medical operation, a satisfied attending physician, a little boy, and his healthy big brother—whose bright eyes and hearty cry engendered enthusiasm and expectation—could refer to something so devastating and destructive of human life. The loaded symbolism represented in the military's appropriation of the actions and attitudes of the medical profession, in this instance, is hard to miss. The significance of such symbolism, however unintended, would only become more pronounced as the doctors continued their unusual contribution to the Manhattan Project in the months ahead. A message clearly intended in the coded cable, though, was that attention had shifted from the successful Gadget in the New Mexico desert to the uranium bomb now headed for Tinian Island.

3

Delivering Little Boy

Does this make you a hero or a villain?
—Alice Blean, note to James F. Nolan

On the morning of July 14, 1945, a closed black truck and seven radio-equipped cars, teeming with security, descended the winding road from Los Alamos toward Albuquerque, New Mexico. In one of the cars were the military couriers of the bomb, James F. Nolan and Robert Furman, who were tasked with carrying a large portion (approximately 60 percent) of the core explosive material (U-235) for the first atomic bomb to be used in military combat. As the convoy wound down the narrow road facing the majestic Sangre de Cristo Mountains to the east, a tire on one of the cars suddenly blew. Armed military guards nervously secured the area while a corporal repaired the damaged tire. Once completed, the caravan continued to Kirkland Air Force Base in Albuquerque, where three DC-3 military planes awaited their arrival.

Nolan and Furman had met for the first time a few days earlier. Furman had recently returned from his work on the Alsos project and was asked to cut short a restful and much anticipated beach vacation. As one of Leslie Groves's most trusted top aides, Furman was assigned to be the security officer and Nolan the science / medical officer for the top-secret transport of the bomb. When Furman first arrived in Los Alamos from Washington on July 11, Nolan invited him to his Los Alamos apartment. Earlier in the day, Furman had met with Robert Oppenheimer in Santa Fe, where, while sitting in a sedan in the parking lot of La Fonda, the scientific director offered more details on their assignment.[1] The tired and emaciated Oppenheimer was on his way to the Trinity test, scheduled for detonation in five days. Oppie wished Furman luck on the mission and then made his way to

Alamogordo, while Furman set out for the thirty-five-mile trek from Santa Fe to the Los Alamos mesa.

Furman arrived at the Nolans' Los Alamos apartment around five o'clock that evening. Ann Nolan served drinks and hors d'oeuvres as the two men got to know each other. Nolan had been given permission to tell Ann about the trip, and she was understandably quite nervous. As more cocktails were served, the small party relaxed. The next day, Furman and Nolan went to the PX at Bruns General Hospital in Santa Fe to procure the necessary accouterments for the false identities they would assume on the mission. Though one was in the Army Medical Corps and the other in the Army Corps of Engineers, Nolan and Furman would masquerade as army artillery officers for this assignment. Artillery insignia, therefore, were among the items they picked up at the PX. Around this time, according to Nolan, they made their "deep and dark cloak and dagger plans for the trip."[2] On the next day, they rehearsed the first part of the anticipated journey, traveling as far as Santa Fe from Los Alamos, in order to assess matters related to timing and security.

With most of the community's attention focused on the Trinity test, the couriers were able to depart on July 14 without eliciting too much attention. The trip, as Nolan remembered, constituted a sort of "secrecy within secrecy."[3] After making the journey from Los Alamos to Albuquerque, Nolan and Furman boarded a military plane at Kirkland, destined for San Francisco, where the USS *Indianapolis* awaited them. The two "artillery officers" were outfitted with parachutes, as was the eighteen-by-twenty-four-inch, three-hundred-pound lead canister of U-235, the core material for the atomic bomb, sitting between them. Soon after, the three DC-3s lifted off from the runway at Kirkland Field, one flying in front and one behind the plane carrying Nolan, Furman, and Little Boy.

It was made clear to the two escorts that protecting the precious cargo was their primary concern, even more important than their own lives. As Furman remembered, "The idea was . . . to keep track of the bomb if the plane crashed. They didn't care about anyone. They just wanted to know where to pick up the uranium."[4] In fact, when Groves briefed Furman on the assignment, he explained that if anything were to happen during the air transport, "we won't be looking for you. We'll be looking for the shipment. You're only the expediter."[5] Richard Newcomb puts it even more starkly: "The instructions were simple—if anything happens to the plane, to hell with the men, save the uranium."[6] After an uneventful flight, the three military planes touched down in the afternoon at Hamilton Army Air Force Base in San Francisco. A convoy of vehicles filled with security was waiting to carry the cargo and the men from Hamilton Field to Hunters Point Navy Shipyard.

The armed guards conducting the ground transport in San Francisco had already rehearsed the route several times, scrupulously observing every detail of the anticipated tour through the city. Leaving nothing to chance, they had tested traffic patterns, made trial runs across the Golden Gate Bridge, and checked train crossings on Third Street and Embarcadero. After picking up Little Boy in the afternoon of July 14, the three-car convoy, whose passengers included two navy captains, headed south across the Golden Gate Bridge. The caravan followed a route that hugged the bay along Mariana Boulevard, to Cervantes, Embarcadero, and Third Street, and then eventually to Hunters Point Boulevard and on to the naval shipyard. Years later, after information about transporting the bomb had been declassified, the *San Francisco Chronicle* published an article focused solely on the San Francisco part of the bomb's journey. A friend clipped and sent the article to Nolan, writing at the top, "Does this make you a hero or a villain?"[7] I suspect my grandfather quietly pondered this provocative question for years after the war.

Nolan and Furman turned over their heavy container, estimated at the time to be worth $300 million, when they arrived at the naval shipyard, where it was temporarily stored in the commandant's office. The next day they checked in at army headquarters, where they were given overseas shots, their military orders, and .45-caliber pistols. Given his antipathy to weapons, Nolan kept his unloaded pistol and ammunition in separate bags, a practice that hardly made his assumed role as an artillery officer convincing. Nolan was also given permission to bring a camera.[8] As the radiological officer for the mission, Nolan carried with him several pocket-pencil-size ionization chambers and a large and somewhat cumbersome ionmeter, an instrument that had been designed to detect potential radiation during the Normandy landings. He also brought a portable Geiger-Muller counter, which was lighter and more fragile than the ionmeter but had a more sensitive range and could be used to measure beta particles.

In the early morning of Sunday, July 15, Charles B. McVay, captain of the USS *Indianapolis,* was summoned to naval headquarters for his final orders. Meeting with Deak Parsons and Admiral William Purnell, he was given instructions for carrying the special cargo. He was told that his ship was to move that day from Mare Island (another naval shipyard about twenty-five miles northeast of San Francisco) to pick up two pieces of top-secret cargo at Hunters Point. The *Indianapolis* was to leave Hunters Point early the next morning. Should anything happen to the ship while traveling, the cargo, even before his ship and his sailors, was to be protected. Little could McVay have realized at the time the significance and ultimate meaning of these portentous instructions.

His ship was to travel across the Pacific at top speed, and neither he nor anyone else on the crew of 1,195 men was to know what they were transporting. In addition to Little Boy, the *Indy* was to take on an extra 100 men (not members of the crew) who would be dropped off at Pearl Harbor before the vessel carried on to Tinian Island. McVay was told further that every day saved in getting from San Francisco to Tinian could shorten the war by the same amount of time. The meeting was direct and lasted all of about half an hour. In keeping with Groves's philosophy of compartmentalization—his belief that no one was to know more than was necessary to complete his or her specific job—McVay was told only what he needed to know in order to carry out his assigned task. He was understandably bewildered by the mysterious instructions, and somewhat nervous about the state of his cruiser.

The *Indianapolis* had been the victim of a damaging kamikaze attack off the island of Okinawa in late March. After limping back across the Pacific, the ship had been undergoing significant repair work at the Mare Island Naval Shipyard, which, when it was selected for the top-secret mission, was a bit behind schedule. After receiving its new assignment, however, the repair work was expedited. With the overhaul barely, or not quite, complete in mid-July, there was little time for McVay to test all of the ship's restored operations and train the approximately 250 new crew members on the routines of his normally well-ordered ship.[9] The rushed schedule, thus, complicated testing and training exercises.

Commander Joseph Flynn, the executive officer on the *Indianapolis* responsible for supervising training exercises, communicated these less than ideal circumstances to Nolan. "By reason of the ship's present mission," wrote Flynn, "our anticipated and needed training period has been deferred" and would have to be conducted while the ship was en route to Tinian. As a consequence, guest officers were asked to stay out of the way while the crew trained "intensively and extensively during this passage."[10] Before departing,

McVay used what limited time he had to test out the repaired (or nearly repaired) vessel. On Saturday, while Nolan and Furman were flying from Albuquerque to San Francisco, McVay and his crew took the *Indianapolis* out for a brief set of sea trials. The cruiser seemed to respond well enough to the tests. After McVay received his final instructions, the *Indianapolis* was moved from Mare Island to Hunters Point on Sunday morning.

Later in the afternoon, after the *Indianapolis* had docked, two army trucks pulled up to the wharf near the ship. From one truck was lifted a large crate, about fifteen feet long, five feet high, and five feet wide. It contained "a collection of bomb casing parts" and was intended to serve as a sort of decoy.[11] From the other truck, two marines lifted the eighteen-by-twenty-four-inch canister of U-235. The canister hung on a metal pole between them as Nolan and Furman followed directly behind. One of the marines, Glover Carter, remembered how "incredibly heavy" the canister was and how they "used a crow bar to lift it."[12] The large crate garnered the most attention and curiosity, such that the smaller shipment, and the two army officers accompanying it, slipped onto the ship with little notice. Lewis Haynes, the ship's doctor, however, did notice the two men. He was standing on the forecastle deck at the time and observed the mysterious cargo and the two fake artillery officers. He didn't recognize either of the men and thought they looked a little nervous, especially Nolan.[13] The container of U-235 was taken to the flag lieutenant's portside cabin and bolted to the floor.

As instructed, Nolan then sought out McVay and informed him that he wasn't an artillery officer but a medical doctor. He assured McVay that nothing they were carrying would cause damage to his ship or to the crew. McVay, more perplexed than relieved, responded, "I didn't think we were going to use bacteriological weapons in this war." Nolan, who had been sworn to secrecy as to the contents of the cargo, said nothing in reply and eventually walked away, or as he put it, "We let it go at that."[14] A little after five o'clock in the morning on Monday, July 16, the *Indianapolis* set sail. In Nolan's words, "We took off like a bat from San Francisco, for Hawaii, in what was purported to be a speed trial." On the very same morning, approximately 1,200 miles to the southeast, the Gadget was detonated at the Trinity Site. Nolan recalled that he was "quite anxious to know whether or not it was successful, but had no way of finding out until we reached our destination."[15]

The USS *Indianapolis*

The *Indianapolis* passed under the Golden Gate Bridge and raced out of San Francisco Bay. By the time the cruiser had reached the Farallon Islands, thirty miles past the bridge, it was clipping along at a speedy thirty-three knots. It would take only 74.5 hours to travel over 2,400 miles to reach Pearl Harbor, a navy record that stands to this day.[16] Upon reaching the Hawaiian base on July 19, the *Indianapolis* quickly refueled while the one hundred extra men got off the cruiser. The one regular crew member to disembark the ship that day was the cruiser's chief engineer, Commander Glen F. DeGrave, who had come up for retirement.

DeGrave, whom Nolan and Furman had gotten to know a bit during the first three-plus days of travel, was not happy about these orders, which he had successfully challenged several times before. While the military had relented in the past, this time his instructions were firm and his forced retirement final. Furman remembered how "indignant" DeGrave was "at the injustice of the orders" and how he "stomped off the ship" at Pearl Harbor while "kicking and screaming."[17] Nolan similarly recollected DeGrave's departure: "He and everyone else seemed to be very sad at the parting and thought it was quite unfair." Alluding to the tragic fate that awaited the rest of the crew and to DeGrave's good fortune, Nolan added, "But he at least avoided the ultimate disaster."[18] The remainder of the crew would not even be allowed ashore, as McVay quickly turned the ship back to sea, less than five hours after arriving at Pearl Harbor.

In addition to his uncomfortable initial interaction with McVay, Nolan endured other awkward moments aboard the *Indianapolis.* Whether because it was broken or because he simply did not know how to wear it, the artillery insignia on his uniform was upside down during the entire trip. Unlike Furman, who had been a Reserve Officers' Training Corps student at Princeton University and thus had some familiarity with military ammunition, Nolan did not know the first thing about artillery. Therefore, he had difficulty responding to queries from the curious naval officers about his assumed role. Nolan remembered, "This got rather embarrassing on several occasions when naval gunnery officers would quiz me about artillery techniques in the Army, of which I knew nothing."[19]

One day, Nolan was on deck with Furman observing target practice. Standing next to the two army couriers were naval officers Donald Blum and Stan Lipski. As the officers surveyed the repeated blasts fired from the

Indy's five-inch guns, Blum turned to Nolan and asked him what size artillery he worked with. Being completely unfamiliar and uncomfortable with weaponry, Nolan paused, then raised his hands, making a circle, and said, "Oh, about this big." Blum and Lipski laughed, as did Nolan and Furman, though Nolan's response was far from a convincing performance. In order to avoid further embarrassment, and because he was generally seasick during the voyage, Nolan spent most of his time with Little Boy in the flag lieutenant's cabin, periodically checking radiation levels of the U-235 with his Geiger counter.

As a doctor, Nolan was understandably interested in learning about the ship's medical facilities. He was, therefore, pleased when McVay arranged a tour of the ship's sickbay. Haynes was proud of his facilities, which may have been larger than Nolan's Los Alamos Hospital, at least during its first months of operation. Haynes's sickbay included about a dozen beds, an operating room, x-ray equipment, a lab, and an office. During the tour, Nolan remained quiet, fearing that if he spoke he might inadvertently use technical language, thus revealing his medical background. Therefore, Furman did most of the talking. Nolan's reticence, however, only deepened Haynes's suspicions. The *Indy*'s doctor justifiably concluded that Nolan was neither an artillery man nor even in the military. Rather, he suspected him of being in the FBI.

Because Nolan spent so much time hiding in the flag lieutenant's cabin, he would not really get to know most of the other men on the ship. In addition to McVay, DeGrave, and Haynes, however, Nolan did recall meeting and talking with the ship's chaplain, Father Thomas M. Conway, a Catholic priest from Buffalo, New York, whom my grandfather described as "a very wonderful young priest."[20] Conway was a good friend of Haynes's. When the *Indianapolis* was under repair in San Francisco, and the crew on leave, Haynes wanted to visit his family in Connecticut but could not afford it. When he told Conway of his plight, the chaplain returned the next day and handed Haynes enough money to make the round-trip journey to Connecticut.[21]

During this same leave period, Conway had also taken the time to fly around the country at his own expense to visit the families of the nine men who were killed during the kamikaze attack off Okinawa. He officiated the Catholic Masses on the ship each Sunday and, with the assistance of Haynes, helped lead the Protestant services as well. As a practicing Catholic, it is likely that Nolan attended the Catholic Mass officiated by Conway on the

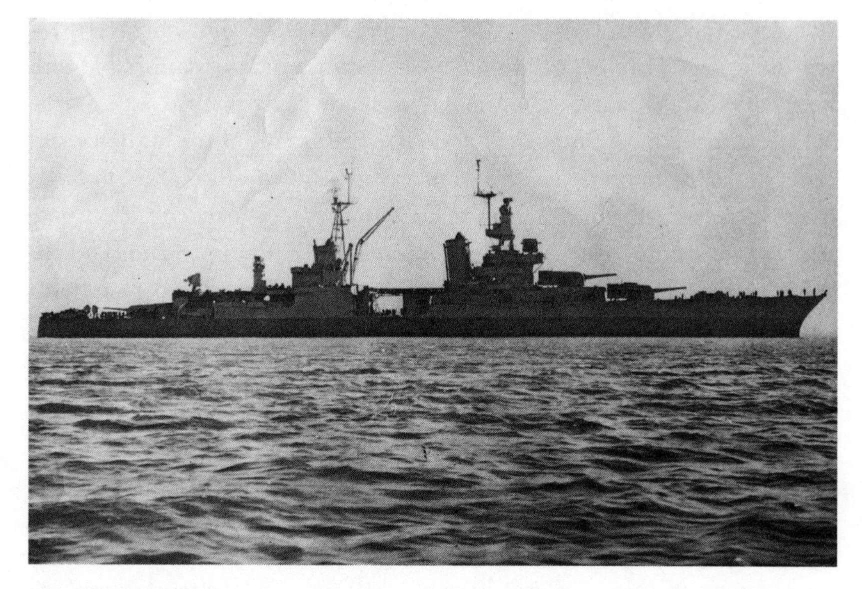

The USS *Indianapolis*.

Indianapolis on Sunday, July 22, a few days before the ship arrived at Tinian Island and one day before the ship passed just north of the Marshall Islands, a destination Nolan would return to after the war, in another chapter in the unfolding drama of the early nuclear age. While Nolan would be spared the ship's ultimate disaster, both Conway and Haynes would act with great heroism in the tragic final days of the *Indianapolis* and its crew.

Given the importance of their cargo, Furman and Nolan took precautionary measures to protect the bomb in the event of an emergency. During his final instructions in San Francisco, McVay was told that if the ship were to go down, the cargo was to be saved at all costs. Nolan and Furman were similarly instructed that "under no circumstances were they to save a life before the U-235. If the ship sank, the U-235 was to have the first motor launch or life raft."[22] Among other measures, therefore, Nolan and Furman practiced "abandon ship" routines with a dummy version of the canister.[23] In these rehearsals, as Nolan remembered, Furman would unlock the straps securing the second cylinder. Then "two large boatswain's mates appeared with a heavy steel bar which they slipped through the handles of the carrying case, and manhandled it into the passage way and out on the deck on the port side." Next, the "boat boom was rigged to swing around and secure the straps." The final step would have been to lower the cargo overboard onto one of the ship's boats steaming alongside the cruiser.[24]

When the *Indianapolis* arrived at Tinian Island on July 26, ten days after leaving San Francisco, the ineffectiveness of this exercise was made clear. Just as they had rehearsed several times during the journey, the canister was unlocked, carried to the deck, and then rigged and lowered overboard. However, when the army landing craft was brought alongside the *Indianapolis* for the transfer, the line holding the precious shipment was revealed to be too short, as the "case was swinging in mid-air about six feet from the deck of the lighter."[25] The large number of army officers on hand enjoyed a good laugh at the navy's expense over this mishap.[26] The canister was subsequently reloaded onto the deck of the *Indianapolis* and the short line was replaced with a longer wire. There were no such hiccups in the transfer of the large wooden crate containing the nonexplosive components. Both items were then quickly and carefully taken ashore and loaded onto a flatbed truck, covered with a tarp, and transported to the staging area on the island.

Nolan and Furman, of course, accompanied the cargo; they were the only men to get off the *Indianapolis* that day. One can only imagine McVay's relief and continuing confusion when he handed Nolan his "change of duty" notice upon disembarking the ship. Issued at eleven in the morning on

CA35/P16-4/00(10:ws) U.S.S. INDIANAPOLIS

26 July, 1945.

1st Endorsement

From: The Commanding Officer.
To : Captain James F. NOLAN, 0522870, FA.

Subject: Change of Duty.

1. You reported on board this vessel at 1430, 15 July, 1945, for transportation.

2. Subsistence was furnished without cost to you while on board this vessel.

3. Transportation completed at 1100 this date. You will proceed and carry out the remainder of your basic orders.

Chas. B. McVay Jr.
CHAS. B. McVAY, III.

Charles B. McVay's "change of duty" orders to James F. Nolan, July 26, 1945.

July 26, 1945, the orders were short and direct, if also notably vague. At this point, McVay still had no idea what Nolan was doing when he instructed the medical officer to "proceed and carry out the remainder of [his] basic orders."[27]

A Naval Tragedy

The rest of the ship's crew departed just six hours after dropping anchor. The fate of the *Indianapolis* represents one of the most tragic and embarrassing disasters in the history of the US Navy. Four days after dropping off Little Boy and its minders, the *Indianapolis* was traveling without escort (though one had been requested by McVay) from Guam to Leyte in the Philippine Sea. It would be joining the rest of the US naval fleet in the region, which was anticipating a land invasion of Japan scheduled for later in the year. Just after midnight on July 30, the I-58, a Japanese submarine under the command of Mochitsura Hashimoto, spotted and fired six torpedoes at the *Indianapolis.* Two of them hit their target, one just below the cabin where Little Boy had been bolted to the floor. The destroyer sank in less than twelve minutes. SOS signals were radioed before the ship went down, though it's unclear whether these were ever received.[28]

Of the 1,195 crew members, it's estimated that between 800 and 900 made it off the ship before it went down. Because one of the ship's engines kept running, the sailors, who abandoned ship at different moments, were spread out over a large area in the Philippine Sea. Many of them were covered in oil, some were in rafts, but most had only a life vest and were without food or fresh water. It would be nearly four days before Lieutenant Wilbur Gwinn, the pilot of a Ventura bomber, on a routine search mission for enemy craft, accidentally spotted the survivors and finally set rescue efforts in motion.

Each day floating in the ocean, men died, some from injuries sustained during the sinking, others from shark attacks, exposure, or dehydration, some from drinking seawater, and still others from suicide or futile efforts to swim toward imaginary islands. Some men were killed at the hands of their own hallucinating shipmates. During these harrowing days, Conway would swim from survivor to survivor offering encouragement, hearing confessions, and praying with the dying men, until finally on the third night in the open sea he himself succumbed to exhaustion. He died in the arms of his friend Haynes. Haynes himself did all that he could to aid survivors, prevent them from drinking the salt water, and dissuade them from acting on their dehydration-, hunger-, and exposure-induced hallucinations.

By the time rescue planes and ships had arrived and plucked the dying men out of the sea, more than 870 men had perished. Several more died in the process of being rescued, or a few days after. In the end, only 316 of the 1,195 crewmembers survived. At the time, none was aware of the secret mission that had spirited them so quickly across the Pacific Ocean in the first place. It would not be until days after the rescue, while recovering in a hospital on Guam, that Haynes and others were told of the actual mission of the *Indianapolis.* Furman, while visiting survivors at the hospital in Guam, found Haynes. He informed the courageous doctor of the atom bomb, of the particular design of the uranium-based Little Boy, and of the role the *Indianapolis* had played in transporting the weapon.[29] Though Haynes was evidently and understandably nonplussed by this information, it finally became clear to him that his suspicions regarding the mysterious army artillery officers had been justified.

The tragic fate of the *Indianapolis* was overshadowed by news of the atomic bomb droppings, Little Boy on Hiroshima on August 6 and Fat Man on Nagasaki on August 9, and the end of World War II. Nevertheless, the navy needed to contact the families of the deceased and explain why such a monumental catastrophe had occurred. What happened next is far from the finest hour in the history of the US Navy. In short, the navy needed a scapegoat, and the venerable Captain McVay was chosen for this unwelcome and undeserved role. McVay had been instructed to zigzag the ship in order to throw off potential enemy vessels, but at his discretion. On the evening of the attack, because it was nighttime and visibility was low, the ship was not zigzagging.

McVay was court-martialed for this ostensible infraction. The ship's survivors supported their captain and many, including Haynes, testified in his defense. The navy was so desperate to pin the calamity on McVay that it took the unprecedented step of bringing Hashimoto, the commander of the Japanese submarine that sank the *Indianapolis,* to Washington, DC, to testify against McVay. His testimony essentially backfired, as Hashimoto stated that because the *Indianapolis* was traveling alone, it did not matter whether it was zigzagging.[30] Still, McVay was found guilty and became another victim of this unparalleled naval tragedy.

Nolan was in Washington during the time of McVay's trial. He was, along with the survivors, deeply sympathetic to McVay's plight and felt that the captain was being treated unjustly. "I thought Captain McVey [*sic*] was a very admirable man, and his crew extremely competent," Nolan recalled. "I happened to be in Washington late in 1945 at the time of the investigation. At that time I felt the greatest sympathy for the Captain, as I can understand how deeply he felt over the loss of his ship and crew."[31] Haynes felt much the same and at the end of his testimony voluntarily stated, "I would like to say that under Captain McVay's command the *Indianapolis* was a very efficient, trim, fighting ship, and I would be honored and pleased to serve under him again."[32] For years after the trial, McVay would receive hate mail from the family members of those who died in the sinking of the *Indianapolis.* He finally had enough, and on November 6, 1968, outside his Connecticut home, with his navy-issued revolver, took his own life.

It would not be until 2000, after decades of protests from the survivors, McVay's family, and others, that Congress finally passed a joint resolution exonerating McVay of any culpability for the loss of his ship and the lives of his crew. Interestingly, it was Hashimoto who would play a pivotal role in urging the Senate to finally take action. In November 1999, Hashimoto wrote a letter to Senator John Warner, chair of the Senate Armed Services Committee: "I have met many of your brave men who survived the sinking of the Indianapolis. I would like to join them in urging that your national legislature clear their captain's name. Our peoples have forgiven each other for that terrible war and its consequences. Perhaps it is time your peoples forgave Captain McVay for the humiliation of his unjust conviction."[33] A year after Congress exonerated McVay, the navy followed suit and, on July 13, 2001, nearly fifty-six years after his court-martial, the following was added to McVay's military record: "The American people should now recognize Captain McVay's lack of culpability for the tragic loss of the USS *Indianapolis* and the lives of the men who died as a result of the sinking of that vessel. Captain McVay's military record should now reflect that he is exonerated for the loss of the USS *Indianapolis* and so many of her crew."[34]

Why did the navy use McVay as a scapegoat in the first place? It appears that a number of mistakes were made by the navy, which, if brought to light, would implicate higher-ranking officers. As Donald Blum, the naval officer who had embarrassed Nolan with his inquiries about artillery, put it, "The whole courts-martial was a put up deal to take blame from the serious mistakes of the higher ups."[35] Not only was McVay denied an escort, there was known intelligence of enemy submarines in the area at the time, about which McVay was not informed. The navy also made errors when personnel failed to record and report that the USS *Indianapolis* did not show up in Leyte as scheduled on August 1, thus resulting in the long-delayed rescue effort.

A thorough investigation and vetting of these errors would bring unwelcome negative publicity to a branch of the military whose very relevance was believed to be in question.[36] Given the effectiveness of air strikes, including the dropping of the atom bombs, the navy began to worry that it might be regarded as an obsolete branch of the military, a concern that would play a significant role, as we will see, in pushing forward the testing of nuclear weapons in the Marshall Islands after the war. Evidence suggests that the navy used McVay as a fall guy, and resisted righting this wrong for years, because it feared bad publicity as well as costly litigation.[37] As we have already seen, similar fears would play a part in the military's efforts to downplay and cover up the full extent of radiation injuries from both experimental and combat use of nuclear weapons.

Tinian Island

Safely situated on Tinian Island, Nolan did not hear about the sinking of the *Indianapolis* until about week after it occurred. Back in the United States, Ann Nolan learned of the tragic fate of the vessel before she heard anything from her husband and did not know whether he was still on the cruiser when it was attacked. Therefore, "when news of the sinking . . . was published in the papers," Nolan remembered, "she was necessarily upset for several days until the mail began to trickle through from Tinian."[38]

Tinian Island, a part of the Mariana Islands in Micronesia, is approximately 1,500 miles south of Japan. Occupied by the Japanese since the end of World War I, the island was taken over by the United States during the Battle of Tinian in the summer of 1944. Among the ships contributing to this successful campaign was the USS *Indianapolis,* in its illustrious days as the flagship of the navy's Fifth Fleet under Admiral Raymond Spruance's command. In the following year, the US military turned the island, curiously code-named Papacy, into one of the world's largest air bases. From Tinian's North Field, by the early summer of 1945, as many as four B-29s would take off simultaneously on the crushed coral surfaces of the mile-long runways for bombing raids on Japan.

It was not uncommon for the hulky planes to crash at the end of the runways. When this occurred, a bulldozer would simply push the wreckage aside, making way for more bombers to take off. Approaching Tinian from the air in the summer of 1945, one could actually make out the piles of debris from the mangled B-29s in what came to be known as "elephants' graveyard," the "resting place for these unfortunate giants of the sky."[39] During these bombing missions, as many as four hundred B-29s would take off from North Field in a period of less than two hours.[40]

Nolan was made part of the Alberta Project or the 509th Composite Group, the military unit sent to Tinian to assemble and deliver the atomic bomb. Nolan recalled his responsibilities: "My duties at the Tinian takeoff point were those of radiation safety for the assembly, loading and takeoff, to ascertain any radiation hazard in case of accident."[41] After Nolan and Furman arrived with their cargo on July 26, they awaited the delivery of the remaining parts of Little Boy, which would be transported by plane under the charge of Peer de Silva. De Silva, who had been the head of security in Los Alamos, would assume the same role on Tinian Island.

At Los Alamos, the security and surveillance efforts that de Silva was responsible for were deeply resented by the scientific community. As noted in Chapter 1, he was the scrupulous and overzealous investigator of Oppenheimer's movements and conversations.[42] Nolan, of course, knew de

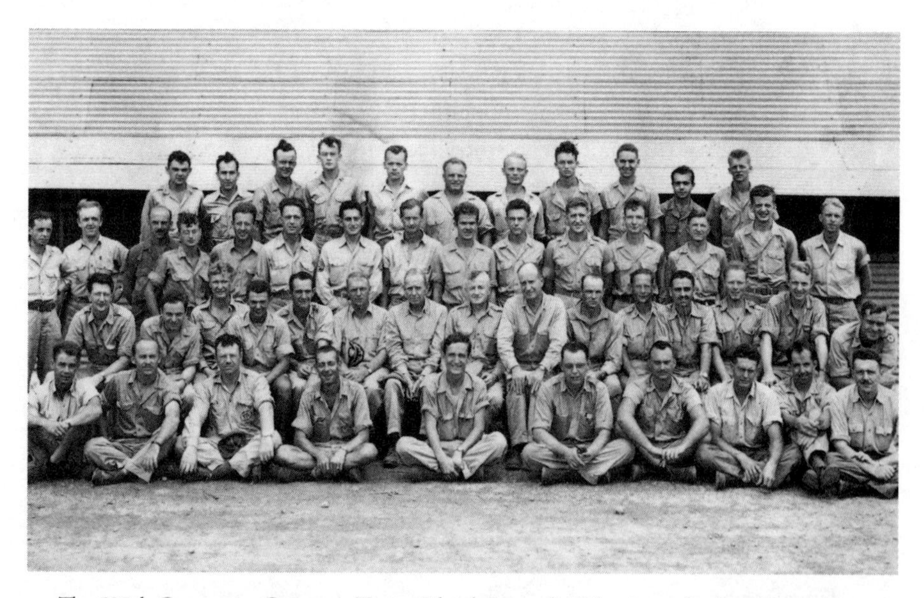

The 509th Composite Group on Tinian Island. James F. Nolan is on the far right in the second row from the bottom.

Silva at Los Alamos. The de Silvas had introduced Jim and Ann Nolan to Eleanor Roensch, a telephone operator on the Hill who would regularly babysit for both families. It was also de Silva who, a week before the Trinity test, first "warned Nolan [that] he was going to Tinian as a courier."[43]

De Silva followed Nolan to Tinian, as he was responsible for overseeing the delivery of the remaining U-235 of Little Boy by air transport. On the same day that Nolan and Furman stepped off the USS *Indianapolis* at Tinian, three Green Hornet C-54s, large military cargo planes, took off from Kirkland Field in Albuquerque. Each C-54 carried one part of the target portion of the fissionable material for Little Boy, or 40 percent of the total

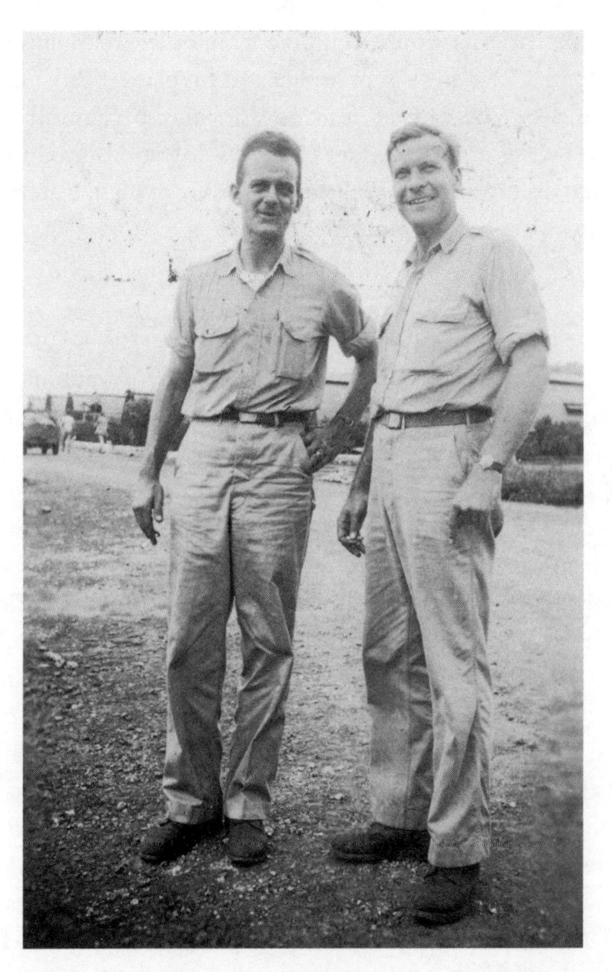

Peer de Silva and James F. Nolan (*right*) on Tinian Island.

U-235 used in the bomb. On the second leg of the journey, the plane carrying de Silva ran into trouble, as one of the Green Hornet's engines failed. In the air for about forty-five minutes, the plane was forced to turn back to San Francisco for repairs; the other two C-54s carried on across the Pacific. By July 28, the planes had arrived at Tinian, and all was now set for final assembly of Little Boy.[44] Transport for the plutonium and component parts of Fat Man, the bomb that would ultimately be dropped on Nagasaki, followed shortly thereafter.

On the day of de Silva's arrival, Nolan sent a secret memo to Stafford Warren updating his medical boss on the safe arrival of their precious cargo and reviewing with Warren his understanding of his duties on Tinian. These would include monitoring the "shipments and assembly operations" and being in charge of "catastrophe equipment" in order "to monitor the scene in case of disaster." Nolan also communicated his plans to "advise local medical personnel on the care of persons who may become ill from over-irradiation." When the remainder of the U-235 and plutonium arrived, Nolan would observe the handling and assembly of these materials, and he promised to report on such activities to Warren later.[45]

Secrecy and Its Consequences

Around this time, Nolan was reminded again of the vital importance of secrecy. This was, of course, a theme that had already been conveyed to him on several occasions. Recall, for example, that secrecy was a primary theme discussed when Nolan first met with Oppenheimer and Groves in Washington, DC, back in February 1943. Recall also that Nolan was made to burn the first security pass issued to him at Los Alamos. Secrecy was one of the reasons Groves objected to Nolan's warnings about radiation fallout from the Trinity test; and Nolan characterized his mission with Furman as a case of "secrecy within secrecy." In case Nolan had somehow missed the message, he was reminded yet again, and in rather forceful terms, about the critical importance of secrecy in a July 30, 1945, letter from Colonel John Lansdale.

The stated intent of Lansdale's letter was to review for Nolan his "obligations in safeguarding the security of classified information concerning work being conducted by the Manhattan Engineer District." Lansdale assured Nolan that this reminder should not be interpreted as somehow questioning the doctor's "integrity or discretion." Rather, the communication was to remind Nolan of the "unusually vital importance of the work" and warn him not to discuss any aspect of it either during or after the mission. "After relief from assignment to the Manhattan District," Nolan was instructed, "you will not discuss the nature of your past work with, or make any unauthorized disclosure of any classified information concerning this District to anyone regardless of status, grade, or rank under the penalties provided by the Articles of War and the Statutes of the United States."[46] So important was the work that Nolan was warned that "disclosure of information cannot be tolerated, and violations of secrecy, whether through intent or carelessness, must be considered as serious." Nolan was made to sign the document and acknowledge that he understood and was aware of "the penalties provided for the violations thereof."[47]

Furman was also reminded more than once about the importance of secrecy, such that he did not tell anyone about his wartime missions for more than three decades after the war ended. As Bendan McNally notes, in an article on Furman, "The Manhattan Project had been a program of such extreme secrecy that Furman was bound by oaths to silence until well into the 1970s."[48] Even after material was declassified and Furman was given more freedom to talk about his wartime service, because the habit of concealment had been so deeply ingrained in him, he remained reluctant to discuss his experiences. Furman himself was aware that this emphasis on secrecy carried over into his personal life in a number of ways.[49] Others have commented on this consequence of the Manhattan Project. Rose Bethe, wife of Nobel Prize–winning German-born physicist Hans Bethe, for example, once observed that "secrecy becomes a habit." She acknowledged that it directly affected the nature of her communication with her husband. "Hans stopped talking about his work. We just stopped talking."[50]

The habit of secrecy also characterized Nolan's life. While in later years he occasionally gave interviews and lectures about his wartime experiences, he was notably reluctant to discuss his various roles. Even close family members recall hearing very little about his unique journey, and concerning some aspects of experience—such as what he saw in Japan—virtually nothing at all. One can only imagine the anguish and psychological toll he endured from keeping hidden and unspoken such life-changing experiences for so long. Yet, given the sort of admonitions communicated to Nolan in Lansdale's letter, it is understandable that he would be reluctant to talk, even among those closest to him.

The *Enola Gay*

Given the frequency with which B-29s crashed at the end of the North Field runways, Deak Parsons and others became concerned about the particular difficulties the *Enola Gay* would face in carrying the extra-heavy (9,700 pounds) Little Boy. An accident in this instance could result in the detonation of the atomic bomb and the destruction of a good portion of Tinian Island. In the case of a mishap, Nolan would be responsible for ascertaining radiation levels before any rescue operations could ensue. Parsons, who was part of the *Enola Gay* crew, was so worried about the hazards of a potential crash that he recommended and then took personal responsibility for completing assembly of Little Boy inside the plane's bomb bay after takeoff.

Nolan was likewise concerned about the possibility of an accident, so much so that he requested additional assistance from Warren. "The danger from catastrophe," he wrote, "is at least directly proportional to the possibility of accident in take-off or landing of aircraft. As this is always a palpable possibility with large 'pay-loads,' it would be advisable to maintain a specially trained person at Destination or else train one of the local physicians (e.g., the radiologist at the General Hospital) sufficiently to take care of possible emergencies."[51]

Just before the *Enola Gay* departed with Little Boy on the morning of August 6, Nolan took a group of military personnel to the end of the runway and instructed them, in the case of an accident, not to go near the crash until he gave them the go-ahead.[52] For some, this was the first they had learned of the actual nature of the bomb. Even some members of the *Enola Gay* crew, though they were aware that they were carrying an important and destructive weapon, would not know that it was an *atomic* bomb until in flight to Hiroshima. Upon their return to Tinian from Hiroshima, the crew was welcomed by a crowd of some two hundred people. After a short congratulatory moment, in which Colonel Paul Tibbets was awarded a Distinguished Service Cross by General Carl Spaatz, the crew was whisked to a debriefing room. The first order of business was a medical examination of the crew by Nolan, which included a medicinal shot of whiskey.[53]

Nolan submitted an account of this examination to Warren the following day. Of particular concern were the eyes of two crew members who forgot to bring and wear their protective goggles. "Although neither one had direct vision," Nolan reported, "they did notice effects of the intense lighting for a very short time."[54] Nolan ran a Geiger counter over the crew members' bodies and over the *Enola Gay.* Thomas Ferebee, the bombardier who released the bomb, raised concerns about sterility. "It's not my eyes I'm worried about, Doc," Ferebee said to Nolan. "It's my manhood." Nolan assured him that his reproductive capacities had not been harmed, evidently with some justification, as Ferebee would go on to father four children.[55]

Another crew member volunteered that he had "noticed a vague but distinctive odor or taste," which Nolan observed was the same sensation "described by Sgt. Kupferberg after the Omega accident."[56] Nolan was referring to an accident that occurred at the Omega Site in Los Alamos on June 4, 1945, in which a number of people had been exposed to high levels of radiation during an experiment measuring the criticality of enriched uranium. Jess Kupferberg was among those who noticed a blue glow when the material approached criticality, and Nolan had been one of the attending physicians who examined the workers after the incident.

Following the return of the *Enola Gay* and its crew, members of the 509th Composite were not given much time to celebrate, as preparations were soon under way for the delivery of Fat Man. The primary target in this case was the Japanese city of Kokura. Cloudy weather on August 9 prevented clear visibility of Kokura. After three attempts to deliver the bomb, Fat Man was dropped on the secondary target city of Nagasaki instead. The two bombs would result in the estimated deaths of 140,000 in Hiroshima and 74,000 in Nagasaki, approximately 95 percent of whom were civilians. Tens of thousands more were injured, in some cases with lifelong and life-shortening, debilitating symptoms. In about a month, Nolan would see on the ground the full extent of the damage wrought by these two destructive weapons.

Waiting to Enter Japan

After *Bockscar,* piloted by Charles Sweeney, took off for delivery of the Fat Man bomb, Nolan gathered with three others on Tinian Island and conspired to initiate an investigative team to enter Japan after its anticipated surrender. As Nolan recalled, "On the evening of August 9th after the 'take-off' for the Nagasaki raid Phil Morrison, Peer de Silva, Bill Penny, and I formulated a plan for the immediate entry of a survey group including medical, scientific, and military intelligence people to operate independently in order to gather data."[57] That same night, the four conspirators took their plot to General Thomas Farrell for his approval. Two days later, Groves put in motion an effort, to be led by Farrell and Warren, for entry into Japan.

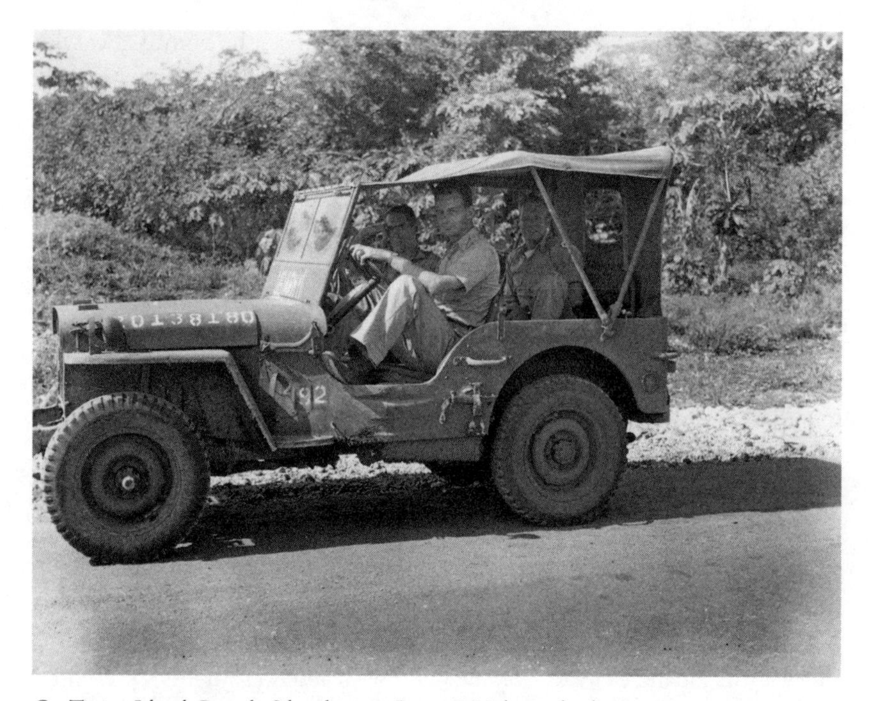

On Tinian Island. Peer de Silva driving, James F. Nolan in back seat.

Though given high priority, it would take a couple of weeks for stateside members of the mission to reach Tinian Island and prepare for transportation into the defeated country. In the meantime, Nolan and Furman had plenty of time to kill on Papacy. As Furman wrote in his diary, "How to spend time, pass it away, becomes an ever present problem for some people." Furman would pass the time reading about physics and Japan, in preparation for the upcoming mission. Others occupied themselves with hand-washing their clothes, playing volleyball, and taking jeep rides around the island. Furman and Nolan took several swimming excursions to Tinian beaches. They found the ocean "warm and exhilarating" and the colorful fish wonderful to look at in the "crystal clear water."[58]

During this period, Furman got a full dose of Nolan's unusual humor. For example, on August 28, about a week before departing for Japan, Nolan publicly celebrated his wife's birthday. Furman recorded Nolan's comic ruminations: "The Captain's wife's birthday is today and we have heard often his prodigious and fervent family feelings expressed as sort of his contribution to her celebration although he is unheard and far away. However well he loves her, it has been evident that he fears she might have bought herself a fur coat. He hasn't decided whether or not to be mad if she did."[59] Nolan's musings, in this instance, were just one example of the way in which the men on Tinian could be "devoured in such thought" as a way of coping with the "bountiful" time afforded them as they waited for their next assignment.[60]

Later, after a group of men went for a jeep ride, Nolan was on his cot "diagnosing and rediagnosing himself." Again, Furman entered into his diary Nolan's curious form of self-entertainment: "Last night he [Nolan] thought he had malaria. Nobody else qualified to know thinks he has a chance of having this mosquito-propagated disease, but he enjoys the game instituted by himself and agrees and disagrees at regular intervals after each review of his case history."[61] Around this time, Nolan also decided that he would grow a mustache, an effort about which he would also offer amusing public commentary. Furman and Nolan, unlike others selected to participate in the forthcoming investigative effort, would not have to wait too much longer for their new assignment, as they would both be in the first group to enter the defeated country.

4

Hiroshima

. . . a trip that seems to have been an unusual mixture of tourism, scientific exploration, and public relations work.

—Daniel Lang, "A Fine Moral Point"

Assembled in an ad hoc manner, three separate American groups were commissioned to enter Japan at approximately the same time. The purposes for the trip were multiple and, as we will see, not entirely aimed at gathering information in a neutral manner. The teams were composed of representatives from the Manhattan Project, including James F. Nolan, under the leadership of Stafford Warren and, for a short time anyway, General Thomas Farrell; an army group directed by Colonel Ashley W. Oughterson; and a navy delegation led by Shields Warren (no relation to Stafford Warren). At first, the separate groups were "all over the place," but they would eventually be merged by General Douglas MacArthur into what came to be called the Joint Commission for the Investigation of the Effects of the Atomic Bomb in Japan, or more commonly the Joint Commission.[1]

Each group, it appears, came upon the idea for the investigative effort independently, though, at least by some accounts, interagency competition was a motivating factor.[2] As it concerns the Manhattan Project, following Nolan's Tinian Island meeting with William Penny, Phil Morrison, and Peer de Silva on the evening of August 9, Leslie Groves sent a memo to Farrell authorizing the investigation on August 12. In the memo he reported that Robert Oppenheimer had suggested that "Nolan, Penny, [Charles] Baker, [Robert] Serber, and Morrison would be good men for the mission."[3] Thus, three of the four original plotters were recommended; only de Silva, the security officer who had so mistrusted and relentlessly surveilled Oppenheimer in Los Alamos, was left off the list. Ultimately, however, he would be made part of the investigating party.

Stafford Warren, who was in Alamogordo at the time looking into radiation fallout issues from the Trinity test, was contacted by Groves on the same day and asked to lead the medical part of this effort. As Warren recalled, "I was tracked down by a GI in a car who said the general wanted to talk to me. So I drove back to the base camp and got on the phone and found it was General Groves calling me from Washington. He said he hated to do this to me but . . . offered me the chance to lead a party into Nagasaki and Hiroshima if we could get there."[4]

After Warren agreed to lead the medical part of the mission, he and Groves hastily recruited other Manhattan Project physicians, including Harry Whipple, Henry Barnett, and Joe Howland, along with intelligence and scientific personnel, to join those at Tinian and prepare for entry into Japan. Much to his disappointment, Louis Hempelmann was not invited to be part of the mission, a decision that was due in part to the earlier choice of having Nolan, Warren, and other physicians enter the military, while Hempelmann remained a civilian. Hymer Friedell, Warren's deputy at Oak Ridge, remembered how upset Hempelmann was: "They wanted only military personnel and that made Hempelmann madder than hell because he was a civilian. And he never went for that reason."[5]

Adding to Hempelmann's frustration, before leaving the United States, Warren's men raided Los Alamos and the other Manhattan District labs of all the Geiger counters and other radiation measurement instruments they could muster, thus making Hempelmann's work in New Mexico all the more difficult. Hempelmann complained that Warren had removed "practically all of our monitors, army men, and taken them away to Japan. So, we were very short handed."[6] The departure of key members of the Health Group, according to Hempelmann, "resulted in a serious breakdown of the health program" both at the Trinity Site and at Los Alamos.[7] It was, in fact, during this time that one of the most serious radiation accidents occurred in Los Alamos. In all, approximately forty men from the Manhattan Project would participate in the Joint Commission, including ten doctors, three physicists, and six intelligence officers.[8]

A couple of weeks after Groves had set things in motion, unaware of the Manhattan Project effort, Colonel Oughterson, then serving as surgical consultant to MacArthur in the Pacific, formulated his own plan of action.[9] After the proposal was approved, Oughterson began recruiting officers and enlisted men for his group. Prominent among them was Lieutenant Colonel Averill Liebow, who would keep an informative and engaging diary of his time on this mission.[10] Liebow would also play a critical role, along with Stafford Warren, in unearthing one of John Hersey's most important sources for his widely acclaimed book *Hiroshima.* The final American military group to make up the Joint Commission was a navy team led by Shields Warren, a pathologist in the Naval Medical Corps.[11] Shields Warren's team would be the last to enter Japan, not arriving to Nagasaki until September 24.

Thus, the Manhattan Project group was the first part of the Joint Commission to enter Japan after the cessation of conflict; and Nolan's team within that company was the first to arrive in the defeated country. Upon entering Japan, the Americans soon learned that Japanese doctors, primarily under the leadership of the esteemed Tokyo Imperial University surgeon Masao Tsuzuki, had already begun extensive efforts studying victims of the bombs in both Hiroshima and Nagasaki. Though at times fraught with misunderstandings and mistrust, there was in general a notable level of goodwill and cooperation between the American and Japanese teams; and, in fact, the Japanese doctors, led by Tsuzuki, would formally be made part of the Joint Commission in early October.[12] The Joint Commission was the precursor to the Atomic Bomb Casualty Commission (ABCC), a more sustained effort to study the biological effects of the bombs. The ABCC would also be a joint effort with American and Japanese doctors and would likewise be characterized by both cooperation and, at times, tensions and misunderstandings.

Some of the disillusionment and resentment in Japan, with both the Joint Commission and the ABCC, stemmed from the reasonable perception that the American doctors treated the *hibakusha* (survivors of the atomic bombs in both cities) as scientific specimens to be studied rather than as patients in need of medical care.[13] Other actions by the Americans during this period—such as the confiscation of more than fifteen thousand feet of film taken by a Japanese film crew in Hiroshima and Nagasaki and the dismantling of two cyclotrons—also caused resentment.[14] In 1975 the ABCC was reformed into the Radiation Effects Research Foundation (RERF), also a collaborative project, though under greater Japanese control. The RERF, which continues to this day to study the effects of radiation in Japan, still has a "no treatment" rule, a policy legacy that extends back to the time of the Joint Commission. Acknowledging ongoing frustration with this legacy, in June 2017 the Japanese chairman of the RERF, Otsura Niwa, expressed regret, though without altering the policy: "I just wanted to stress to the survivors how deeply sorry we are."[15]

Unlike the participants in the longer and more concentrated ABCC and RERF efforts, members of the Joint Commission, and especially those from the Manhattan Project, were, as journalist Daniel Lang put it, "sent to only make a spot check."[16] Indeed, Nolan was only in Japan for five weeks, from September 5 to October 12. What was the purpose of this spot check? To what extent were the doctors acting as doctors, or was it a more purely scientific mission? Were the doctors seeking to ascertain, in an objective manner, the medical effects of a nuclear explosion, or were they simply helping the military advance a predetermined narrative about the impact of nuclear radiation? Lang, based on an interview with the Manhattan Project physicist Phil Morrison, perceptively concluded that the trip was "an unusual mixture of tourism, scientific exploration, and public relations work."[17] The last aspect appears to have been the driving factor motivating Groves to get his men into Japan as quickly as possible.

Negative Press and Groves's Reaction

Days after the bomb was dropped on Hiroshima, news accounts started coming out of Japan of ongoing radiation poisoning. Groves was evidently shaken by this news, not so much because of the harmful biological effects on the Japanese but because of how these reports might affect public perceptions of the Manhattan Project's production and use of the atom bomb. Radiation could be likened to biological or chemical warfare, and Groves feared having to give an account for what could justifiably be seen as an inhumane (and illegal) form of combat. In the summer and early fall of 1945, there was little public understanding of radiation and, in particular, of the differences between *initial* and *residual* radiation.

Initial radiation refers to human exposure, primarily from neutrons and gamma rays, received in the seconds immediately after the detonation of the bomb. *Residual* or *secondary radiation,* on the other hand, refers to radioactive materials that remain in the environment for some time after the explosion. Residual radiation comes in the form of induced radiation—the penetration of neutrons and gamma rays into the soil or other substances on the ground following a nuclear explosion, resulting in the creation of new radioactive isotopes. Residual radiation can also come in the form of fallout, such as occurred at Trinity—that is, radioactive material raised up into the atmosphere by the fireball of the bomb and distributed unevenly based on weather conditions, sometimes eventually falling to the ground (including in the form of "black rain").

With reports out of Japan of ongoing radiation sickness, Groves turned to one of the military doctors at Oak Ridge to seek reassurance. On August 25, the nervous Groves placed two calls to Major Charles Rea, a University of Minnesota–trained physician and Nolan's counterpart at the Oak Ridge hospital. In his conversation with Rea, Groves read directly from one of the problematic articles: "Radioactivity caused by the fission of the uranium used in atomic bombs is taking a toll of mounting deaths and causing reconstruction workers in Hiroshima to suffer various sicknesses and ill health."[18]

Seeking to assuage his worried boss, Rea implausibly speculated that the injuries were really just the lingering effects of "thermal burns" and that what was needed was a direct response to this "hokum" and "good propaganda."[19] Groves continued, "This is the kind of thing that hurts us—'The Japanese, who were reported today by Tokyo radio, to have died mysteriously a few days after the atomic bomb blast, probably were the victims of a phenomenon which is well known in the great radiation laboratories of America.'" "That, of course," stated Groves, "is what does us the damage."[20] The articles, in other words, made the case that not only were the ongoing fatalities a consequence of exposure to radiation in Japan, but American officials had been fully aware of this effect.

Though the Manhattan Project doctors' understanding of the biological effects of nuclear radiation, given the nascent nature of the field, was incomplete, they were clearly among the most knowledgeable and informed about the phenomenon. However, as was evident in the case of the Trinity test, their warnings and concerns were not always welcomed or heeded. In a 1986 interview, Hempelmann was asked directly whether he had expected radiation from the Hiroshima and Nagasaki bombs. "Yes," was his unequivocal response. He added, though, "I don't think too much thought was given to it. The main idea was to use them and end the war."[21] In late August 1945, however, in response to Groves's agitation, Rea did not tell Groves that the doctors, or anyone else, expected radiation injuries; rather he recommended publicly refuting the "propaganda" from Japan and getting "some big-wig to put out a counter-statement in the paper."[22]

Groves also had to contend with public statements from one of his own Manhattan Project scientists. On August 7, the day after the Hiroshima bomb, the thirty-three-year-old Columbia University geneticist Harold Jacobson told a reporter that the radiation effects of the bomb would be substantial and predicted that it would take seventy years for the deposited radiation in Hiroshima to fully decay, a statement that is still remembered and cited in Japan today. Groves called both Oppenheimer and Stafford Warren in order to prepare a statement to discredit Jacobson's claims. "This is, of course, lunacy," Oppenheimer said to Groves after being read Jacobson's statement over the phone. "Based on the test in New Mexico," he added, "there would be no appreciable activity on the ground and what little there was would decay very rapidly."[23] Stafford Warren confirmed Oppenheimer's assessment, thus equipping Groves to publicly refute Jacobson.

The Manhattan Project radiologist Robert Stone, head of the health division at the Met Lab in Chicago, was surprised when he read Oppenheimer's categorical denials in the press. After seeing these statements, he quickly sent a letter to his former student Hymer Friedell at Oak Ridge expressing his incredulity: "I could hardly believe my eyes when I saw a news release said to be quoting Oppenheimer, and giving the impression that there is no radioactive hazard. Apparently, all things are relative."[24] In fact, both Oppenheimer and Warren knew about the possibility of radioactive damage in Japan and had warned both Groves and General Farrell accordingly.

Three months before the Hiroshima and Nagasaki bombs, Oppenheimer had, in a top-secret memo, explicitly warned Farrell that radioactivity was to be expected from the explosions: "During the detonation, radiations are emitted which (unless personnel is shielded) are expected to be injurious within a radius of a mile and lethal within a radius of about six-tenths of a mile." Oppenheimer even acknowledged, contingent on weather patterns, the conceivability of residual radiation, especially in the case of rainfall following the detonations.[25] Likewise, a couple of weeks before the Hiroshima and Nagasaki bombings, based on calculations from the Trinity test, Warren had sent Groves a top-secret memo (which was not declassified until 1981) warning him about potential exposure to troops who would be entering the cities immediately after a nuclear detonation. He even proposed a table of possible levels of exposure and the corresponding seriousness of injuries that would result for "normal active troops." These levels of exposure were not insignificant and ranged from thirty to five hundred roentgens of exposure depending on the length of time spent within the detonated areas. At the higher levels, he even anticipated "permanent damage" to troops.[26]

As for Jacobson, he was forced to publicly amend his comments. When military counterespionage agents interrogated him in his office, threatening imprisonment, he collapsed. Jacobson's exaggerated predictions, inasmuch as they focused on residual radiation, would, in the final analysis, serve Groves's purposes. Because of confusion about the differences between initial and residual radiation, by publicly discrediting Jacobson's overstated comments on the long-term effects of residual radiation, the military was able to tamp down concerns about radiation more generally.[27] As would become clear over time, much more dangerous and consequential than residual radiation were the penetrating—though often delayed and not immediately observable—injuries caused by initial radiation.

An important goal of the Joint Commission (especially for the Manhattan Project group) was to get a firsthand assessment of the effects of radiation and to counter the so-called propaganda about its dangerous and widespread effects.[28] Among those recruited by Groves and Warren to participate in the effort was Lieutenant Donald Collins. Collins had graduated from Michigan State University with a BS in physics. Sometime after joining the Army Air Forces, he was assigned to the Met Lab in Chicago and later transferred to Oak Ridge. On the morning of August 12, 1945, literally on the same morning Collins and his family had arrived to their new apartment in Tennessee (with moving trailer still unpacked), Collins was awakened by three military police officers. "They gave me 15 minutes to pack for an extended trip," Collins recalled.[29] Collins was ordered to take his measuring instruments and join Stafford Warren for the new assignment. While en route to Tinian Island aboard a large C-54 transport plane with other Manhattan Project recruits, he learned that the war had ended.

Once at Tinian, Farrell explained the operation to the assembled doctors and scientists. As Collins recollected, "We were addressed by Gen. Farrell who told us more specifically that our mission was to prove there was no radioactivity from the bomb."[30] Collins, who regarded himself as more of a scientist than a military man, then impertinently asked, "I thought we were going to measure the radioactivity."[31] Farrell "sputtered and stammered" in response, and Stafford Warren had to quietly warn Collins about talking back to a superior officer.[32] Collins perceived that Farrell was "concerned about public relations" and that their findings were predetermined. With biting irony, he concluded, "While we were sitting, waiting to get into Japan . . . we read in the Stars and Stripes the results of our findings!"[33]

Farrell's instructions were especially surprising to Collins in that he originally understood, as conveyed to him by Warren before arriving at Tinian, that not only were they meant to investigate levels of radiation in a more objective manner, but this information would be for the purposes of helping "medical officers in treating the casualties." In other words, he assumed that medical care was a central part of the operation. In fact, he believed the assignment was first "a humanitarian effort to assist the Japanese victims."[34] Given this perception, one can understand his surprise at hearing Farrell's instructions.

Traveling into Japan

Once the stateside component of the Manhattan Project group arrived at Tinian on August 14—and had subsequently been briefed on their mission by Farrell—the men were divided into three main groups. One group would go directly to Tokyo with Farrell and General James B. Newman Jr.; another with Stafford Warren to Nagasaki via Okinawa; and a third with Friedell by way of Guam (and then Zamboanga, Philippines) to Hiroshima. Nolan, along with Peer de Silva and Robert Furman, were part of the first group.

Furman, Nolan's partner in escorting Little Boy to Tinian Island, wasn't really part of the three main teams assessing the biological and structural damage of the bombs. He had his own special mission. As in his earlier work with the Alsos Project, Furman was part of a metallurgical group tasked with determining how far along the Japanese were in producing an atom bomb. Thus, his investigative work took him not into Hiroshima or Nagasaki but to various factories, corporations, research universities, and mining facilities, both in Japan and in Korea, to determine Japanese knowledge of and capacities for making a nuclear weapon. He soon learned that the Japanese were not remotely close to having the necessary intelligence, metallurgical resources, or facilities to make a nuclear bomb. In fact, Japan had "made even less progress than the Germans and had come nowhere near the attainment of an atomic bomb."[35] Having rather quickly assessed the situation, Furman would be among the first members of the Manhattan Project group to return to the United States.[36]

The Tokyo contingent, led by the generals, with whom both Nolan and Furman traveled, landed at the Atsugi airport, about thirty-five miles southeast of Tokyo, on September 5 "amid a scene of tremendous activity."[37] When they landed, it was only three days after Japan's formal surrender aboard

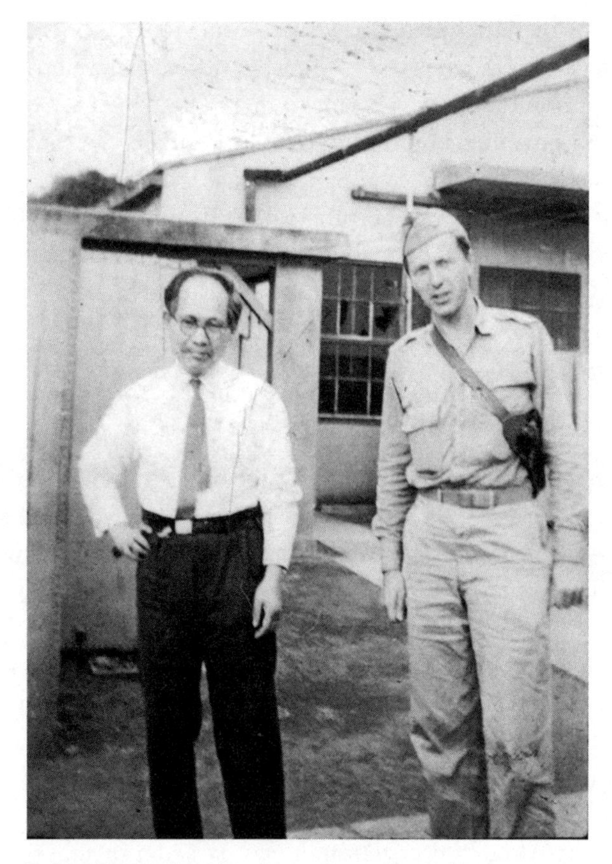

Robert Furman (*right*) in Japan, September 1945.

the USS *Missouri*. Nolan remembered the day well, as it marked his thirty-first birthday, a commemoration he was sure to make known to his coinvestigators. In addition to such entries as "Weather like Virginia in September" and "American POWs board planes for home," Furman also entered into his traveling notebook on September 5 Nolan's humorous, and no doubt oft-repeated, rendition of "Happy Birthday to Me."[38]

From the Atsugi airport this advance party entered Yokohama, a prefecture approximately twenty-five miles south of Tokyo, and began negotiating with general headquarters about starting the groups' forays into Hiroshima and Nagasaki. At this point, while the two other Manhattan Project groups were still awaiting entry into Japan, a Swiss Red Cross doctor, Marcel Junod, requested permission to ship relief supplies into Hiroshima. Junod had just received an alarming and urgent telegraph from a Red Cross delegate recently sent to Hiroshima: "Situation horrifying . . . 80% of town razed. All hospitals destroyed or severely damaged. . . . Conditions indescribable. . . . Deaths occurring in great numbers. . . . Immediate action necessary."[39] MacArthur approved Junod's humanitarian mission and Farrell capitalized on this authorization. That is, Farrell saw joining Junod as "an opportunity to get to Hiroshima," and thus sent for Stafford Warren to be flown to Tokyo immediately. Leaving his group in Okinawa, Warren joined the Tokyo group on September 6. At this point, Nolan contacted Colonel Oughterson, now in Tokyo with MacArthur, to coordinate and make arrangements for the group's entry into Hiroshima.[40]

The assembled party met the next day with Tsuzuki, who briefed the Americans on what he and other Japanese doctors had discovered in their early investigations. The fifty-two-year-old Tsuzuki spoke good English, as he had spent time at the University of Pennsylvania as a student and researcher two decades earlier. The respected Japanese surgeon, though largely cooperative with the Americans, could also be acerbic and critical. During one meeting with the American investigators, he handed to Phil Morrison his 1926 study of the damaging effects of radiation on laboratory animals.[41] After Morrison scanned and returned the document, Tsuzuki slapped the American physicist on the knee and said, "Ah, but the Americans—they are wonderful. It has remained for them to conduct the *human* experiment."[42]

On September 7, even before departing for Hiroshima, Farrell held a press briefing in an effort to dispel notions of ongoing radiation sickness. Farrell was feeling pressure from Groves to put out some kind of public statement, as Groves had been sending frantic memos requesting reports that he could use to dispel the "Japanese propaganda" finding its way into the American press. On September 5, for example, Groves sent a panicky message to Farrell asking when "our parties [would] reach Hiroshima and Nagasaki." He informed Farrell, "News stories by newspaper men who visited Hiroshima recently are causing considerable trouble here." Groves continued, "We need preliminary cable reports from Warren and Friedell covering radioactive angle from which we can extract data for use here." Groves was particularly anxious about reports "getting a big play in the American press concerning tiny and apparently harmless burns which result in death after several days. . . . Need any information you now have by immediate cable."[43]

Groves was so desperate to get some kind of report out of Japan that, while awaiting his teams' entry in early September, he even proposed having low-flying planes equipped with Geiger counters pass over Hiroshima to take measurements. General Newman consulted with Morrison about the feasibility of such a mission and then diplomatically responded to Groves: "Mechanical adequacy of instruments, and successful operation under the conditions stated, can not be guaranteed."[44]

An example of the sort of press accounts upsetting Groves was that of the Australian journalist Wilfred Burchett. Just a few days before Farrell's press briefing, after a bold and stealthy journey by train into Hiroshima, Burchett had surreptitiously transmitted via Morse code an article for the British newspaper *Daily Express* published on September 6. In the article, Burchett referred to the mysterious and continuing deaths of Japanese bomb victims as "the atomic plague." At the conclusion of Farrell's September 7 briefing, the disheveled Burchett, who had just stumbled back into Tokyo from his Hiroshima excursion, challenged the general's assertions that ongoing deaths were due only to the blast and heat effects of the bombs. Burchett asked Farrell whether he had been to Hiroshima. Farrell, of course, had not, as his group would not be leaving until the next day. Then Burchett described some of the radiation-related deaths and injuries he had just witnessed in Hiroshima, including his firsthand observations of fish swimming into a tidal river affected by the bomb and dying from contamination. As when challenged by Collins a few weeks previously, Farrell "looked pained" at Burchett's confrontation. "I'm afraid you've fallen victim to Japanese propaganda," he finally said to Burchett. Farrell then closed the briefing and sat down.[45]

Burchett was later taken to a hospital, where it was found that his white blood count was low.[46] He was told that it was likely due to a knee infection, for which he had been given antibiotics, though he later concluded that it was a consequence of radiation sickness. When he was released from the hospital, Burchett discovered that the photographs from his camera had been confiscated and that his press accreditation had been revoked. He was expelled from Japan by general headquarters and banned from doing further reporting.[47] One week later, MacArthur imposed a moratorium on any information going out of Japan. The censorship order, put in place on September 19, strictly prohibited publications on atomic bomb damages, including information about medical injuries.[48]

The morning after the press briefing, on September 8, the party, which included Warren, Oughterson, Nolan, Junod, and Tsuzuki, along with Generals Farrell and Newman and Colonel R. C. Wilson, boarded several military planes, carrying with them fifteen tons of medical supplies destined for

Hiroshima. A day or two earlier, a party that included Nolan and Warren had flown over Hiroshima to have an initial look from the air and take some aerial photographs of the city. As the DC-4 plane passed over Hiroshima, one of the photographers, likely Kurt Kasznar, "wanted to lie down on the floor and stick his camera out the cargo door." To facilitate this perilous effort, Nolan and Warren "had to sit on his feet," which made the doctors quite nervous. "We didn't like this," remembered Warren, "because this was while the plane was making turns up on one wing a bit, and we were all looking straight down to the ground through the open hatch." Warren feared that with any sudden change in movement, "we could have just nicely slid right out."[49]

On the September 8 trip, however, the planes transporting the larger group landed on an airstrip outside Hiroshima—a precarious endeavor, given that the runway was riddled with wreckage, potholes, and bombed-out craters.[50] After a three-hour flight, and several passes over Hiroshima, the American team landed around noon at the Iwakuni Airport (located about twenty miles southwest of Hiroshima). Awaiting them was a delegation of Japanese, who had prepared a small welcoming ceremony, outfitted with arranged chairs, tea, and baskets of beer.[51] Anxious to get to work and wanting to protect their delicate measurement instruments from the elements, the Americans declined the extended hospitality and quickly boarded a bus for a cumbersome journey toward Hiroshima. The decrepit, charcoal-powered bus proceeded slowly, as it had to stop every twenty minutes for refueling. As a consequence, it took nearly five hours for the group to travel fifteen miles to the Chugoku Military Headquarters outside Hiroshima. Because of this, and the limited boarding options in the bombed-out city, the group did not make it into Hiroshima that day.

Instead, the Americans were ushered to a ferry and escorted to a small island in the Hiroshima Bay called Miyajima, the home of the ancient Itsukushima shrine and a romantic vacation destination. Miyajima, about halfway between the airport and Hiroshima and far enough away to have been largely untouched by the direct impact of Little Boy, was described by Warren as "a deserted Coney Island," and by Morrison as "simply sybaritic," a place "where couples used to go for their honeymoons."[52] The party was "bivouacked in what was a very famous restaurant and hotel" and "installed in bridal cottages in a cypress grove next to a brook."[53] The strange juxtaposition of (and the glaring contrast between) this romantic holiday spot and the rancid, dusty, rubble remains of Hiroshima, some twelve miles away, is hard to envisage.

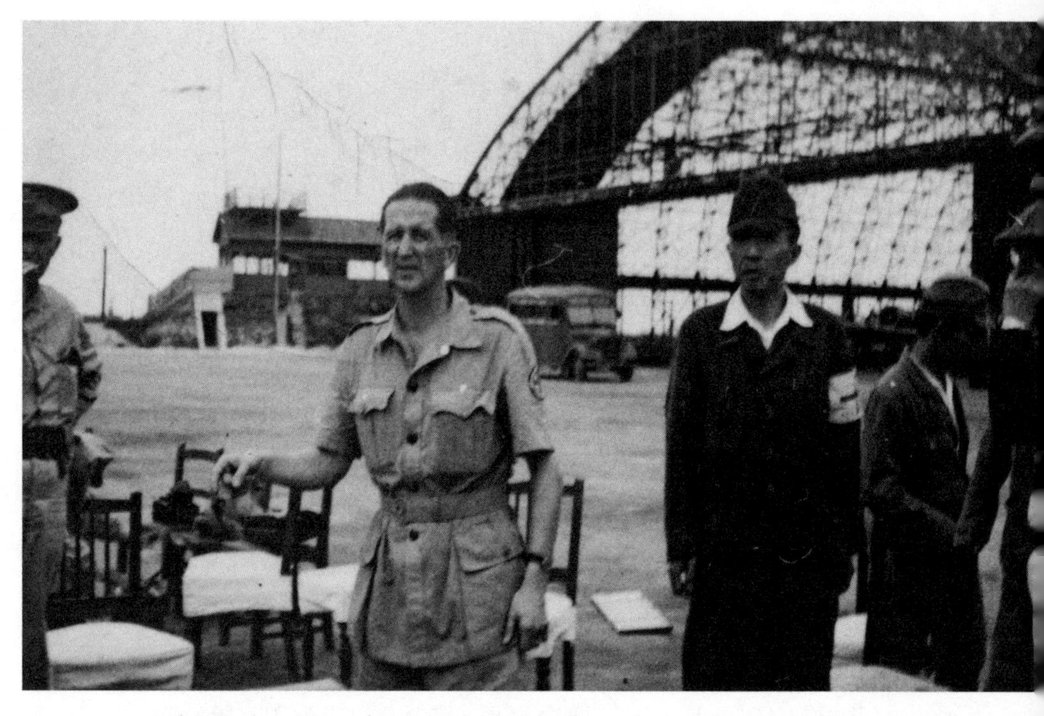

Red Cross doctor Marcel Junod (*center*) and others at Iwakuni Airport on September 8, 1945. Note the awaiting bus in the background.

Thus began, in almost comical form, the tourism part of their journey. After arriving at the resort, baths were prepared for the traveling military party of approximately twenty doctors, GIs, and officers. Members of the party were outfitted with *geitas* (wooden slipper-type shoes) and kimonos in preparation for bathing. The American officers walked to the baths on gravel with the uncomfortable *geitas* and kimonos, which on some of the taller officers only went to mid-thigh. Matters became even more awkward when the amused Japanese maids employed at the hotel stayed on hand to help the visitors bathe. The Americans also had difficulty adjusting to the Japanese "bathrooms" on the resort island, which required them to assume a squatting position on the floor and relieve themselves into a *benjo,* a ceramic bowl situated just beneath a small mosquito-infested hole in the floor. The contents of the *benjos* at the resort were gathered each day and hauled to a central location, where local farmers would collect their allotment for use as crop fertilizer.[54] Fearful that news of the surrender had not reached all parts of Japan, some of the American officers slept anxiously with .45-caliber revolvers stuffed under their pillows.

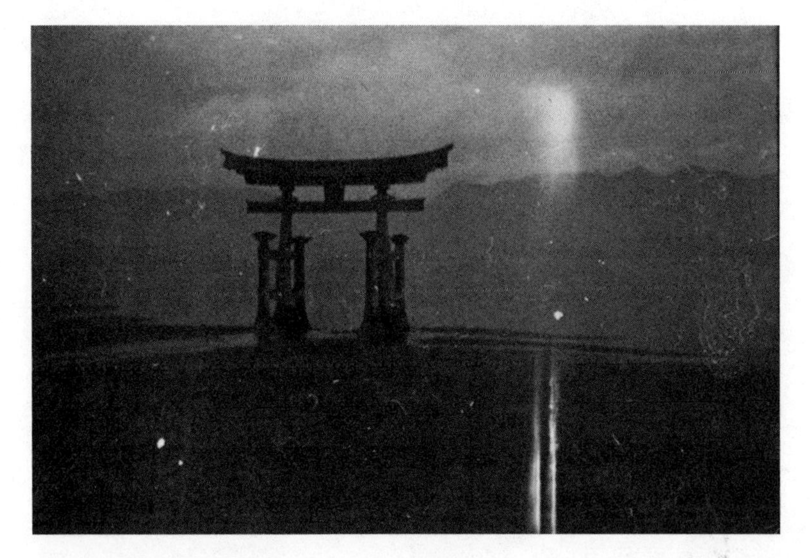

Temple gate of the Itsukushima shrine on Miyajima Island.

Entering Hiroshima

The next morning, September 9, Nolan, Warren, and the others set out for Hiroshima. With the incoming tide lapping against the large pillars of the shrine's iconic temple gate, the traveling party boarded a small steamer, which took them from Miyajima across the bay. After reaching the opposite shore, they loaded into awaiting cars for final transport into Hiroshima. As they moved closer to the center of the city, even four miles out, they began to witness the utter destruction caused by the bomb. At three miles from the epicenter, they saw fallen roofs and beams jutting from the wrecked walls of destroyed houses. At two and a half miles from ground zero, all the buildings had been obliterated and burned. The only visible signs of the once-thriving port city were portions of some of the houses' foundations and the charred remains of crumbled ironwork. Just under a mile from the epicenter, there was virtually nothing to be seen at all.

Amid an eerie silence, the first official party of Americans to see, on the ground, the direct effects of Little Boy climbed out of their cars and began to walk toward the center of the city. Not a bird or any other animal could be heard or seen. The quiet and stillness were only broken by the words and gesticulations of Tsuzuki, who, acting as the group's guide, pointed to the locations of once-bustling hospitals, banks, and other sites. While the physicists made measurements (to determine the location and height of the

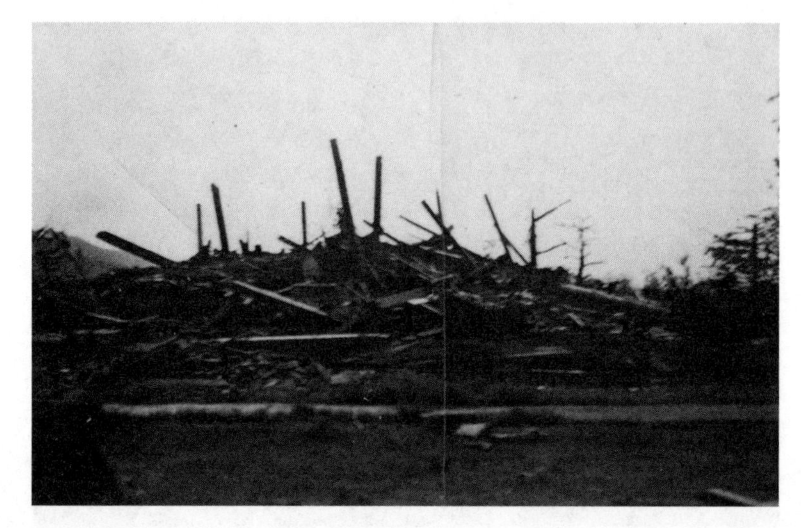

Hiroshima, September 1945.

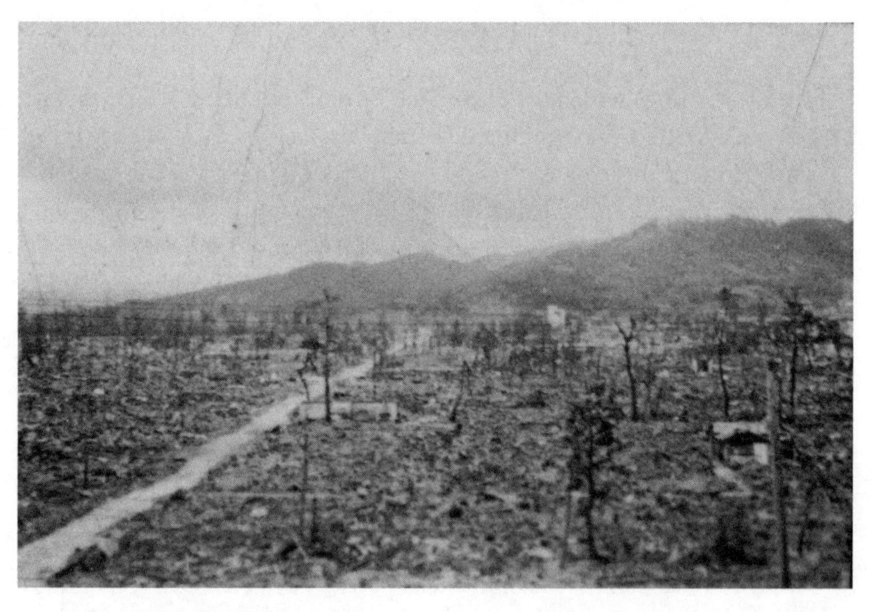

Hiroshima, September 1945.

bomb's explosion), Tsuzuki took the doctors to makeshift hospitals on the outskirts of the city where, as Junod recalled, "the most terrible sights of all awaited us."[55] What the doctors witnessed was horrifying: "the thousands of helpless, suffering bodies stretched out on the ground; the thousands of

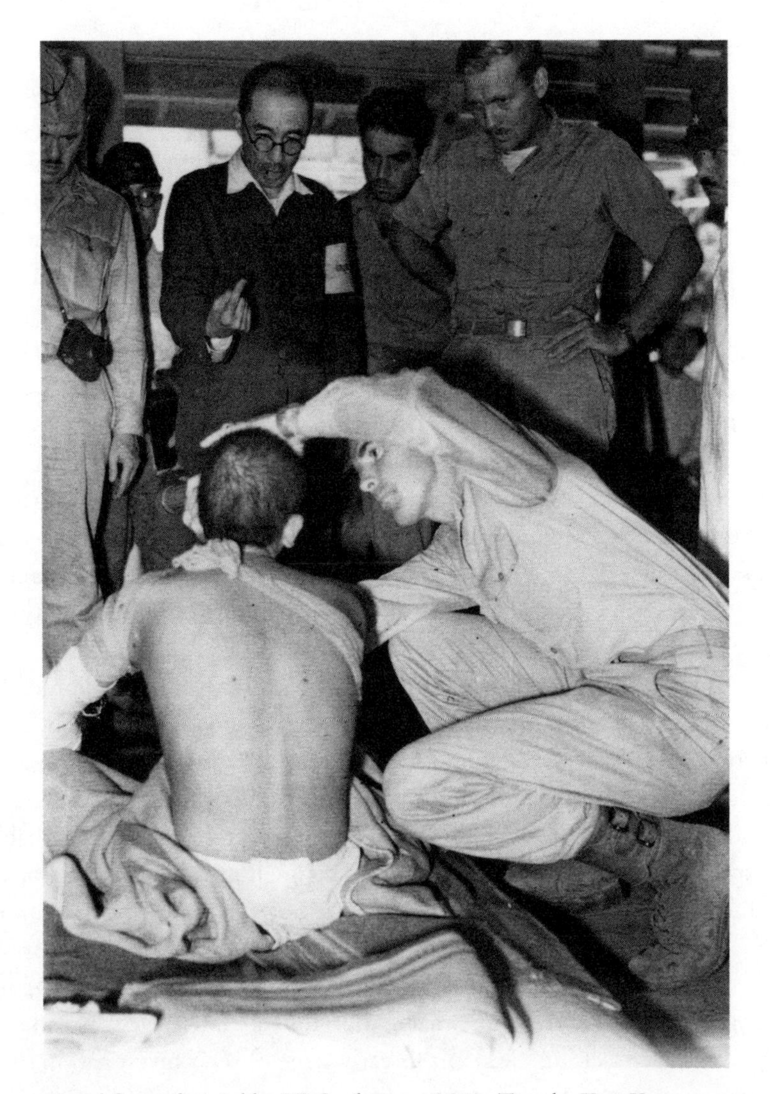

From left, standing: Ashley W. Oughterson, Masao Tsuzuki, Kurt Kasznar, and James F. Nolan. Examining patient is the ophthalmologist John J. Flick. Ono Army Hospital, September 10, 1945.

swollen charred faces; the ulcerated backs; the suppurating arms raised up in order to avoid contact with any covering."[56]

The doctors were told that about one hundred Japanese were still dying each day.[57] Tsuzuki's explanations of their surroundings and of the victims' conditions could be direct and uncompromising. He pointed to one semi-conscious woman, for example, who had suffered burns and had signs of acute radiation sickness. "Infection of the blood," Tsuzuki announced. "White corpuscles almost entirely destroyed. Gamma rays. Nothing to be done about it. She'll be dead this evening or tomorrow. That's what an atomic bomb does." At another location, Tsuzuki held up a dissected brain from a recent autopsy and, referring to his earlier studies on the effects of radiation on animals, stated bluntly, "Yesterday it was rabbits; today it's Japanese."[58]

In addition to visiting hospitals, the American group moved about the ruins with their Geiger counters in compliance with Farrell's instructions. Junod was struck by the Americans' apparent determination and certainty. "The experts from the American commission did not remain idle," Junod remembered. "They placed their detectors almost everywhere amongst the ruins. They were adamant: one month after the explosion of the bomb, the place was perfectly safe and there was no longer any danger of radioactivity for human beings."[59] For his part, Junod made his way to the Japanese Red Cross Hospital, the least damaged of the Hiroshima hospitals, for a longer visit, and then met with the director of public health in Hiroshima to arrange for the distribution of the medical supplies.[60]

As Tsuzuki explained the conditions of the various victims examined by the investigation team, the Japanese noted the difference between the posture of the American doctors and that of Junod. Where the American doctors looked on with the "cool and collected attitude" of scientific observers, Junod insisted that medicine be quickly distributed to the "indescribably sorrowful figures" he saw laid out in rows before him.[61] Junod's medical assistance, which included treating "many citizens who had fallen victim to the A-bomb," is still recognized and memorialized in Hiroshima today.[62]

Because of the rain and humidity, the American doctors' measuring instruments may have been somewhat compromised. Nevertheless, Nolan and Warren could ascertain, even at this early stage of their investigation, that "there was no doubt that there was gamma-radiation injury" (that is, initial radiation) and that there was a "very slight amount of radioactivity on the ground" (that is, residual radiation).[63] As Warren recalled, "Our Geiger counters had gotten wet and weren't working. We knew there was some radioactivity there, but we couldn't measure the amount. We could just get an indication."[64] The two Manhattan Project doctors, aided by Tsuzuki and Major Hitoshi Motohashi (another Japanese doctor and translator), continued like this for several days.[65] As Warren remembered, "We divided our day in half. In the morning we would go around to see casualties. In the afternoon, we would look over the destruction and the ruins, try to make measurement to

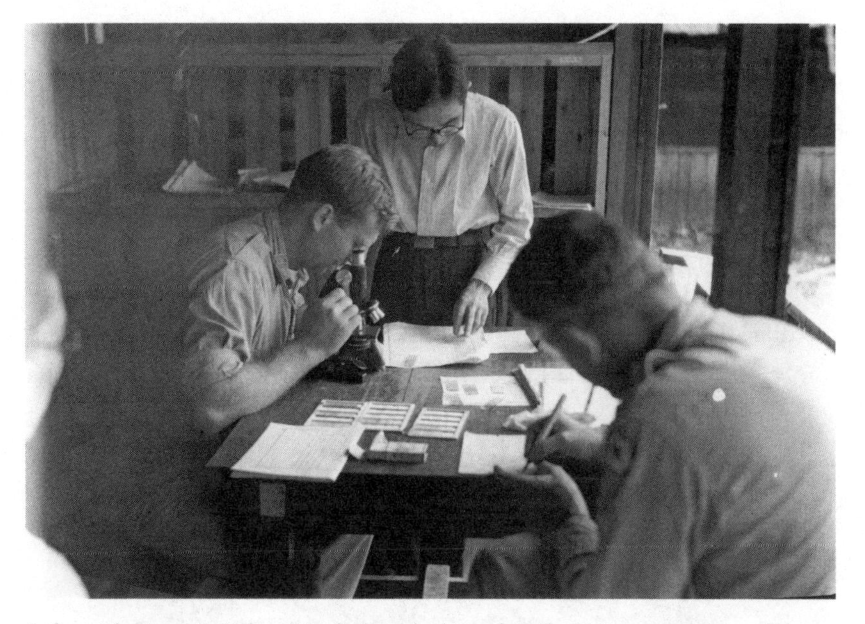

Left to right: James F. Nolan, Hitoshi Motohashi, and Stafford Warren examining slides at Ujina Army Hospital, September 9 or 10, 1945.

see where the center was, and what the distribution of downwind contamination might be."[66] On their rounds, they would also examine autopsied specimens, blood samples, and other data collected by the Japanese doctors.

Farrell, on the other hand, departed with plans for a quick trip to Nagasaki before returning to Tokyo. On September 10, he sent Groves a secret message supplying him with the counterpropaganda he was seeking. Referring to what he called "Warren's preliminary report," Farrell communicated to Groves, "Number dead or injured from radiation unknown, but preliminary survey indicates that there are only a small percent of injured survivors," to which he added, "Warren found no measurable radioactivity on preliminary measurements under detonation site or elsewhere on ground, streets, ashes or other materials."[67] This, of course, was not exactly what Warren and Nolan found. Though slight, they did find a measurable amount of radiation on the ground. Even with their ostensibly imperfect measuring instruments, they "knew there was some radioactivity there." Moreover, though Warren may have reported that radiation injuries were likely only a small percentage of the overall casualties, it was far too early to make such a determination, and his preliminary estimates on this score would prove to be considerably below the mark.

Farrell closed the communication by informing Groves that, though his plans were to travel to Nagasaki in the next few days, "Warren, Nolan, Oughterson, and Flick are remaining 2 days for further study."[68] These further studies, which would end up taking more than two days, included a visit to the Ono Army Hospital south of Hiroshima. The ophthalmologist John Flick, who was part of Oughterson's group, examined victims at this hospital, which was a former tuberculosis sanatorium. Among the patients at the hospital were "two moribund Japanese soldiers with blood diarrhea, bleeding from the gums, covered from head to foot with petechiae," all classic symptoms of "radiation sickness."[69] Less than a week after the group's

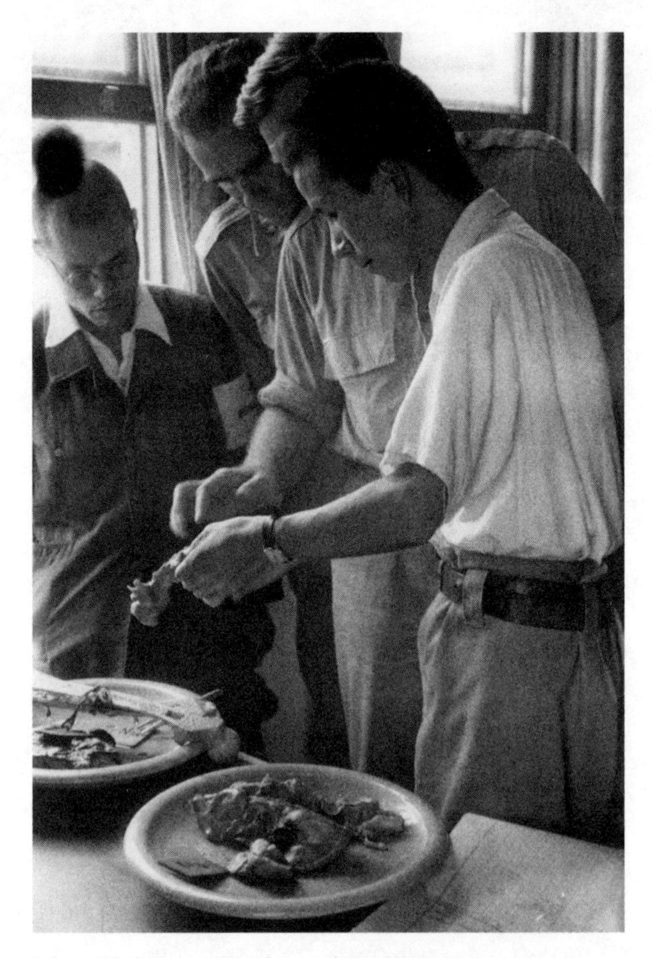

John J. Flick, James F. Nolan, and two Kyoto University researchers examining autopsied specimens at Ono Army Hospital, September 10, 1945.

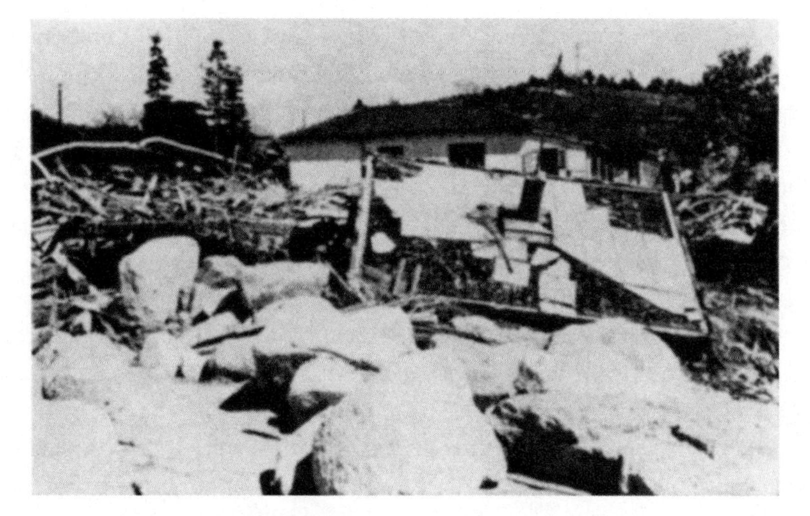

Ono Army Hospital after the September 17 typhoon.

visit, on September 17, Hiroshima was hit hard by the Makurazaki Typhoon, which resulted in dangerous floods and mudslides, including one that destroyed the Ono Hospital, killing more than 150 patients, staff, and researchers, including the two Kyoto doctors pictured on the previous page.

After his very short trip to Hiroshima, Farrell held a press conference in Tokyo on September 12 in which he "denied categorically that [the bomb] produced a dangerous lingering radioactivity in the ruins of the town or caused a form of poison gas at the moment of explosion." In contrast to what Warren remembered finding, Farrell stated that his group "found no evidence of continuing radioactivity in the blasted area on September 9, when they began their investigations." Invoking the authority of his "chief medical officer" (that is, Warren), Farrell argued that the largest number of casualties came from the blast of the bomb and the resulting fires. With this statement, the doctors were essentially used to provide cover for the military in their advancement of a false and unsubstantiated (or, at best, very incomplete) narrative about the effects of radiation. During this press conference, Farrell did acknowledge that Japanese doctors had found that some survivors "were dying from a marked decrease in the number of white corpuscles required to sustain life," which, though he did not articulate it as such, is a direct consequence of radiation exposure.[70]

Farrell's essential denial of the effects of radiation in this instance not only aided Groves in his advancement of a preferred and predetermined narrative, it also had the consequence, perhaps unintended, of discouraging official

Japanese efforts to provide medical care for the survivors of the atom bombs. If there were no ongoing harmful effects from radiation exposure, and if the Japanese government was in a position of wanting (or needing) to comply with American occupation interests, then government-sponsored medical care for such victims could be viewed as problematic. Thus, as Japanese scholar and *hibakusha* Hirotami Yamada argues, Farrell's public denial of the harmful effects of radiation on September 12 resulted in the abandonment by the Japanese government of providing "relief for the atomic-bombing victims."[71]

Concerning this predetermined narrative, Warren himself later tipped his hand as to the pressure, legal and otherwise, he was under to downplay the effects of radiation in both Japan and the New Mexico desert. After the war, when he wanted to return to an area near the Trinity test—a stretch in the direction of Gallinas Peak—to explore possible fallout, he was discouraged from doing so "because the lawyers and everybody were against doing anything." In this instance, according to Warren, the military objected to further investigations on the grounds that no residual radioactivity had been found in Japan, so it was not worth looking further. "Aw, you're nuts," they told Warren. "There was nothing in Japan." Warren disagreed: "Well there was; it was all of academic interest, but we found it."[72]

In fact, after Friedell's party finally arrived in Hiroshima on September 26, they found and investigated a trail of measurable fallout for a considerable distance to the west of the epicenter. They traced the contamination to the top of a hill adjacent to the edge of the city and were only prevented from going farther because of a lack of roads and an "impenetrable bamboo forest."[73] Shortly after Friedell arrived in Tokyo by train from Hiroshima, Warren sent a top-secret message to Groves stating the measurements of these findings: "Friedell found radio-activity at Hiroshima 8 to 10 times background immediately under 0. Rest of area 2 to 4 times background, also verified Japanese physicists finding 3 kilometers southwest, 2 to 3 times background."[74] Thus, residual radioactive fallout had clearly been detected, though, as Warren was careful to note, it was "very minor and not hazardous, being almost at the lower limit of sensitivity of their instruments."[75]

In the late 1960s, Warren summarized what his team had found in Japan and, though he still tried to downplay and nuance their findings, he did not deny the presence of residual radiation, of both the fallout and induced varieties. "We found, first, that there was some fallout that we could trace" and, second, that there "was some neutron activation of radioactive materials in the immediate target area."[76]

The Trinity Photo Op

Groves did not even wait for Farrell's September 12 press conference to launch his own public relations effort. On Sunday, September 9, the same day Nolan, Warren, and company finally trudged into Hiroshima, Groves and Oppenheimer assembled a group of some thirty-one news correspondents and photographers, along with a handful of scientists, doctors (including Hempelmann), and a dozen military men, at the site of the Trinity test. The purpose of the gathering was, in part, to counter the disturbing news coming out of Japan—that is, the "Japanese propaganda . . . that Americans won the war by unfair means."[77] The assembled news reporters were told, "The Japs admit that there is not harmful X-ray activity now."[78] The accounts of various Japanese doctors, as we will see, make clear that they had not come to any such conclusion.[79]

During this press gathering, Groves and Oppenheimer did not communicate a clear understanding of the differences between initial and residual radiation, thus enabling the American officials to deny the dangerous effects of radiation outright. Groves and Oppenheimer did claim to reporters that while the Gadget at the Trinity Site was detonated at only 100 feet above the ground, the Hiroshima and Nagasaki bombs were exploded much higher (about 1,950 and 1,650 feet, respectively) in order to avoid depositing residual radiation on the ground. "The Japan heights of explosion," Oppenheimer stated to the assembled reporters, "were picked so that there would be no indirect chemical warfare due to poisoning the earth with radioactive elements and no horrors other than the familiar ones due to any great explosion."[80]

This was a misleading statement in two respects. First, the radiation horrors, as such, were not avoided in Japan; and, second, the real purpose for the higher explosions was to cause the greatest amount of damage from the blast. In a recent and careful summary assessment of this contested issue, historian Sean Malloy persuasively concludes that "there is no evidence that concerns about limiting radiation exposure played any role in setting the blast height."[81] With respect to the effects of initial radiation, Groves admitted that some Japanese may have died from radioactivity but asserted that "the information now available indicates that this number was relatively small."[82] It's important to highlight here that Groves made this statement on the same day that the first members of his team had finally arrived in Hiroshima. In other words, the investigators' spot check had only just commenced.

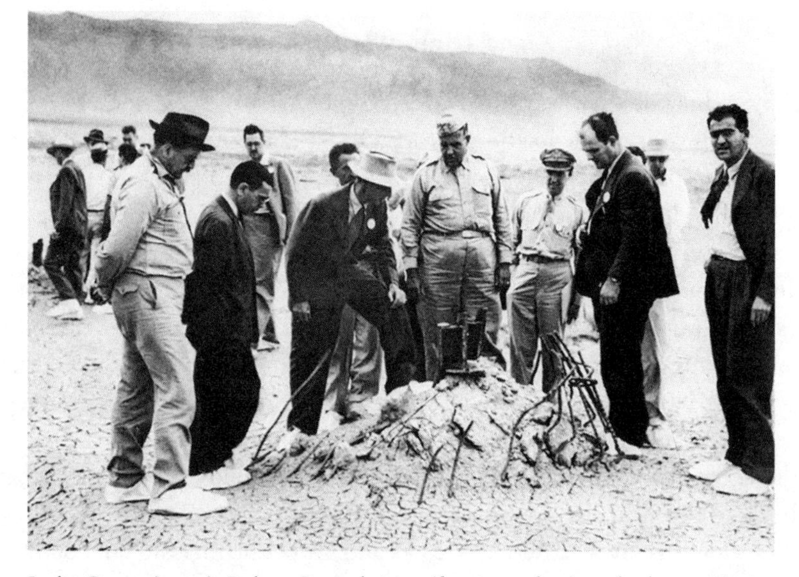

Leslie Groves (*center*), Robert Oppenheimer (*leaning on knee*), and others at Trinity Site near one leg of the tower, September 9, 1945.

The public relations stunt at the Trinity Site itself nearly backfired. Part of the reason for discussing the detonation heights of the Hiroshima and Nagasaki bombs while standing at ground zero in the New Mexico desert was to demonstrate that even in a place where the atomic bomb had exploded only one hundred feet above the earth's surface—and where the radioactive contamination on the ground was presumably much greater—it was safe to walk around. However, as seen in the above photo, those attending the Trinity photo op were encouraged to wear protective white booties, a safety measure recommended to Groves in the not very well received document presented to him by Nolan back in June 1945.

Two weeks before the event, Groves had asked Hempelmann whether it would be safe to bring newspaper reporters to the Trinity Site. Hempelmann stated that "they wouldn't be so safe." He explained that "initial intensities were quite high; about 250 [roentgens] on the ground but they fell off rapidly at first but not so fast right now."[83] Ignoring Hempelmann's cautionary words, Groves went forward with the press briefing anyway. During the briefing, Hempelmann and Joe Hoffman, a Cornell-trained physicist who worked in the area of health physics, were carrying monitoring meters and were becoming increasingly nervous about the whole ex-

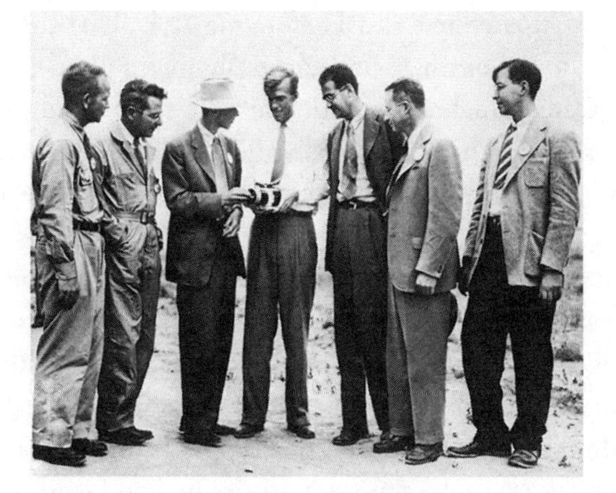

From left: Kenneth Bainbridge, Joe Hoffman, Robert Oppenheimer, and Louis Hempelmann (holding a radiation monitoring meter) at Trinity Site on September 9, 1945.

ercise. As recounted by Hempelmann, "Joe Hoffman and I were there with our meters and trying to keep things under control. And Oppie chose to hold an informal press conference near one of the legs of the tower. People were just like ants all over the place. Joe and I were trying to keep up with them, but we really couldn't."[84] When Hempelmann detected that the radiation level on his meter read fifteen roentgens per hour, he nervously approached Oppenheimer. "So, I went over to Robert . . . and I said to him, 'I think you better talk to these men some other place.' And he [Oppenheimer] said, 'How high is it?' And I said, '15.'"[85] Hempelmann worried that a journalist standing nearby had overheard this encounter.

Departing from Hiroshima

After several days journeying between Miyajima Island and Hiroshima, Nolan and Warren returned to Iwakuni to await air transport back to Tokyo. On their final morning on Miyajima, Tsuzuki arranged for the American party to participate in a ceremony at the Itsukushima shrine. First established at the end of the sixth century, the ancient shrine became a World Cultural Heritage site in 1996 and remains a popular tourist destination. The American doctors entered the impressive building, took off their shoes, and "were admitted to the inner Shrine." Tsuzuki and the high priest, dressed all in white, participated in a ritual before the idol. Two other men entered the scene, also dressed in white, and "furiously waved plumes" to drive away "evil spirits." Ceremonial dishes and sake were served and the two American leaders of the group, Oughterson and Warren, were invited to make statements. Oughterson "paid his respects to the local factotum who had treated us so courteously."[86]

Stirred by the experience, Warren then "gave a toast to the future peace between all nations and the hope there would be no more war again," an emotional tribute that "surprised the Priest greatly." Both the Americans and the Japanese, moved by the solemnity and goodwill of the ceremony, were evidently able to dispense with some of their prejudices regarding the other. Warren, for example, put aside stories he had heard that the shrine was the premission consecration site for departing kamikaze pilots. And the priest was grateful not only for the kind words offered by Oughterson and Warren but also for knowledge of the fact that the Americans, during their stay, did not "rape or pillage his community."[87] As another member of the Manhattan Project group put it, "The Japanese propaganda had prepared them to expect the worst from Americans."[88]

After the group crossed Hiroshima Bay for the final time and made their way to Iwakuni, their plans for a return to Tokyo were forestalled for two reasons. First, the weather did not cooperate, making plane travel from the crater-pocked Iwakuni runway impossible. Second, both Warren and Nolan came down with bad cases of diarrhea. Diarrhea, as the doctors on the Joint Commission quickly learned, was one of the most common symptoms of radiation exposure. However, Warren attributed their cases to Japanese food: "This fish or something gave most of us a violent, crampy diarrhea for three days. . . . The whole party lost weight."[89] In Nolan's recollections, "It was during this time that Warren and I got the diarrhea and subsisted on hard tack and Port wine for several days."[90]

During this delay in more concentrated investigative activity, the two Manhattan Project doctors, along with Tsuzuki, Motohashi, Oughterson, Flick, and Kasznar (an army photographer, who would become a rather successful Broadway and film actor after the war), were billeted at the Iwakuni branch of the Naval Academy, near the airport. Among other souvenirs picked up during their travels, Nolan acquired a Japanese folding fan, which he decided would be a nice gift for his wife, Ann. On the day before their departure from Iwakuni, Nolan asked both the Japanese and American components of the group to sign the fan for her. This was just one of several souvenirs—which also included small hand-carved wooden frogs, dolls, rifles, paper cards of Japanese artwork, and samurai swords—that the American party collected during their investigations, or, again in Lang's words, their unusual journey of "tourism, scientific exploration, and public relations work." After several days at the Iwakuni Naval Academy, Nolan and Warren finally gave up on air travel and procured tickets for a crowded and suffocating train ride back to Tokyo.

5

Tokyo and Nagasaki

It was a scene right out of hell.
—Raisuke Shirabe, *A Physician's Diary*

As James F. Nolan and Stafford Warren traversed the four-hundred-plus-mile train ride between Hiroshima and Tokyo, they passed through "one bombed out city after another," interspersed between acres of beautiful countryside. Taking in the incongruous scenery was made difficult by the conditions of the "old style coach" in which they traveled, with its tattered and "filthy dirty" straight-up seats and the pungent "perfume" emanating from the train's platform-style *benjo.* After an "arduous" journey, the two Manhattan Project doctors finally arrived back in Tokyo on September 15, where they received word that "our wandering generals had already been into Nagasaki."[1] They also soon learned that Warren's group—which the colonel had left behind in Okinawa nine days earlier—had finally made it into Nagasaki. Nolan and Warren then set about making their own arrangements to get to Nagasaki and succeeded in securing a morning flight for September 19, two days after the rest of Warren's men had reached the city.

After their arrival and a brief survey of the damages in Nagasaki, Warren stayed with his group "to spur their investigations," while Nolan returned the next day "to push the arrival of the second group under Friedell."[2] Hymer Friedell's team, still stranded in Zamboanga, had been delayed because of several typhoons. They would not get to Hiroshima until September 26, thus making this group's overall stay in Japan relatively short, about ten days in total.[3] It was during this time in Tokyo, before returning to Nagasaki, that Nolan first met Averill Liebow, who, like John Flick, was part of Ashley W. Oughterson's army general headquarters group. Liebow's diary recounts the September 21 meeting in Tokyo of these two army doctors: "Captain Nolan of the Manhattan District, a tall and very affable young man[,] . . . gave us some preliminary details concerning Hiroshima." Interestingly, on this occasion, Nolan, like Warren, offered an understated and somewhat ambiguous account of their findings, though it was still substantively distinct from that presented by Farrell a week earlier. Nolan reported that their "Geiger counters and other detection equipment . . . had found no significant residual radiation." Nolan, however, also told Liebow and company that it had "rained twice after the catastrophe"—a factor, as acknowledged by Robert Oppenheimer, that can intensify radioactive fallout—and that "many" Japanese victims "had multiple petechial hemorrhages and injury to the bowel," direct effects of radiation exposure.[4]

As far as I know, my grandfather maintained until the end of his life a full belief in the dominant narrative about the use of the atom bombs—that is, that these destructive weapons were necessary to end the war and that their use saved thousands of American (and even Japanese) lives.[5] Interestingly, Nolan and other Manhattan Project members of the Joint Commission played a significant, albeit indirect, role in advancing a counter-narrative to this official view, one that gave more attention to the horrific and ongoing effects of radiation and other injuries in Japan, and that raised important moral questions about the use of the bomb.

During his time in Tokyo, Nolan and other Joint Commission doctors made trips to the Pathological Institute of the Imperial Tokyo University in order to examine "microscopic sections" of specimens prepared for them by Masao Tsuzuki. The doctors would eventually take many of these specimens back with them to the United States for further study, a move that troubled some of the Japanese doctors.[6] In addition to examining biological specimens, during one of these trips to the Pathological Institute, the Joint Commission doctors also "absconded with the Geisha girl in the tin can" (another act of souvenir-collecting tourism).[7]

While in Tokyo, Nolan and other Joint Commission doctors "investigated Fr. Siemes."[8] Father John Siemes, a German Jesuit priest, had been living at his order's novitiate house in the hills of Nagatsuka, about three miles outside Hiroshima, when the bomb exploded on the morning of August 6. In the weeks that followed, Siemes wrote a compelling account of the impact of the bomb and of his community's heroic rescue and aid efforts. More than a hundred injured survivors were given shelter at the novitiate house in Nagatsuka, where they received care from, among others,

Sept. 17. '45
1230.

東京帝國大學

Col. Warren and other Gentlemen:
Many microscopic sections are ready for you in our Pathological Institute.
I myself have a lecture for medical students between 1300–1400, after the lecture see you in path. Institute.
Dr. Miyake, Vice-chief of the path. Institute will take care of you, until I come.
Yours
Prof. M. Tsuzuki.

Dr. Tomio Ogata

Takeo Tamiya
Tokyo Imperial University

Dr Kaiti Mu

Dr. Masao Tsuzuki
Surgical Clinic
Imperial University
Tokyo, Japan

Note from Masao Tsuzuki to Joint Commission doctors, scheduling a meeting at the Pathological Institute, September 17, 1945.

the medically trained Father Pedro Arrupe, another member the community and the future superior general of the Jesuits.

On August 7, the day after the bomb, Arrupe said Mass at the novitiate house in a room filled with the wounded, "who were lying on the floor very near to one another, suffering terribly, twisted with pain." When he turned around from facing the altar (in pre–Vatican II style) at the end of the Mass, he was overwhelmed by what he saw. "I can never forget the terrible feeling I experienced when I turned toward them and saw this sight from the altar. I could not move. I stayed there as if I was paralyzed, my arms outstretched, contemplating this human tragedy—human science and technological progress used to destroy the human race. They were all looking at me, eyes full of agony and despair as if they were waiting for some consolation to come from the altar. What a terrible scene!"[9] Four of the priests in the order, including Father Wilhelm Kleinsorge, were actually residing in the center of

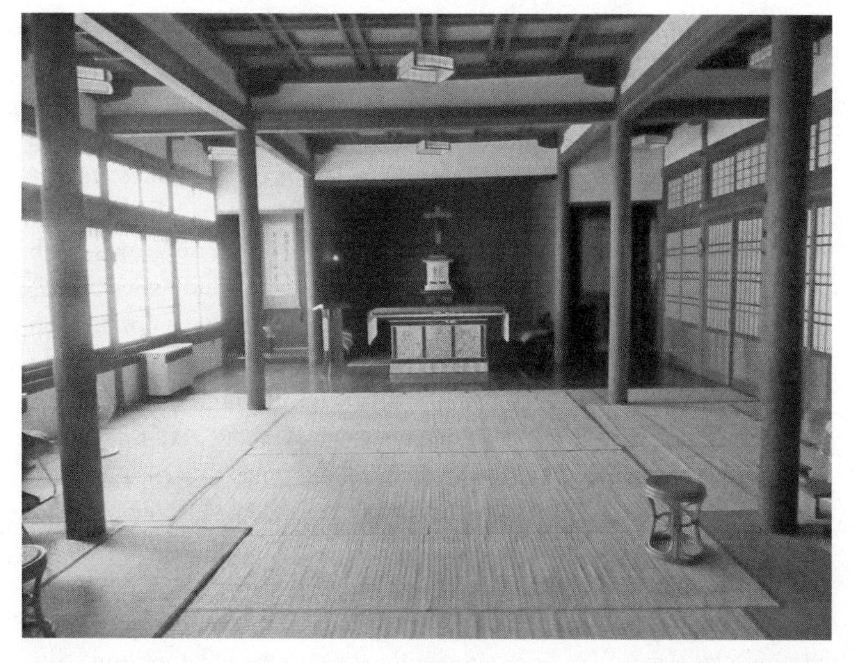

The room in the Nagatsuka novitiate house where Pedro Arrupe said Mass on August 7, 1945, in front of more than one hundred injured victims. Glass from the windows on the left had been shattered by the force of the bomb.

Hiroshima at the parish house of the central mission church, about eight blocks from the hypocenter, on the morning of the bomb.

After meeting with the Manhattan Project group in Tokyo, Siemes gave Warren a copy of his account, written in German. Warren handed the manuscript over to Liebow, who knew German, and asked him to translate the document into English. Siemes's written testimony became an important source for John Hersey's best-selling book *Hiroshima.* Hersey had read Liebow's translation of Siemes's account before arriving in Hiroshima in April 1946.[10] Having done so, Hersey's "first move in arriving was to get in touch with the Jesuit mission in Hiroshima."[11] There he met Kleinsorge, who became one of the six accounts featured in Hersey's riveting on-the-ground description of real people affected by Little Boy. The book, which was originally published as a long article in the *New Yorker* in late August 1946, gave many Americans, for the first time, a vivid picture of the devastating human consequences of the atom bomb.

When Liebow read and translated Siemes's "remarkable document," he was "spellbound and horrified" by Siemes's "stirring, beautifully and modestly written description."[12] While in Tokyo, Liebow read his English translation aloud to one of the army sergeants traveling with Warren's group, who skillfully typed up the dictated testimony. Inspired by the account, the Joint Commission doctors visited the ailing Kleinsorge, whom Liebow described as a "keen kindly man, thin and pale," at the St. Luke's International Catholic Hospital in Tokyo.[13] Hersey, in fact, notes in *Hiroshima* that during this first of numerous hospitalizations, when Kleinsorge was exhibiting many of the classic signs of radiation sickness, including leukopenia (low white blood cell count), "American doctors came by the dozen to observe him."[14] For Liebow, who had yet to visit either Hiroshima or Nagasaki, this was his first direct contact with an atomic bomb patient.[15] After completing the translation of Siemes's account, Liebow gave the English version to Warren. On October 2, while waiting for a table with Nolan at the Dai-Ichi Hotel in Tokyo, Warren communicated to Liebow his "pleasure at the Siemes translation."[16]

Warren's positive response is interesting for several reasons. First, Siemes discussed the effects of radiation from the bomb in a manner not fully in keeping with Farrell's public statements. Siemes noted, for example, that in some cases in which the "prognosis seemed good," the victims "died suddenly." While he was a little skeptical about the exaggerated effects of residual radiation, Siemes understood that "gamma rays had been given out at the time of the explosion, following which the internal organs had been injured in a manner resembling that consequent upon Roentgen irradiation," which "produces a diminution in the number of the white corpuscles," as occurred with his fellow priest Kleinsorge.[17]

In addition to these observations on the effects of radiation exposure, Siemes also reflected on the morality of the bomb, which he and his community had evidently contemplated together in the days and weeks after August 6. "We have discussed among ourselves the ethics of the use of the bomb," he wrote.

> Some consider it in the same category as poison gas and were against its use on a civil population. Others were of the view that in total war, as carried on in Japan, there was no difference between civilians and soldiers, and that to bomb itself was an effective force tending to end the bloodshed, warning Japan to surrender and thus to avoid total destruction. It seems logical to us that he who supports total war in principle cannot complain of a war against civilians. The crux of the

> matter is whether total war in its present form is justifiable, even when it serves a just purpose. Does it not have material and spiritual evil as its consequences, which far exceed whatever the good that might result? When will our moralists give us a clear answer to this question?[18]

This exact quotation from the English translation of Siemes's account is included in Hersey's *Hiroshima.* Interestingly, after returning to the United States, Warren would give a copy of the document to General Leslie Groves. Groves would subsequently quote selectively from it in his testimony before Congress in November 1945.

What did Warren and Nolan make of these reflections? Did they also question the morality of the bomb, witnessing as they did the direct consequences of its power and lingering deathly effects? Were they also confounded by the destructive capacities that humans had produced through scientific and technological progress? Apparently, they did have occasion to reflect on these questions, though they seem to have come to different conclusions from those of Siemes. While awaiting their return trip to Tokyo, the American and Japanese members of the Joint Commission grounded at the Iwakuni Airport engaged in a long discussion one evening about the "ethics of the bomb" that lasted "far into the night." According to Warren, the group collectively "came up with the following arguments" (though he conceded that the Japanese were less communicative than the Americans on this occasion).[19]

First, according to Warren, it was agreed that even before the bombs were dropped, the Japanese realized that they were defeated; yet they were still prepared to fight for a couple of months following the initiation of an anticipated land invasion. With the utter devastation from the atomic bombs, however, further resistance was made impossible, thus enabling the Japanese to save face and surrender without having to commit hara-kiri, which would otherwise have been expected of them. Second, a land invasion "would have killed perhaps as many as several million Japanese" and "as many as five hundred thousand American boys." "Was it not better," the group reportedly concluded, "to extinguish two cities instantaneously and bring the matter to an abrupt stop by what amounted to a surgical operation, the net result of which saved many more lives?"[20]

These, of course, are arguments characteristic of the dominant narrative—that is, that the Japanese were not prepared to surrender in the summer of 1945 and that the only viable alternative to dropping the bombs was a bloody land invasion that would cost hundreds of thousands of both American and Japanese lives. Years later, Warren elaborated on this perspective and, like Siemes, compared the atom bombs to the "total war" attacks in places like Tokyo. However, rather than questioning the morality of total war itself, as did Siemes, Warren concluded that the quick and "surgical" nature of nuclear warfare was comparatively more "merciful." Consider his reasoning: "Very few people realize the fact that more people were killed by the fire bombing in Japan—at Tokyo and Yokohama—than were killed by the two bombs at Hiroshima and Nagasaki. The difference was that it took a week or more in the former cases for the fire bombing, and people were subject to the terror of the attack and the fire. If there is any such thing as that any kind of killing is more merciful, the atom bomb is more merciful."[21]

Given this perspective, it is ironic that, though Warren and other Manhattan Project doctors maintained their allegiance to the official narrative, they actually contributed to the development of an important and foundational text in the "counternarrative" canon, one that unnerved American officials. General Farrell, for example, was so troubled by Hersey's article that, just a few days after its publication, he wrote a letter to Bernard Baruch, then serving as the US representative to the United Nations Atomic Energy Commission, urging him to produce and publish an equally compelling article in the *New Yorker* about the mistreatment of prisoners of war in Japan.[22] Discomfort among American officials only intensified when, shortly after reading Hersey's article, the journalist Norman Cousins penned a response in the *Saturday Review* in which he articulated, through a series of questions inspired by Hersey's piece, essential tenets of the counternarrative: "Do we know, for example, that many thousands of human beings in Japan will die of cancer during the next few years because of radioactivity released by the bomb? Do we know that the bomb is in reality a death ray, and that the damage by the blast and fire may be secondary to the damage caused by radiological assault upon human tissue? Have we as a people any sense of responsibility for the crime of Hiroshima and Nagasaki?"[23] Cousins additionally questioned why the physicists' proposal for a demonstration test was ignored, and he challenged the official and oft-stated view that use of the bomb saved "numberless thousands of American lives."[24]

Hersey's article and Cousins's response to it alarmed US officials. American leaders also had to contend with the findings of their own US Strategic Bombing Survey, which were released in early July 1946. The civilian-led survey team, comprising more than one thousand military and civilian personnel, "interviewed more than 700 Japanese military, government, and industrial officials."[25] Based on its thorough investigative work, which began in the fall of 1945, as well as testimonies collected from Japanese leaders, the survey team concluded, "It is the Survey's opinion that certainly prior to 31 December 1945, and in all probability prior to 1 November 1945, Japan would have surrendered even if the atomic bombs had not been dropped, even if Russia had not entered the war, and even if no invasion had been planned or contemplated."[26]

Following these various counternarrative publications in the summer of 1946, a concerted and coordinated effort was initiated to put forth a clear and convincing articulation of the dominant narrative, the final result of which became a famous *Harper's* magazine article, "The Decision to Use the Atomic Bomb," published in February 1947. The *Harper's* article was assembled and written by a number of people, including Groves, though strategically published under the authorship of the esteemed former secretary of war Henry Stimson. Regarded as "the most influential article ever published on the atomic bomb," its persuasive presentation of the official narrative effectively stemmed the tide of growing sympathy with the counternarrative.[27] Significantly, the Stimson article makes no mention of the effects of radiation, residual or otherwise.

While the article succeeded in muting the public potency of the counternarrative engendered by Hersey's *Hiroshima,* the debate represented in these early missives has far from subsided, as the heated controversy over the Smithsonian's proposed 1995 exhibit of the *Enola Gay* made clear. Had the originally planned exhibit gone forward, it would have included information, visual and otherwise, about the effects of the bomb in Japan. However, heated opposition from veterans' groups, among others, resulted in the jettisoning of such "revisionist history." About a year after the publication of the Stimson article, Warren himself observed that ethical concerns about the morality of the bomb had "quieted down both in Japan and the United States," though, tendentiously, he also lamented that "our own people frequently bring the subject up as a sort of neurotic self-flagellation."[28]

Nagasaki

Nolan's second trip to Nagasaki was somewhat limited (September 29 to October 2), though it was meant to be longer. As Nolan recalled, "We returned to Nagasaki for the first group and it was during this flight that another typhoon caused us to be three days late for a three hour trip."[29] After finally arriving on September 29, Nolan joined the rest of Warren's group at Omura Naval Hospital, about twenty-two miles north of Nagasaki, where a large number of the injured survivors (along with doctors from Warren's team) had been relocated. One of the Japanese doctors collaborating with the Americans in Omura was Raisuke Shirabe, a surgeon from the Nagasaki Medical School.

On the morning of August 9, Shirabe had been in his office at the medical school reviewing a student's thesis when the second atomic bomb used in warfare was dropped. Originally intended for the primary target of Kokura, the B-29 *Bockscar,* piloted by Major Charles Sweeney, was redirected to its secondary target, Nagasaki. Here, too, cloud cover prevented a clear view of the city. As *Bockscar* approached Nagasaki from the north, the clouds briefly opened and the plutonium bomb Fat Man was released, a mile and a half north of the intended target, over the prefecture of Urakami, rather than the center of Nagasaki. The bomb detonated at 11:02 a.m. about 550 yards from the Nagasaki Medical School and about 650 yards

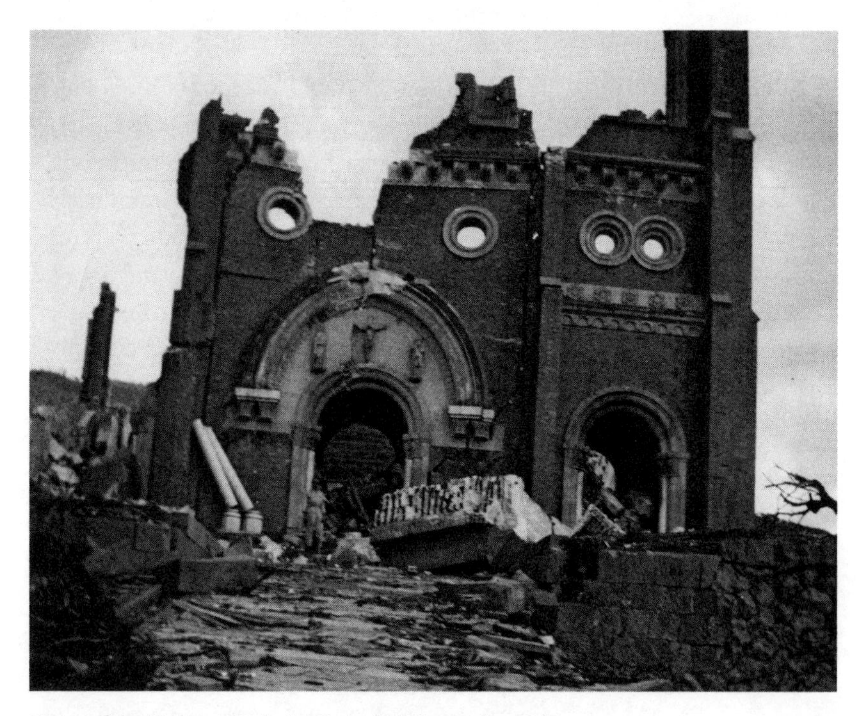

Ruins of the Urakami Catholic Cathedral, September 1945.

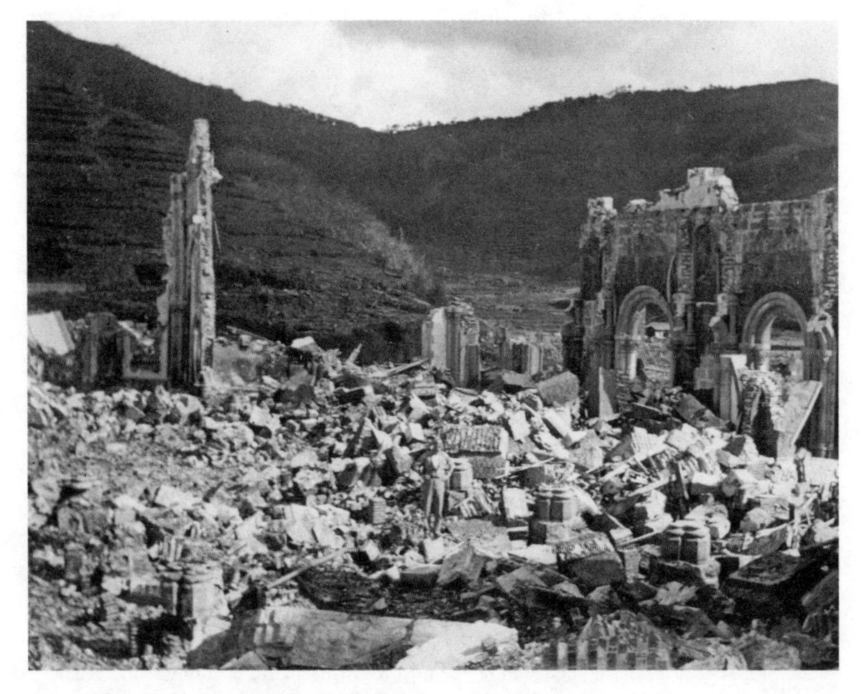

Ruins of the Urakami Catholic Cathedral, September 1945.

from the Urakami Catholic Cathedral, for centuries the center of Japan's long-suffering Christian community. Of the approximately 12,000 Christians living in Urakami at the time, 8,500 were killed, including several dozen parishioners and two Catholic priests, who were hearing confessions in the cathedral that morning.

Members of the Manhattan Project team, surveying the destruction of Nagasaki in September, took immediate notice of the damaged cathedral, large photographs of which are included in my grandfather's files.[30] In fact, even before landing in Nagasaki on September 17, as Warren's group circled the city in a C-54, they observed and commented on the ruins of the cathedral.[31] Once on the ground, Donald Collins was struck by the destruction of one of the cathedral's belfries, which he described as a "dramatic indication of the tremendous force of the blast." He and his colleague, the Oak Ridge civil engineer Captain Walter Youngs, observed that the fifty-ton bell tower had been blown into a ravine nearly "fifty meters distant from the church."[32] The relocated belfry remains in the ravine today, not far from the reconstructed cathedral.

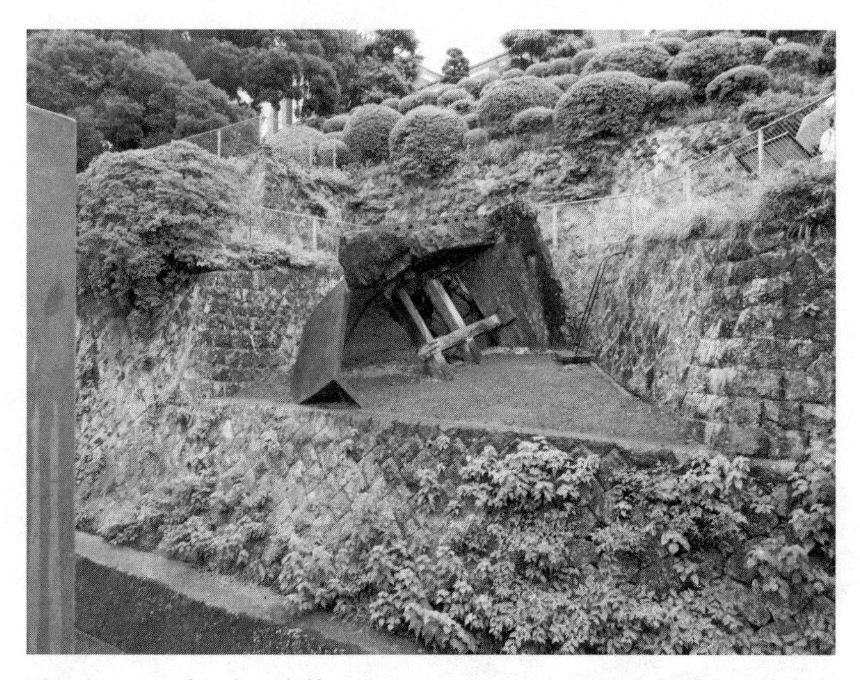

Blasted remains of displaced belfry in ravine near reconstructed Urakami Cathedral.

The destruction of the Urakami Cathedral and the high number of fatalities among the Nagasaki Christians is ironic for several reasons. Not only was another city, Kokura, the intended primary target for Fat Man on August 9, but Kyoto had previously been on the list of potential targets. Kyoto was, in fact, one of General Groves's preferred targets. Following a somewhat tense struggle between Groves and Stimson, Kyoto was ultimately removed from the list. Having visited the city in the 1920s, Stimson strongly objected to Kyoto because of the city's religious and cultural significance. In a curious twist of fate, Nagasaki, also a place of religious significance—in fact, for centuries, the epicenter of Christianity in Japan—would become the ultimate target for the plutonium bomb. The Urakami Cathedral had been intentionally built on a site where the persecuted "hidden Christians" had endured severe forms of torture for many years. The Christians finally emerged from more than two centuries of hiding when Japanese authorities loosened restrictions on religious freedom in the second half of the nineteenth century, a development that was itself a consequence of Western influence. The Urakami Cathedral was the largest Christian structure in the Asia-Pacific region at the time of the bombing.

As illustrated in this case, Nagasaki, the setting for the famous opera *Madame Butterfly*, had long been a port city open to Western influence. The tragic paradox that Nagasaki then became a target of a Western-produced weapon of mass destruction is not lost on the Japanese. The very first descriptive caption one encounters upon entering the Nagasaki Atomic Bomb Museum highlights this paradox. "Nagasaki, where the curtain of history opened with the arrival of Portuguese ships in 1571. Nagasaki, which through its relations with Holland and China was Japan's only open port from 1641 to 1859. Nagasaki, where Japanese students gathered to draw from the well of Western Knowledge. Nagasaki, [where] Western style buildings stood side by side and the foreign settlements bustled in the late 19th century. . . . Nagasaki, surrounded on three sides by mountains and boasting a colorful history of 374 years, greeted the summer morning of August 9, 1945."

The French-influenced neo-Romanesque cathedral in Urakami, the construction of which began in 1895 and was completed in 1925, was one of the most renowned and visible Western-style buildings in Nagasaki referenced in the museum's display caption. Images of the cathedral ruins, which are prominently featured in the museum and elsewhere, were (and remain) one of the most well-known and recognized symbols of the destruction of Nagasaki. So iconic were the images of the cathedral ruins—often compared to the A-Bomb Dome in Hiroshima—that there was strong resistance among many Nagasaki citizens to removing the crumbling remains of the church and rebuilding the cathedral on the same site. City officials preferred maintaining the ruins (as was done with Hiroshima's A-Bomb Dome) as a memorial to the historical significance of the August 9 bombing. The Christian community, however, very much favored reconstruction of the cathedral, and on the same site, because of its important history to their community. In the end, the Urakami Catholics prevailed, and the new building, completed in 1959, looks much like the original structure.[33]

Early Rescue Efforts

A prominent member of the Christian community and parishioner at the Urakami Cathedral was Takashi Nagai, a colleague of Shirabe's at the Nagasaki Medical School. Nagai, dean of the Radiology Department and an adult convert to Catholicism, had married Midori Moriyama, the great-granddaughter of the last *chokata* (or headman) of the "hidden Christians" in Urakami. Midori died in the blast, though their two children, Makoto and Kayano, had recently been relocated to the countryside and were thus spared. Nagai had contracted leukemia before the bombing, because of his work as a radiologist. He dutifully provided x-rays for patients in wartime conditions that afforded him little protection from radiation exposure.

Nagai was in the Radiology Department preparing a lecture on the morning of August 9. When the bomb exploded, the windows in his office shattered and he was blown a distance of ten feet. In addition to his receiving radiation from the explosion, a piece of shattered glass severed an artery in his right temple. Within fifteen minutes of the blast, while the medical school complex was engulfed in flames, Nagai, two nurses, and other surviving staff from the Radiology Department began treating the many injured in the area. Nagai's head injury eventually had to be addressed. After several failed attempts by his team to stop the bleeding, Shirabe was summoned for assistance. Improvising with what supplies were available to him, Shirabe placed a tampon on Nagai's wound and sutured the laceration over it, which finally stopped the bleeding.[34] With impressive serenity, Nagai and his team then walked down the hill to set up camp and carry on with their work among the other injured survivors.

Shirabe and Nagai were two of only twelve professors from the medical school who survived the bombing. Though both would suffer from radiation sickness in the weeks following August 9, shortly after the explosion they set about searching for and treating the many victims of the bomb in the area. Even though the hospital, with its reinforced concrete walls, was stronger and more resistant than other structures to the force of the bomb, it had still been largely destroyed, and 80 percent of the staff and patients in the hospital killed. It was therefore not a viable location for treating the injured in Nagasaki.

That the medical school hospital was no longer suitable for the care of patients is made clear in Colonel Warren's description of the complex, which he discovered during the American team's entry into Nagasaki: "I shall never forget walking into the Medical School in Nagasaki about five weeks after the detonation, and, on the landing of the second floor, stepping over the body of a young female partly burned, going down the corridors . . . [and] finding in room after room . . . more bodies, partly burned, entangled in window frames, and twisted under the benches. . . . Outside was a pile of bones from the cremated bodies. The pile was about three feet deep and fifty feet in diameter."[35]

In his detailed diary documenting the days after the bomb, Shirabe described the scene at the hospital in the moments after the atomic explosion, some five weeks before Warren's visit to the same location: "The place had turned into a scene of terrible confusion, and it was more than just a gruesome scene. There were burned, naked, blackened faces staring eyes, tinted red with blood. It was a scene right out of hell."[36] Nagai offered an equally graphic and disturbing account of what he witnessed around the medical school hospital after the detonation:

> The horrific scene has been branded in my mind. I will never forget. It is far beyond my ability to describe. This must have been the Apocalypse or a scene right out of hell. How awful was the sight of groups of people climbing the hills on the far side to avoid the fire. The injured also pulled their dying friends. Children carried their dead parents; parents held the corpses of their children, as they desperately climbed the hill. Their skin was stripped, stained with fresh blood. Everybody was naked. They kept looking back at the spreading flames, as they sought safety.[37]

Because of the hospital's condition, Shirabe and Nagai were forced, after their initial triage efforts, to establish relief missions in other parts of Nagasaki—Nagai in the Mitsuyama district, about three miles north of the epicenter, and Shirabe, first in the Nameshi neighborhood (about two and a half miles from the epicenter) and then eventually at the Omura Naval Hospital, where he met and worked directly with the American doctors from the Manhattan Project group, including Harry Whipple, Birchard Brundage, and Joe Howland. The American doctor with whom Shirabe interacted the most was Henry Barnett, the St. Louis–based pediatrician and medical school classmate of Nolan's and Louis Hempelmann's, whom they had recruited to take care of the many newborns in Los Alamos. Shirabe and Barnett established a friendly working relationship, which was emblematic of a number of the collaborations between the American and Japanese doctors during this period.

Making Sense of Radiation Sickness

During this time of close contact with American members of the Joint Commission, Shirabe had a number of interesting conversations with

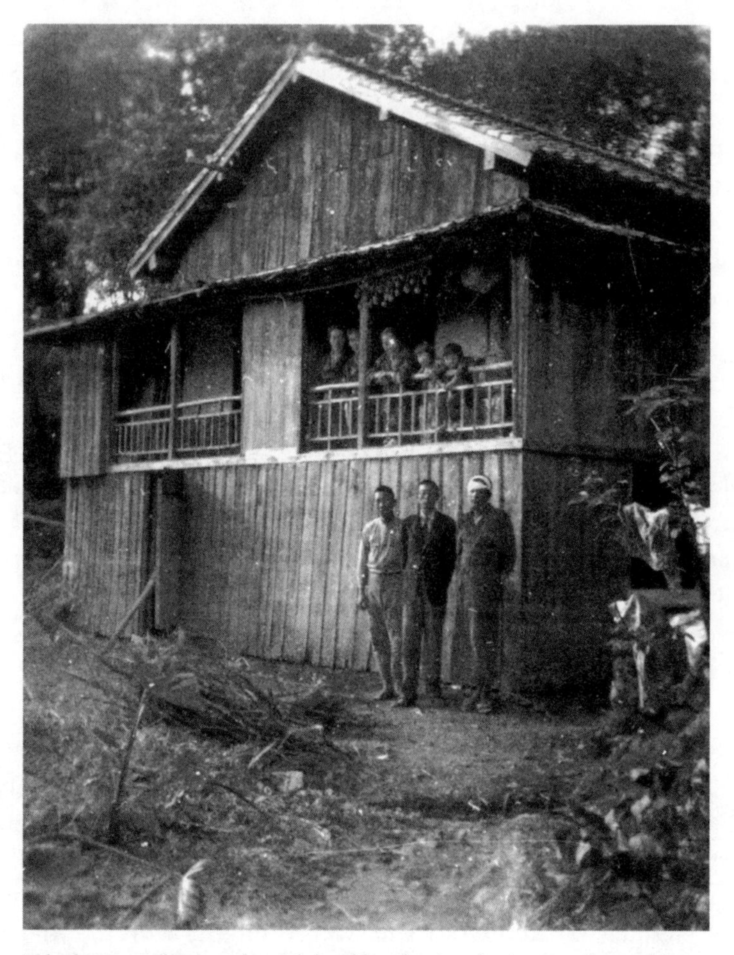

Takashi Nagai (lower right with head bandage) and other members of the relief team in Mitsuyama.

Manhattan Project doctors about a range of topics, including the issue of residual radiation. In a revealing discussion with physicist Robert Serber, Shirabe observed to the American physicist that "people from the countryside who came into the hypocenter area after the bombing suffered from atomic sickness." Serber was surprised to hear of this and insisted that "the atomic radiation at the hypocenter would only be temporary." Not entirely persuaded, Shirabe noted the clear differences in the nature and extent of atomic sickness among those who stayed in the hypocenter for extended periods and those who left more quickly.[38]

Before the Americans arrived at the Omura Naval Hospital in late September, the Japanese doctors had witnessed firsthand the lethal effects of radiation, initial and residual, among the victims in their care. It was a sort of sickness with which most had had little previous experience. The wounded who had been transported to Omura with relatively minor injuries began to display the symptoms of radiation illness, including hair loss, diarrhea, petechia (small purple bleeding spots on their skin), fevers, fatigue, and blood oozing from their gums. For example, on August 11, Dr. Masao Shiotsuki approached the bed of a female patient at Omura who had not been seriously injured. She showed the doctor how, when using a comb, clumps of her hair would fall out. Shiotsuki, in an attempt to put her at ease, proposed that hair loss sometimes occurs in burn cases and that it would likely stop after a few days. By midnight of the next day, the patient had died.[39]

This was not an isolated case. Many of the injured at Omura, even those "with only mild symptoms who seemed to be on the road to recovery[,] suddenly began dying." Even some of the ostensibly uninjured rescue workers serving at the hospital, who had helped bring victims out of Nagasaki, began showing similar symptoms; "one after another," they also began to die.[40] The same was happening at rescue and aid stations in other parts of Nagasaki. Dr. Tatsuichiro Akizuki, for example, an expert in the treatment of tuberculosis, who was working at the Urakami First Hospital, less than a mile northeast of the epicenter, observed, "There were many whose hair fell out overnight, who excreted blood from their noses and mouths, and who suffered from diarrhea accompanied by blood. Even people without any visible wounds, who thought that they had been miraculously spared, later died one after the other from radiation, which vitiated the entire body."[41] At Omura, it was even reported that a doctor who had not been in Nagasaki on August 9 and had not entered Nagasaki at any time after the explosion temporarily showed signs of radiation sickness, "because of his continuous and direct contact with victims who had been exposed to high levels of radioactivity."[42]

Of the various doctors in Nagasaki, the radiologist Takashi Nagai was uniquely prepared to make sense of the bomb and its effects. His biography represents the antithesis to compartmentalization, as his life and work demonstrated a seamless integration of the roles of scientist, doctor, and humanitarian. For this reason, there was no inherent conflict, for this doctor, in both studying the effects of the bomb and providing medical care for the injured. Before the bomb, he had been part of a research group studying nuclear physics and was well versed in the field, which included knowledge of the groundbreaking discoveries of Enrico Fermi, Niels Bohr, Albert Einstein, Arthur Compton, and others.[43] When a member of his team picked up a leaflet, dropped by American planes, announcing delivery of the atomic bomb and encouraging immediate surrender, Nagai and others stopped to contemplate how, in reference to recent discoveries in nuclear physics, Americans had achieved the remarkable feat. Moreover, as a radiologist, he was all too familiar with the effects of radiation. He himself had contracted leukemia and had written and read about the biological effects of radiation, including Tsuzuki's experimental work with rabbits.[44]

He understood the dynamics of initial and residual radiation and was less surprised than others by the variety of symptoms he witnessed around him. One reason he finally left the relief station at Mitsuyama and moved back to his home near the epicenter on October 8 was to study the effects of residual radiation. He observed that the remaining radioactivity in the environment was caused by both induced radiation and fallout, including in the form of black rain, which he directly observed. So intense was the residual radiation in the days after the bomb, according to Nagai, that those who came back to live near the epicenter within the first three weeks after the explosion "began gradually to experience nausea and injury to the digestive organs. . . . They also suffered from severe diarrhea." Those who dug among the ruins—either searching for the remains of loved ones or looking for personal items in burned-out homes—experienced even more serious symptoms, not unlike those "who had been profoundly irradiated during the explosion itself." Some people even "got diarrhea just from passing through Urakami during the first ten days of the explosion."[45]

As time went on, Nagai observed, the radiation decayed and the danger decreased. However, even among those who moved into the city a month after the bomb, such symptoms as nausea, diarrhea, a decrease in white blood cells, and the development of pus from insect bites and small cuts were still "much in evidence." After three months, symptoms were less obvious, but "a very tiny amount of radioactivity" remained, which, according to Nagai, is "exactly what the Americans warned us [about] at the time of the explosion."[46] While Nagai regarded Jacobson's "seventy-five-year theory" as "not tenable," he also observed that, even a year after August 9, though it had dissipated considerably, there was still radioactivity on the ground. "Yet even now—one year after the explosion—a small amount still remains and continues in a weak manner its work of irradiation."[47] The observations of

Nagai and the other Japanese doctors directly contradicted Groves's assertion, offered at the Trinity Site on September 9, that the "Japs admit that there is not harmful X-ray activity now."[48] Clearly, as these multiple accounts demonstrate, the Japanese doctors had made no such admission. In fact, at the time of Groves's statement, as Takemae Eiji argues, "Japanese physicians were documenting overwhelming evidence to the contrary."[49]

Indeed, the Japanese doctors' findings in this regard were precisely what General Farrell reported to Groves after investigating Nagasaki in early September 1945. After his brief excursion into Nagasaki—which followed his quick trip through Hiroshima—Farrell sent another message to Groves on September 14, in which he acknowledged that "Japanese officials report that any one who entered the blast area from outside after the explosion has become sick." The Japanese doctors also reported, according to Farrell, that a "number have died up to September 1st who did not seem to be wounded originally" and that about twenty wounded were still dying daily. In this case, because Nolan and Warren were still in Hiroshima, he did not have the doctors' ostensible imprimatur to refute these reports. "Warren and Nolan have not yet arrived from Hiroshima," Farrell wrote, though he assured Groves that a report "will be sent to you as soon as Warren can make a detailed check."[50]

In his "detailed check," Warren learned that many of the injured from Nagasaki were evacuated by "relief trains," a rescue effort that, remarkably, began operating just a couple of hours after the detonation of the bomb. Four "relief train" runs carried some 3,500 wounded on August 9 between the burning city and the northern outskirts of Nagasaki toward Omura. Packed like sardines, many victims died even before getting off the train.[51] When told about these evacuation efforts, Warren agreed that the deaths "were due to a combination of shock and a high dose of gamma radiation." Even those with lower doses would eventually die, many of them around the time that the American doctors arrived on the scene. "And then there were those who had lethal doses of a less amount [*sic*], which had produced bloody diarrhea and the small intestine then fell apart. Four to six week later the bone marrow was destroyed and bleeding and the pallor were evident." These later deaths, according to Warren, occurred "about that time when we arrived."[52]

Thus, it was not only the Japanese doctors who observed the serious consequences of radiation among the injured in Nagasaki. Another Manhattan Project doctor working in Nagasaki, Birchard Brundage, observed

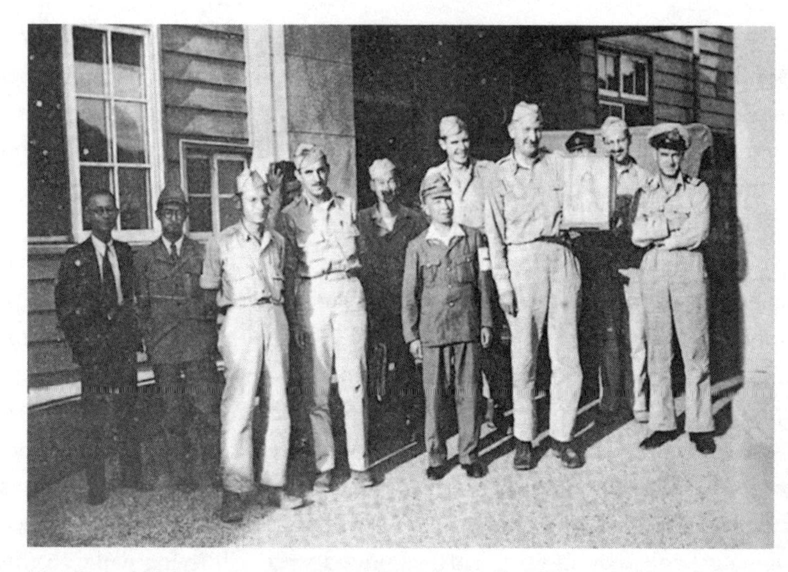

Members of the Joint Commission in Nagasaki, Stafford Warren holding doll.

three types of injuries during his time in the city: injuries from flying debris and falling buildings, skin burns, and internal injuries when there was little or no evidence of external injuries. The latter two, and especially the last, can be attributed to radiation exposure. Many patients with these injuries, according to Brundage, "died and had to be cremated without autopsy examinations."[53] Thus, the full extent of radiation injuries will never be fully known, as many victims were cremated before any kind of formal medical assessment could be made of their cause of death. That is, many died and were cremated before any Americans had arrived on the scene. The number of cremated bodies was high, as illustrated in Warren's encounter with the enormous pile (three feet deep, fifty feet wide) of cremated remains outside the Nagasaki Medical School Hospital.

Even after their arrival, Warren's team witnessed at other places in Nagasaki the continuing practice of cremating radiation-induced fatalities. Daily, the American doctors would visit the various rescue and aid missions set up by Japanese physicians around the city. One of these locations was a small building where a medical school doctor and two nurses received patients. In the thirty-by-forty-foot building, the injured were spread out very close to one another, side by side on the floor. Warren and his team visited this spot each day and observed many patients suffering from radiation sickness.

> Outside there was a pile of ashes from bodies incinerated the day before. This went on day after day. We would come and look at these people. Many would have purpura, or little bleeding spots about an eighth of an inch in diameter, on various parts of the body. These were mostly on the face, chest, and arms. Any spot that was slightly bruised had a hemorrhage. They would be a sickly yellow color. We did a few white blood counts and found 50 cells instead of 5,000. The next day when we'd come back, they'd be gone and replaced by others. Their bodies had been incinerated.[54]

Shirabe remembered when Nolan and the others arrived at Omura from Tokyo on September 29. That evening, he was introduced to Warren, who offered general instructions about the Joint Commission's efforts. Warren emphasized the cooperative nature of the enterprise and urged the Japanese doctors to continue with their research, including documenting the location of victims and indicating any structures that might have inhibited, even partially, exposure to the blast.[55] Shirabe enjoyed his collaboration with the American doctors, especially with Henry Barnett. One evening, he and Barnett, along with Shirabe's colleague Kanehiko Kitamura, a dermatologist from the Nagasaki Medical School, discussed the mechanics of the atomic bomb and the probability of residual radiation from Fat Man. Admitting the possibility of radioactive fallout, Barnett noted that "gamma rays attached to the dust" may have moved in a cloud following the explosion "to the east of the hypocenter in Nagasaki." Shirabe confirmed that "the wind was blowing from the west immediately after the bombing"; it was agreed that this should be investigated further.[56]

At the time of this conversation, Donald Collins, an expert on the mechanics of measurement instrumentation, was investigating fallout in Nagasaki. Collins found radioactivity in keeping with the fallout pattern discussed by Barnett, Shirabe, and Kitamura. Evidently, Collins still resisted the stated purpose of the mission as articulated to him by General Farrell on Tinian Island. Far from proving there was no radiation, as Farrell directed, Collins was able to trace "fallout from the bomb some 32 miles out to sea in one direction." The residual radiation detected, though negligible when compared with the dangerous impact of initial radiation, was, according to Collins, "about three times the normal background at that point."[57] Moreover, even in his makeshift Nagasaki laboratory, Collins found "radiation levels" that "were measurably higher than normal for

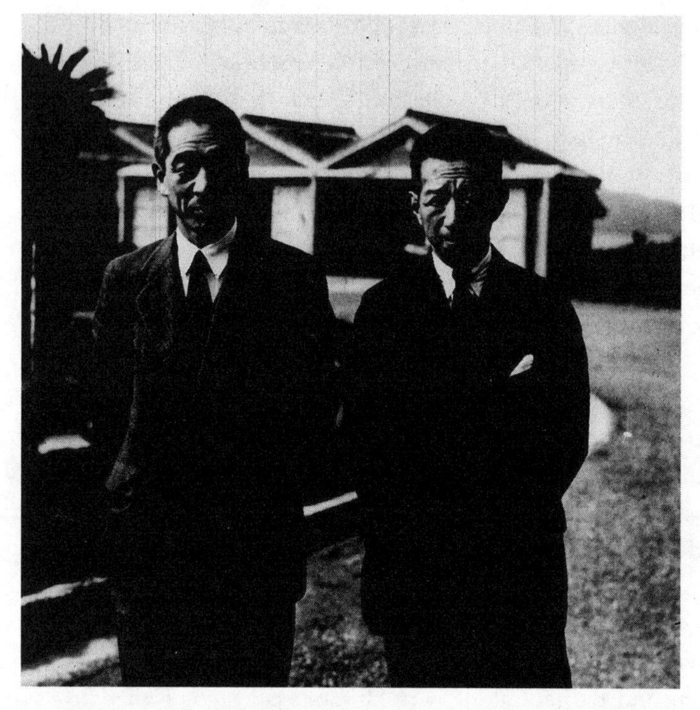

Nagasaki Medical School doctors Raisuke Shirabe and Kanehiko Kitamura.

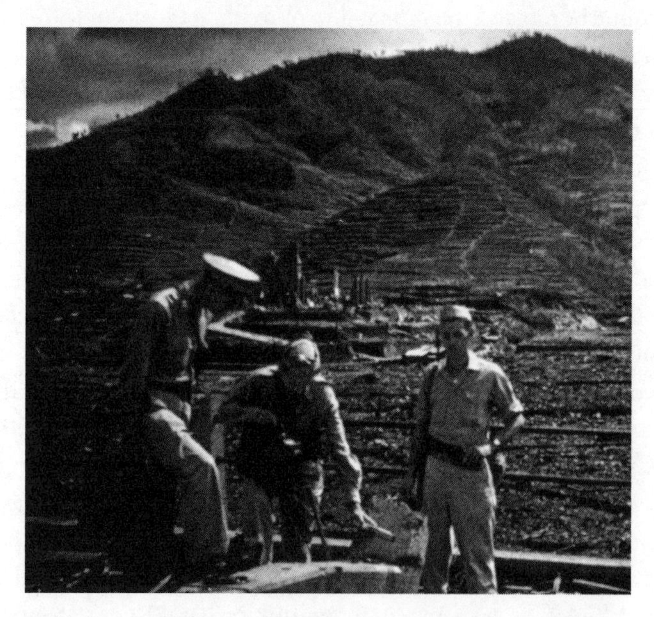

Walter Youngs (*left*), Donald Collins (holding Geiger counter), and A. T. Greenwood, with Urakami Cathedral ruins in background, September 1945.

Japan, due to fall out of debris from the bomb and to radiation induced by the neutrons emitted by the bomb."[58]

The Nagasaki Medical School doctors Shirabe, Kitamura, and Nagai would all be made part of the Joint Commission, though, because of their location at Omura Naval Hospital, Shirabe and Kitamura had a more direct and formal association.[59] In early October, doctors from the army and navy teams, including Shields Warren with the navy and Elbert DeCoursey with the army group, would take over at Omura as the Manhattan Project doctors prepared for their return to the United States. In an interesting, microlevel example of competing narratives, Shields Warren recollected his encounter with Nagai. He learned that Nagai had contracted leukemia before the August 9 bombing, which he correctly understood to be a consequence of Nagai's "failure to protect himself because he felt it was unpatriotic, while others were sacrificing their lives, to slow down his [x-ray] work by taking precautions." Incredibly, Shields Warren somehow concluded that Nagai was "actually helped by the bomb," in that the estimated three hundred roentgens of exposure he received from the August 9 blast had the positive effect of shrinking his spleen and lowering his white blood cell count.[60]

Nagai and his community, not surprisingly, had a very different explanation for his remarkable recovery. Around September 8, when members of the American team were first making their way into Hiroshima, Nagai began to manifest the symptoms of severe radiation sickness. Nagai correctly understood that the radiation he received from the bomb did not suppress but "added to [his] chronic radiation illness."[61] His temperature rose to 104 degrees, where it remained for a week. His face swelled and the wound on his temple reopened and began to bleed again. Three Nagasaki doctors confirmed that he was dying. In preparation for his death, Nagai gave a general confession and received communion from a Catholic priest. In accordance with Japanese custom, he also penned a traditional farewell song. Soon after writing his sayonara poem, he fell into a state of semiconsciousness.[62]

At this time, his mother-in-law, Gram, brought water from the Lourdes grotto of the Hongochi Monastery, located in the southern part of Nagasaki, a place where Midori Nagai had regularly gone to pray. As Gram applied the water to his lips, the barely conscious Nagai prayed to Father Maximilian Kolbe, the Polish Franciscan priest and founder of the Hongochi Monastery. Nagai had known Kolbe during the priest's time in Nagasaki, even x-raying him to test him for tuberculosis. Unbeknownst to Nagai,

Kolbe had, after returning to his native Poland, perished in Auschwitz four years earlier. The saintly Kolbe had famously offered his life in the place of that of another prisoner who had a family and had been selected for execution. Almost immediately after the Lourdes water was put on Nagai's lips, the bleeding stopped and the thirty-seven-year-old Japanese radiologist recovered.

Beyond the expectations of many, Nagai would live for almost six more years, dedicating himself to the reconstruction of the medical school, hospital, cathedral, and city and spreading a message of peace and forgiveness. During these years, Nagai wrote a number of books, including *The Bells of Nagasaki,* one of the very few early accounts of the bomb that got past Douglas MacArthur's censorship, but only after long delays and after Nagai agreed to add an appendix describing Japanese atrocities in the Philippines. *The Bells of Nagasaki,* which has been compared to Hersey's *Hiroshima,* became a national best seller and was later made into a popular movie.[63] Unlike Shields Warren, Nagai attributed his miraculous recovery not to the atom bomb but to divine intervention and to the intercessory prayers of Kolbe.[64] In an interview with Nagai's grandson, Tokusaburo Nagai, in Nagasaki, I asked him about Shields Warren's curious account of his grandfather's recovery. He laughed and stated that he too had heard this explanation, which he "could not believe." In a serious and pointed manner, he added, "I do not believe the atomic bomb helped him."[65]

This individualized example of competing narratives regarding the merits of the atomic bomb calls to mind "nuclearism"—that is, an enthusiasm about the bomb that attributes to it almost transcendent qualities. We've already encountered such religious references as the use of the word *trinity* as the name of the test site in Alamogordo, Oppenheimer's quotation of the lines from the Bhagavad Gita after witnessing the Trinity test, and the use of the term *papacy* as the code name for Tinian Island. Somehow, only religious concepts and images were adequate to capture the awesome power of this new technology.

Nuclearism, as such, is perhaps best represented in the person and rhetoric of William L. Laurence, the *New York Times* journalist who observed both the Trinity explosion and, from the air, the Nagasaki bomb.[66] Recall Laurence's divinized description of the Trinity test. He again invoked a sense of the transcendent while flying aboard one of the instrument planes during delivery of the Fat Man bomb. On the flight toward the primary target, Kokura, Laurence celebrated the unique opportunity he was given to witness the bombs: "And here I am. I am destiny. . . . There's a feeling of a human being, a mere mortal, a newspaper man by profession, suddenly has the knowledge which has been given to him, a sense—you might say—of divinity."[67] When "destiny chose Nagasaki as the ultimate target," Laurence observed, from the instrument plane accompanying *Bockscar,* the mushroom cloud, which he described as "a living thing, a new species being born right before our incredulous eyes."[68]

One could say that Shields Warren took nuclearism and the transcendent qualities of the bomb to another level. Not only was the bomb lifelike, it was life giving; it had the power to heal. Nagai clearly attributed his recovery to the healing power of another source, one that compelled him toward a tireless and sacrificial advocacy for peace and for the total elimination of nuclear weapons. His influence is still felt deeply in Nagasaki today.

To Treat or Not to Treat

One of the contested issues regarding the Joint Commission, as well as the collaborative investigative entities that would follow (the Atomic Bomb Casualty Commission [ABCC] and Radiation Effects Research Foundation [RERF]), was the practice of doctors interacting with patients for scientific purposes but not providing medical treatment. As Eileen Welsome succinctly puts it, "Warren's job was not to minister to the sick but to find out whether the two bombs had left any residual radiation."[69] A number of justifications for this policy have been offered over the years, including the arguments that to provide treatment would take away work from Japanese doctors; that it was difficult for American doctors to get medical licenses to legally practice in Japan; and that the ABCC and RERF were more exclusively scientific endeavors, making direct medical care inappropriate. Susan Lindee, in her comprehensive and enlightening analysis of the ABCC, however, argues that the no-treatment policy was determined in a more fundamental way by the issue of atonement. That is, if American doctors were to offer medical care to the victims of the bomb, they would be acknowledging moral responsibility for the plight of the *hibakusha* in both cities. In allegiance to the official narrative, this was not something Americans were willing to admit.[70]

However, Lindee also observes that the public no-treatment policy was not always followed in practice. On occasion, both Japanese and American doctors working with the ABCC did provide some medical care, even as officials knowingly looked the other way.[71] Moreover, it has been argued that the diagnostic services offered by the ABCC were themselves an important part of the overall treatment process. With a proper evaluation of their conditions, *hibakusha* were in a better position to seek more informed and appropriate medical care, and ABCC and RERF doctors were free to refer patients to Japanese doctors elsewhere who could provide medical treatment.

Even in the case of the Joint Commission, one discovers instances when the American doctors ignored the no-treatment policy. Consider, for example, Shields Warren's recollections on this point: "Under the terms of the treaty we were not allowed to treat any Japanese ourselves. This was reserved for the Japanese physicians, but we could advise the Japanese physicians as to what to do. Of course, sooner or later this broke down and we were treating them just like the Japanese were. But on a theoretical basis we could, under the treaty, only investigate and advise."[72]

Averill Liebow reported instances when the American doctors gave vitamins to Japanese patients, but this was less a form of necessary medical care than it was a means of complying with custom and fulfilling the expectations of Japanese patients.[73] Hiroshima *hibakusha* Tomiko Morimoto West, who was thirteen years old at the time of the bombing, remembers being given "some kind of pills" by the American doctors, though she didn't "know if they helped."[74] While staying at Miyajima, the American doctors learned that some of the bombing casualties had been relocated to the island. According to Stafford Warren, these victims, for whatever reason, did not want to be seen by the Americans. Nevertheless, Warren did propose help, including offering to provide the injured with some of the penicillin and plasma the doctors were carrying with them.[75]

Interestingly, while the American doctors were not supposed to medically treat the Japanese victims, there was at least one occasion when an American doctor benefited from the medical care of Japanese doctors. While at the Omura Naval Hospital near the end of their time in Nagasaki, Stafford Warren sought treatment for an infection on his leg. "I was a little worried about it," Warren remembered, "because the purulent material was white, and I thought I had a staphylococcus alba infection." As with diarrhea—which Warren experienced after several days of traipsing through the ruins of Hiroshima—evidence of a pustule, as noted by Nagai, was also a symptom of residual radiation, and a type of symptom that corresponded with the time frame in which Warren was in the bombed-out cities. Warren sought out the Japanese doctor, a bacteriologist, in charge of the Omura Naval Hospital, who carefully and successfully treated the infection. Warren was grateful for the good care he was given.[76]

The Occupation Troops and Preparing for Departure

In late September, as the Manhattan Group was winding down its work in Nagasaki, a large contingent of American occupation troops entered the city. Their arrival would change the dynamics of the city and, in some cases, the way the Americans were able to relate to the local Japanese population, which until that point had been, in the main, amicable and cooperative. When the marines landed in the port and began to move into the city, the local population noticeably withdrew. The troops entered "enemy" territory not quite knowing what they would encounter, but they were, as Warren put it, "expecting trouble and hoping there would be trouble."[77] One of the marines who entered Nagasaki at this time acknowledged the difficulty of switching from a combat to an occupation mentality: "We had been fighting these people. We could not just flip a switch and turn off all the instincts of battle. Hate was very deep-seated and very obvious."[78]

The leadership of the occupying troops did not know what to make of the Joint Commission, which did not fall directly under their jurisdiction. They seemed to resent the fact that the Manhattan Project group had been in the city several weeks before their arrival. Collins was even admonished by a marine commander for "collaborating with the enemy."[79] Near the end of the Manhattan Project group's time in Nagasaki, the prefectural governor invited them to a local geisha house for a little going-away dinner party. On the way to the venue, the group was stopped by a recently erected barricade set up by US Marines. After some haggling about rank and jurisdictional authority, the marines refused to allow the Manhattan Project doctors and scientists to pass through. Warren, Collins, and the others simply ignored their proscriptions and proceeded to the event. During the evening, as had been the practice throughout their time in Japan, little attention was paid to distinction or rank. Recall that most of the members of the Manhattan Project group were not proper military to begin with. Therefore, the party at the geisha house was a colorful mixture of Americans and Japanese, military and civilians, enlisted men and officers, all enjoying the food, sake, and entertainment together.

Miffed by the flagrant disregard shown to their authority, a group of marines stormed the party, "brandishing arms," and placed the Americans under arrest, though only Warren was ultimately charged. The colonel was "accused of violating blockade orders, of behavior unbecoming an officer, of fraternizing with enlisted men, fraternizing with the enemy, and of being drunk in a whorehouse." The men with Warren, including Collins, testified in his defense and assured the marines that Warren "definitely was not drunk" and that, as far as they were aware, "the Geisha house was a legitimate establishment, not a whorehouse." The charges were dropped, though, to his apparent embarrassment, Warren was verbally chastised for his actions.[80] This was not the only conflict the Manhattan Project group had with the newly arrived occupying forces.

On a more serious note, Collins recalled an episode during the occupation that brought considerable ignominy to the American forces in Nagasaki, an incident that suggests that the Itsukushima priest's prejudices toward the Americans were not entirely without merit. Even though the troops had been given strict orders regarding their behavior, these instructions were evidently not always heeded.[81] One day during the occupation, "a sailor who had obtained shore leave went berserk. He is reported to have entered a private home, shot the old man who lived there, then raped his wife and daughter." Members of the Joint Commission were told that the offending American sailor was "promptly court-martialed and sentenced to death."[82]

Given some of the tensions with the occupying forces, members of the Manhattan Project group likely were not disappointed that their time in Nagasaki was coming to an end. As Shields Warren and other members of the army and navy components of the Joint Commission began to take over, they looked to Stafford Warren's team to gain a fuller understanding of radiation and its effects. The Manhattan Project doctors, however, were less than fully forthcoming about their knowledge of radiation. One justification offered for this reticence was, once again, concerns about secrecy, a trope, recall, that was similarly advanced by Groves to resist health and safety measures at the Trinity test. In his well-regarded biography on Groves, Robert Norris highlights the manner in which Groves continued to invoke secrecy as a way of controlling the postwar narrative about radiation.[83]

One finds evidence of this essential strategy employed by the leaders of the Manhattan Project group as well, when other members of the Joint Commission were seeking a deeper understanding of nuclear radiation and its effects. For example, in contrast to what the Japanese doctors observed,

Hymer Friedell downplayed the potency of traveling neutrons. In a discussion with Oughterson's team, Friedell asserted that induced radiation was not a "major hazard"; he claimed the same concerning the harmfulness, or lack thereof, of radioactive fallout. When asked to provide "specific information" to back up these assertions, Friedell declined because it "was considered classified."[84] On another occasion, Averill Liebow—acknowledging the relative lack of knowledge among the non–Manhattan Project members of the Joint Commission—had hoped to learn more about radiation from those more closely involved with the development of the bomb. He was particularly interested in knowing more about "the spectrum and intensity of the radiation at the source." In response to this inquiry, Stafford Warren deferred, claiming that "this was still considered secret." He "would provide no information," wrote Liebow, except to say, unhelpfully, "that there was a soft mixture of hard and soft gamma radiations."[85]

Their lack of a deeper understanding about radiation notwithstanding, the army and navy components of the Joint Commission, led by Oughterson and Shields Warren, would carry on their investigations in Japan for several more months, while the Manhattan Project group, nearing the completion of their "spot check," began preparations for their return to the United States. At this point, Stafford Warren and the Manhattan Project group were prepared to pass along to Groves the more "detailed check" that had been promised to him by Farrell on September 14. Because Farrell had already returned to the States, it would instead fall to General James B. Newman Jr. to communicate the team's Nagasaki findings.

Newman's October 5 communication is difficult to decipher. On the one hand, he acknowledged much that had been found by both American and Japanese doctors, information that would presumably not be viewed favorably by Groves. For example, Newman reported that radioactivity had been traced in a zone east of the city that was two to six times background levels and even as high as ten to fifty times background in some places. He also made reference to Warren's belief that "radioactivity could be explained as the result of neutron bombardment near 0 and subsequent spread by dust and ashes arising from city in thermal columns"; and he noted Warren's findings that measurements of certain materials near the epicenter "indicate[] strong neutron bombardment."[86]

Newman reported, moreover, that "many late cases of severe gamma ray injury found up to 2000 meters. Milder injury at 2500 meters." Of an estimated forty thousand injured, he would guess that about five thousand were "injured by gamma rays without other serious injury." Given all of this information, it's hard to make sense of one line on the third page of the five-page memo: "Warren says without qualification that there never was a dangerous amount of radiation anywhere in the city of Nagasaki or its environs." One imagines that, despite the other data, this line would please and be used by Groves. Wrapping up the memo, Newman communicated to Groves that Oughterson, of the army general headquarters team, and Shields Warren, of the navy team, would stay longer in Japan to conduct further research and follow up on the work begun by the Manhattan Project team.[87]

A Friendly Farewell

On the following day, October 6, the Manhattan Project group departed from Omura to begin their journey back to the United States. Before leaving, Shirabe met up with and exchanged gifts with Henry Barnett, Joe Howland, and some of the other American doctors. Shirabe gave Japanese color prints and fans to the Americans, while Barnett offered to Shirabe and Kitamura large packages of cigarettes. Shirabe noticed that the American doctors were "excited about going back to their homeland." In his view, the collaboration had been a success: "I think we accomplished the objective of American-Japanese friendship." In particular, Shirabe remembered Barnett as a "friendly person" who always remembered his name.[88]

While tensions clearly lurked in the background and while certain actions—for example, the absconding of autopsied specimens, the destruction of Japanese cyclotrons, and the no-treatment policy—caused some resentment, the friendship between Shirabe and Barnett could also be seen in other working relationships among the various members of the Joint Commission. Stafford Warren, for example, told the story of being presented with ancient samurai swords by Tsuzuki and Hitoshi Motohashi in Tokyo in the days just before the Americans' return trip to the United States. When asked whether there was any hostility between him and the Japanese doctors, Warren replied, "No, not a bit. . . . We had been together almost six weeks with these two Japanese officers in our party, and we liked each other."[89]

The forty-two-year-old Japanese pathologist Michihiko Hachiya, at the Teishin Hospital in Hiroshima, remembered fondly working alongside Captain J. Philip Loge, a physician from Oughterson's group. "Dr. Loge was a young medical officer who came to my hospital every day and spent all his spare time examining patients," Hachiya wrote in a postscript to his *Hiroshima Diary.* "Though we could not speak the same tongue, we understood each other's feelings. He was a gentleman, and all my staff and patients became fond of him." Generalizing as to the benefits of this successful collaboration, Hachiya concluded, "There is no boundary where sympathy and understanding are present."[90]

Likewise, Liebow found in the Japanese pathologist Zenichiro Ishii a "firm and helpful friend." Liebow described working and traveling with Ishii as among the "most cherished memories" of his assignment in Japan.[91] As one indication of their friendship, toward the end of Liebow's time in Japan, Ishii generously gave Liebow a blue-and-red obi (a sash worn around the waist of a kimono) to take home to his bride, which Liebow treasured. Liebow's colorful and insightful diary is filled with positive references to Ishii and expressions of appreciation for the time the two worked together in Japan.

Beyond his warm reminiscences about working with Ishii, Liebow, writing the conclusion of his diary, entered into a deeper reflection about the meaning of the bomb, based on his four-month-long experience in Japan as well as his work with Barnett, Oughterson, and three others compiling material for a six-volume final report on the Joint Commission's investigations. According to Liebow, the experience of thinking and writing about the bomb and its effects "filled us with revulsion."[92] His thoughtful reflections, offered at the end of his diary, come much closer to the sentiments expressed in Father Siemes's account, John Hersey's book, and Norman Cousins's short essay than they do to the justifications offered by Warren or presented in Stimson's defense of the official narrative.

For example, Liebow, like Hersey and Cousins, wondered whether Americans had been "accessories to a crime against humanity." He also considered, along the lines suggested by Leo Szilard and other Manhattan Project physicists, whether a demonstration test would have been a preferred course of action. Additionally, he questioned whether, even if the atomic bombing of one city was "necessary," one could "justify the devastation of another." He was profoundly affected by what he saw in Japan and admitted to feeling "guilt and shame" in witnessing "the pitifully crippled and maimed" victims of the bomb. Significantly, far from downplaying the effects of radiation, he was deeply worried about what he saw regarding "the nature and extent of radiation injury in man. Never before had human beings been exposed en masse to this force that surely would have to be lived with, or even lived by."[93]

He also acknowledged the uncoordinated and chaotic nature of the genesis of the Joint Commission, observing that it could have been better anticipated and better organized. In deference to the respect and appreciation he felt for Ishii and the other Japanese doctors with whom he worked, he acknowledged that the Joint Commission only accomplished as much as it did because of the "expert knowledge, ingenuity, ideas, and unflagging efforts of our Japanese colleagues." In conclusion, he recognized that while the last chapter of the Joint Commission report may have been written, the final chapter of what the Manhattan Project had set in motion "remains unfinished." Rather, "it continues as a haunting memory. May the evil of which it tells never come back!"[94]

Concerning the final chapter of the Joint Commission, the majority of the Manhattan Project team departed from Tokyo on October 12. The final days before leaving included, for Nolan, "a secondary junket to Kyoto for investigation of the [pathological] material transferred there from Hiroshima." In Kyoto, he met up with "other boon-dogglers including the Tinian group from the 509th." The end of Warren's time in Japan included a harrowing flight to Hiroshima, with Tsuzuki and Motohashi, in a failed effort to pick up Friedell's group. The terrifying flight, which Warren regarded as the most frightening experience of his life, had to be cut short because of weather and lack of visibility. Warren, Nolan remembered, "only got back to Tokyo by the skin of his teeth and Tokyo Rose."[95] The group's less eventful return trip to the United States would include stops in Iwo Jima, Tinian, and Honolulu before landing in San Francisco on October 14. From San Francisco, Warren headed back to Oak Ridge, while Nolan took a week's leave to visit his family in Los Angeles. On the day they touched down on American soil, it had been exactly three months since Nolan and Furman had departed from Los Alamos with Little Boy in tow.

6

Managing Radiation and the Radiation Narrative

From the first, the hazards of radioactivity were hopelessly obscured in a flurry of vague, optimistic, and downright misleading pronouncements.

—Paul Boyer, *By the Bomb's Early Light*

After touching down at Hamilton Army Air Force Base in San Francisco, James F. Nolan boarded a train for an overnight trip to Los Angeles. There he was reunited with his wife and two children, from whom he had been absent for more than three months. In Los Angeles, the family prepared for their return trip to Los Alamos. After a week's stay with the Reynoldses, they traveled by car back to Los Alamos. Resituated in their army-issued Sundt apartment by the end of October, the next few months would be a busy and chaotic time for Nolan. With the war over, many features of the once-secret Site Y were now in a state of flux. Nolan was asked to take over from Louis Hempelmann as head of the Health Group in the Los Alamos lab. Since February 1945, before his time overseas, Nolan had been serving as the alternative group leader to Hempelmann, with most of his responsibilities dedicated to setting up the safety and evacuation procedures at the Trinity Site.

As the new leader of the Health Group, Nolan would, like Hempelmann before him, serve in this role as a civilian. Therefore, after returning from Japan, he began the process of securing a discharge from the army, something he was evidently keen to achieve. Though he was highly commended for his military service—in the fall of 1945 he was awarded both a Legion of Merit citation and a Bronze Service Star—he was nevertheless eager to get out of the military.[1] As his daughter, Lynne, recalls, "He couldn't wait to get out of the army."[2]

Second, Nolan would work with Stafford Warren to prepare a report on their findings for Leslie Groves, who was scheduled to testify before Congress in the next month. After staying in Los Alamos for less than three weeks, Nolan again boarded a train destined for Oak Ridge. It had been five months since his last trip, when he had traveled to warn Groves about potential fallout from the Trinity test. This time, he was in Oak Ridge to prepare a report on fallout and the other effects of the bombs that they had discovered in Japan. After a week in Tennessee, Nolan then journeyed to New York and finally to Washington, DC. He and Warren were in Washington during Groves's two days of testimony (November 28 and 29) before the Special Committee on Atomic Energy. On the day before his first day of testimony, Warren supplied Groves with a completed preliminary report of their findings.

Presenting the Joint Commission's Findings

In preparation for his testimony, Groves had read the preliminary report supplied to him by Warren, along with a draft of Father John Siemes's translated testimony, which Warren included for "its value as background material and its narrative interest."[3] While presenting his opening remarks—which focused primarily on the structural damage caused by the bombs—Groves was interrupted by Vermont senator Warren Austin, who asked whether the general could report on the presence of any radioactive residue in Hiroshima or Nagasaki. Groves responded without the slightest equivocation, "Yes, sir: and there is none. That is a very positive 'none.'"[4]

Minutes later, Senator Richard Russell from Georgia asked Groves to elaborate on this point, to which the general responded, "There was no radioactivity damage done to any human being excepting at the time that the bomb actually went off, and that is an instantaneous damage." In other words, there was no residual radiation ("none"), and any injuries caused by radiation were from the initial detonation of the bombs; and "the number of casualties from that [was] relatively small," Groves added. So exceptional were these limited cases, he testified further, that it "would take an accident for a man, the average person, within the range of the bomb to be killed by radioactive effects." In the rare (or accidental) instances in which people did die from radiation alone, Groves argued, "I understand it from the doctors" that they did so "without undue suffering." Invoking the purported authority of his physicians' expertise, he then shockingly added, "In fact, they [that is, the doctors] say it is a very pleasant way to die."[5]

Eileen Welsome does not overstate matters when she characterizes Groves's testimony here as "patently untrue."[6] In fact, though he summoned the authority of his Manhattan Project doctors, as did Thomas Farrell two months earlier in Tokyo, Groves's statement was not even commensurate with the material supplied to him by Warren—even though the report itself appears to have been constructed in such a manner as to be as favorable as possible to Groves's preferred narrative. A close reading of the document, however, shows that the preliminary findings of the Manhattan Project doctors did not, in substance, support Groves's testimony.

The report, for example, did not say there was no residual radiation. Rather, it indicated that though "the intensity of radiation is quite low, it is measurable with the very sensitive instruments used." Warren even conceded that, in some cases, the acceptable tolerance dose "is exceeded slightly," and in reference to radioactive fallout, he cited, without refutation, Japanese data showing "evidence that patients in Nagasaki as far away as 4 kilometers did show effects of radiation." Moreover, rather than radiation casualties being "relatively small," as Groves testified, Warren reported that of the "approximately 4000 patients admitted to hospitals, 1300 or 33% showed effects of radiation and of this number approximately one-half died."[7]

In the report, Warren once again noted the limitations of the group's measuring instruments. He admitted that his group, in the end, only measured the effects of gamma rays. Attempts were made to measure alpha and beta particles, but these were not calibrated because of "technical difficulties and inaccuracy in evaluating the readings." Most significantly, no measurements were made (or reported) of neutron activity. Warren wrote, "The additional role that neutrons may have played in the production of these symptoms can not be evaluated from the data."[8] This was a significant omission, because, as David Bradley, a physician who would work with Warren and Nolan in the Marshall Islands after the war, explained, "it is likely that most of the damage done specifically at Hiroshima and Nagasaki was done by neutrons."[9] In a later interview after the war, Warren admitted to the significance of this omission: "Not too much was known about the effect of neutrons except we knew that they were destructive. We had a hard time measuring them."[10]

Recall that what the doctors accepted as a maximum permissible dose of radiation exposure in 1945 would eventually be seen as far too high. While the doctors regarded one-tenth of a roentgen as a safe maximum tolerable dose of radiation at the time, Nolan acknowledged, "no one knew really how much radiation a human could stand." While planning for the Trinity test, Los Alamos scientists negotiated with Nolan to accept a higher limit, finally settling on five roentgens, which, less than twenty years later, would be regarded as eight hundred times higher than the accepted standard.[11]

During his testimony before the Senate subcommittee, Groves also selectively and strategically used Siemes's written account to support his arguments concerning the effects of radiation. He read directly from it: "It was also noised about that the ruins of the city emitted deadly rays and that many workers who went there to aid in the clearing died, and that the central district would be uninhabitable for some time to come. I have my doubts as to whether such talk is true, and myself and others who worked in the ruined areas for some hours shortly after the explosion suffered no such ill effects."[12] Groves, however, skipped over sections of the document that would have heavily qualified, if not directly contradicted, his constructed narrative. While Siemes may have been somewhat skeptical about the effects of residual radiation, he did observe the severe consequences of initial radiation. He knew, for example, of several cases in which individuals "who did not have external burns died later." He also observed, "There seems to be some truth in the statement that the radiation had some effect on the blood." Specifically, his colleague Father Wilhelm Kleinsorge, who did not suffer burns, remained very weak and was found by an attending physician at the time to have leukopenia.

Though Siemes was, in the summer and early fall of 1945, inclined to attribute his fellow priest's frailty to his "generally weakened and malnourished condition," John Hersey's more long-term view, put forth in a later edition of *Hiroshima,* found that Kleinsorge's health struggles, including leukopenia, would persist for years. The ailing Jesuit priest returned regularly to the hospital for treatment, sometimes for prolonged stays, and struggled for the rest of his life with many of the common symptoms of radiation sickness.

It should also be noted that Warren's report offered no empirical support whatsoever for Groves's assertions about no "undue suffering" and the "very pleasant" dying process of fatal radiation injury. In fact, Warren's report is full of references to such unpleasant radiation-induced symptoms as fever, nausea, vomiting, loss of appetite, diarrhea, petechiae, "epilation, severe ulcerative lesions of the mouth and throat[,] . . . rapid and extreme emaciation[,] . . . destruction of the bone marrow and the lymphatics, ulcerative lesions of the colon and rectum," and so on.[13]

During his testimony, the senators perceived a notable defensiveness on Groves's part in the manner in which he repeatedly denied the harmfulness of radiation exposure. After Groves falsely asserted that the limited damage from radiation took place only at the moment of explosion, the chairman of the committee, Senator Brien McMahon from Connecticut, interjected, "General, you don't make any point of congratulations on that result, the fact that that didn't happen, do you? If there was radioactivity, there wouldn't be anything morally wrong with that?" McMahon was prompted to ask these questions given how often Groves and other military officials asserted the relative absence of radiation damage in Japan. "Its very reiteration," McMahon stated, "seemed to me to indicate that there was some feeling on the part of the War Department that there was something morally wrong if it had [caused significant radiation damage]."[14]

Given Groves's anxiety, apparent as early as mid-August when reports first started coming out of Japan of radiation poisoning, the senator correctly perceived a notable defensiveness on Groves's part. In response to the senator's questioning, Groves again stated that ongoing radioactive damage in Japan had been avoided. Then, putting forth what could only be regarded as a vague and questionable dichotomy, he added, "If it was a choice between radioactivity on a few Japanese or even a number of thousands of Japanese or a case of saving 10 times as many American lives, I would go the American way on that question without any hesitation. . . . There would be no feeling, as I say, on my part on anything that would have shortened this war by a single day."[15] At the time of his testimony, however, Groves was clearly aware of the harmfulness of radioactivity, even beyond its effects on "a few" or even "thousands of Japanese." In other words, "the American way," as such, included Americans.

The Blue Glow at the Omega Site

In addition to the descriptions of the agonizing symptoms of radiation sickness presented in Warren's report, Groves was also fully aware of the suffering of one of his own scientists who had died from radiation exposure in an accident at Los Alamos just ten weeks before his Senate testimony. In late August, while Warren, Henry Barnett, Harry O. Whipple, and the other Manhattan Project doctors were en route to Japan, the understaffed Hempelmann was struggling to maintain safety standards at Los Alamos. During this time, Harry Daghlian, a young scientist who had studied particle physics at Purdue, was conducting an experiment popularly known as "tickling the dragon's tail."

The dangerous experiment, which took place in the Pajarito Canyon at the Omega Site, about three miles from the main Los Alamos lab, involved measuring criticality with a 6.19-kilogram, nickel-plated sphere of plutonium. Daghlian was working alone on the evening of August 21, 1945, though a military guard named Robert Hemmerly was also in the room, reading a newspaper with his back to the assembly. The twenty-four-year-old Daghlian was building layers of tungsten carbide bricks around the smooth sphere of subcritical plutonium. The bricks, or tamper material, had the effect of reflecting neutrons back into the plutonium. The young physicist was attempting to measure just how much tamper material was necessary to reach criticality. As Daghlian was laying the last brick in the fifth and final layer of the assembly, a monitoring device signaled a notable uptick in neutron activity. As Daghlian tried to pull the brick away, it slipped out of his hand and fell into the middle of the assembly. At that moment, an eerie blue flash filled the room, noticeably lighting up Hemmerly's newspaper.

Daghlian removed some of the bricks from the assembly, including the one that had slipped out of his hand. As a consequence of the accident and Daghlian's efforts to disassemble the layers of tungsten carbide, he received a harmful dose of neutrons and gamma rays. He was taken to the hospital for examination and treatment by the Los Alamos medical staff, including Hempelmann. Some thirty minutes after the accident, "he complained of numbness and tingling of the swollen hands."[16] In the days that followed, his condition worsened and his suffering increased. He experienced violent vomiting, severe diarrhea, and the blistering and shedding of skin, especially on his heavily exposed hands. In fact, the skin on Daghlian's hands and forearms was eventually lost, progressing to the point of "actual dry gangrene" on his fingers, all of which was clinically observed and documented photographically.[17] Exhibiting many of the same symptoms as the victims in Hiroshima and Nagasaki, he died twenty-five days after the accident.

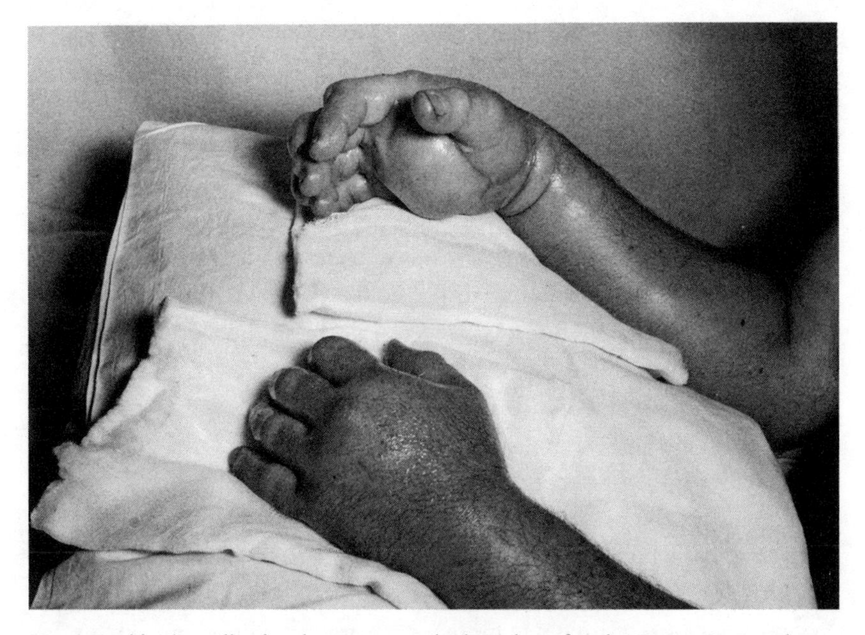

Harry Daghlian's swollen hands approximately three days after the Omega Site accident.

Hemmerly, who was about twelve feet from the assembly at the time of the accident, received a lower dose of radiation. He stayed in the hospital for two nights before being released. After a couple of months, he appeared to have recovered from his relatively mild symptoms, though later in life he would be diagnosed with acute myeloblastic leukemia. Following more than a year of unsuccessful treatment, he died at the age of sixty-two. In a 1979 follow-up study of the accident, Hempelmann admitted to the likelihood that Hemmerly's death had been caused by the radiation he received in the Omega Site accident.[18]

This was not the first time the blue glow had been seen in the labs of Los Alamos. About two and a half months before the Daghlian accident, on June 4, 1945, another incident occurred at the Omega Site in which several people, including Harold Hammel, Jess Kupferberg, and James Bistline, received large doses of radiation. In this case, briefly mentioned in Chapter 3, the experiment involved slowly adding water to a tank containing enriched uranium. During the test, water had been added too quickly and, as occurred in the Daghlian case, a monitoring instrument indicated a sharp and dangerous rise in neutron activity. Kupferberg and Bistline responded by cutting further water intake, as well as releasing some of the excess water from the tank. In these brief moments, an observable blue glow could be seen around the water tank. Those closest to the tank, including Kupferberg, also "noticed a deepseated tingling sensation in their bodies."[19]

Nolan, who was in Los Alamos during the June 4 accident, would hear another account of this particular symptom while stationed at Tinian Island. In the memo he sent to Stafford Warren, written the day after the Hiroshima bomb, Nolan recorded that one of the *Enola Gay* crew had experienced a similar sensation. As conveyed in the summary account of his medical examination of the crew, Nolan wrote, "One crew member at seven miles noticed a vague but distinctive odor or taste. This was purely voluntary information and was not suggested. The sensation was the same as that described by Sgt. Kupferberg after the Omega accident."[20]

As for those exposed during the June 4 incident, blood samples were taken from all who had been in the room at the time of the accident. The four closest to the water tank were taken to the hospital for further observation. In a report written one month after the accident, Hempelmann indicated that "there were no untoward symptoms of any kind," although all four of the hospitalized workers experienced reduced blood pressure. Additionally, Bistline reported a loss of appetite and was found to have a lower white blood cell count, and Hammel's "initial count . . . showed some leucocytosis and relative lymphopenia." The four hospitalized workers were instructed to avoid further radiation exposure and to stay out of the sunlight. The accident resulted in the implementation of (or the attempt to implement) more stringent rules for the Omega group "concerning the handling of critical assemblies."[21]

With full awareness of these earlier accidents and with the lab in a state of chaotic transition following the end of the war, Nolan was presented with the challenging task of collecting data from departing workers—many of whom were less than fully cooperative—while also establishing more rigorous and routinized safety measures to better protect those who remained at the lab. With the war over, there was no longer any excuse for a cavalier attitude toward the protection and safety of those handling radioactive materials.[22] Nolan noted a change in attitude among the plutonium workers: "With the lifting of security and the lack of pressure afforded by the war, employees at this laboratory now have many qualms about the special hazards."[23] No longer, for example, would anyone tolerate the high levels of plutonium excretion detected among the workers at the time of the Trinity test.

With many leaving Los Alamos "to return to peacetime pursuits," the Health Group determined to collect and record data, including blood and urine samples, as systematically as possible from departing workers. This created an "enormous load" and "major headaches" for the Health Group, as there "was little cooperation on the part of individuals about to be discharged." Nevertheless, "great pains" were taken to get these data, and Wright Langham was charged with obtaining "urine assays on plutonium workers who were terminating." The physicians even set up a "milk-route" to collect specimens from individuals in their homes because of their lack of cooperation in furnishing them otherwise.[24]

In addition to instituting termination procedures, the Health Group, under Nolan's leadership, sought to increase the protection and safety of those still working at the lab, or at least to give the impression of showing greater concern for workers' health. Implementation of these new measures was complicated by the involvement of Manhattan Project doctors in other activities, including continuing follow-up work with the Trinity test (for example, monitoring cows exposed to radiation) and preparing for Operation Crossroads, an emerging plan to test more atomic bombs in the Marshall Islands in the summer of 1946. All three of the leading Manhattan Project doctors—Nolan, Warren, and Hempelmann—were scheduled to be part of the radiation safety (radsafe) team of Operation Crossroads and had to devote some time to preparing for this new venture.

In spite of these distractions, new safety and monitoring practices were implemented during the interim period (November 1945–May 1946), which included assigning nurses to first-aid stations at some of the outlying sites and employing an additional nurse in the Tech Area. Joe Hoffman was tasked with more comprehensively distributing and collecting film badges to measure radiation at various locations around the lab. Additionally, in light of the earlier accidents, Nolan attempted to establish tighter supervision over the critical assembly group. Toward this end, following a conference meeting with the doctors, Canadian-born physicist Louis Slotin agreed to assign a man from his critical assembly team to report on monitoring activities to the Health Group.[25]

This was a tragically ironic choice, as the thirty-five-year-old Slotin, who had been a close friend and colleague of Daghlian's, would soon be involved in the most famous radiation accident to occur in Los Alamos. On May 21, 1946—exactly nine months to the day after Daghlian's accident—Slotin was working with plutonium materials scheduled for use in the upcoming nuclear tests on the Bikini Atoll in the Marshall Islands. In fact, Slotin was scheduled to take part in Operation Crossroads. Working at the Omega Site in the Pajarito Canyon, he was demonstrating to a group of six other scientists the steps involved in "tickling the dragon's tail." As in the Daghlian case, a security guard was also present in the room.

This time the experiment involved slowly lowering a half sphere of beryllium over a plutonium core. Slotin had conducted the experiment more than forty times before and had become a bit too comfortable and incautious with the exercise. The famous Italian physicist Enrico Fermi once warned Slotin, "Keep doing that experiment that way and you'll be dead within a year."[26] On the afternoon of May 21, using a screwdriver, Slotin gently lowered the beryllium tamper closer to the plutonium core while listening to the clicks of the Geiger counter sitting beside him. Suddenly, the screwdriver slipped and the hemisphere of tamper material came into direct contact with the plutonium. Slotin instinctively separated the two spheres with his bare hands, an action that likely saved the lives of the others in the room, though it exposed Slotin to a dangerous and ultimately lethal dose of radiation.

Once again, a distinctive blue glow emitted from the radioactive substances. As the security guard, Patrick Cleary, recounted, "I saw the sphere come off the assembly, and saw the blue glow all around the sphere uniformly, like a halo."[27] In keeping with the prevailing policy of compartmentalization, Cleary, unlike the scientists in the room, had no understanding of the materials or the experiment that was taking place at the Omega Site that afternoon. "I did not actually know what the material or sphere was at the time, or anything about it," Cleary recounted.[28]

Slotin, along with the others at the Omega Site, who had received lesser doses of radiation, were rushed to the Los Alamos Hospital. Hempelmann and Nolan were among the attending physicians. Warren, having been told of the accident, flew immediately from San Francisco (where he was preparing for Operation Crossroads) to Albuquerque. Other medical specialists from around the country also traveled to Los Alamos. The triage efforts that followed were both medical and scientific in nature. Regarding the latter, the exposure of eight individuals to varying levels of radiation provided a valuable opportunity for scientific investigation of the effects of radiation exposure on humans. Unlike in Japan, there were no blast or fire burn injuries to disentangle from the radiation injuries; the injuries were entirely caused by radiation. Scientific analysis began immediately. When Norris Bradbury,

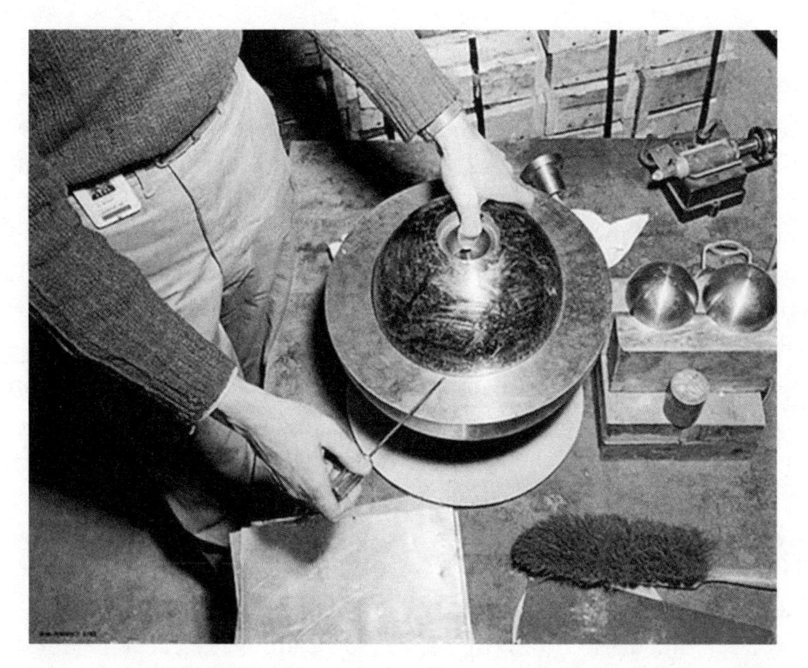

Reenactment of the "tickling the dragon's tail" experiment that resulted in Louis Slotin's death.

Robert Oppenheimer's successor as head of the Los Alamos lab; Phil Morrison; members of the Health Group; and others converged on the scene of the accident, they "started making measurements and collecting samples," and the "night was spent counting coins, badges, blood and urine samples, and trying to get an understanding of the extent of the dose."[29]

In addition to the medical and scientific activities, Manhattan Project officials also worried about how to handle the public relations dimension of the accident. Two days after the accident, Bradbury assembled a meeting, which included Nolan, Hempelmann, and Paul Hageman—the new post surgeon at the hospital—to "coordinate the many immediate things to be done concerning the injured men." Notably, the "things" requiring attention mainly had to do with how the lab would manage public information about the accident. Among the six points considered in the May 23 meeting of doctors and scientists was whether to issue a press release, who would make any public statement, and "how many next of kin should be notified immediately." None of the six points for this hastily assembled meeting—which included four Los Alamos physicians—mentioned anything about the medical treatment of the injured men.[30]

This is not to say that nothing was being done medically. Noting the seriousness of Slotin's case, in particular, Bradbury acknowledged the work of the doctors in attending to their patient: "Nolan and Hempelmann are both here and the former will remain as long as needed. Col Warren has come. . . . I feel that all is being done that can be done."[31] However, there was little the doctors could do. Slotin's body deteriorated even more quickly than did Daghlian's, and once again in ways that approximated the frightful effects of radiation experienced by the victims of the Hiroshima and Nagasaki bombs. On May 30, just nine days after the accident, Slotin died. It was an agonizing and painful death, only partially relieved by the morphine administered to him by the doctors. In terms of scientific observation, Slotin (as had Daghlian before him) willingly allowed his injuries to be measured, examined, and photographed, including full-length pictures of his naked and decaying body.

The accident did nothing to slow preparations for the Bikini tests, Bradbury assured his superiors. Once again Hempelmann would be asked to stay home and manage the crisis, while Nolan and Warren departed for the Marshall Islands.[32] In fact, both Warren and Nolan left Los Alamos several days before Slotin died. Hempelmann, on the other hand, remained to attend to the aftermath of the accident, which included meeting Slotin's parents, Alexander and Sonia Slotin, when they arrived at Los Alamos and traveling back with them, and the casket carrying their deceased son, to Winnipeg on May 31. The army moved quickly to settle with the Slotin family, offering $10,000 in compensation, but while requiring Slotin's mother to sign a release form denying that the army had any liability for the accident. The army also covered all of the Slotins' travel, room, and board expenses for the trip to and from Los Alamos.

As for the others who were in the room during the accident, it was estimated that, after Slotin, the physicist Alvin Graves received the next highest dose of radiation. Following the accident, he manifested some of the acute symptoms of radiation sickness, including high fevers and vomiting. He subsequently lost most of his hair, became temporarily sterile, and struggled with debilitating fatigue for several months.[33] Graves and his wife, Elizabeth (or Diz, as she was commonly known), had been two of Nolan's monitors for the Trinity test. Diz, who was seven months pregnant at the time of the Trinity test, and thus also Nolan's patient, had "raised hell" with him "to get in on the TR test." She and her husband were finally "allowed to perch in the motel in Carrizozo" as part of the team monitoring fallout from the test. In retrospect, Nolan confessed that, had he known about the prospect of the Omega Site accident, he would never have allowed them to participate, as the May 21, 1946, accident might have prevented the couple from having any more children, thus making the baby with whom she was pregnant in June 1945 "the last Graves baby."[34] In 1966, at the age of fifty-four, twenty years after the accident, Graves suffered a fatal heart attack while skiing. His heart condition, Hempelmann later acknowledged, can be "assumed to have been the result of the radiation exposure."[35]

After Slotin and Graves, Allan Kline received the next highest level of radiation, an estimated dosage of one hundred roentgens.[36] Four days after the accident, Bradbury sent a letter to Kline's mother, June Kline. In it, he claimed that her son "was not seriously affected by his accidental exposure to radiation." Bradbury quoted directly from Hageman's medical report: "S. Allan Kline experienced only minimal symptoms and no objective evidence of radiation disease. Laboratory data is equivocal. To be kept under observation. Prognosis is good."[37] After the accident, Allan Kline was terminated from the Manhattan Project and moved back to Chicago. He would suffer from the effects of radiation exposure for years. His hair fell out, he had to avoid exposure to the sun for a long time, he struggled with severe lassitude (and would sleep sixteen hours a day), and he was sterile for two years.

While in Chicago and then later in New York, he initially sought medical care from doctors connected with the Atomic Energy Committee (AEC), the civilian-controlled entity that took over the work of the Manhattan Project on January 1, 1947. However, Kline eventually realized that he was not really being given medical care but, like the victims studied by the Joint Commission and the Atomic Bomb Casualty Commission (ABCC) in Japan, was rather being examined for the purposes of collecting scientific data. About three years after the accident, Kline wrote, "I was actually used as a guinea pig during this whole period as no medication or treatment was given me for my recovery, nor was any advised. All any of the physicians did was to check my physical condition and subject me to very long, uncomfortable tests and the results of these tests then became the property of the U.S. Government, and I was not given access to them."[38]

Kline eventually stopped cooperating with AEC physicians and turned to private doctors instead. He sought unsuccessfully for years to retrieve his medical records from Los Alamos and to secure some kind of settlement for his injuries. As late as March 1951, nearly five years after the accident,

Kline was still trying to retrieve medical information from the AEC, including data from blood and urine samples, a sternum puncture, blood coagulation data, and radiation measurements from coins, his watch, his belt buckle, and so on, which had been collected during his stay in the Los Alamos Hospital after the accident.[39] In response, Kline was told the following: "There are certain data which you request such as calculations of radiation emitted from objects on your person which are apparently nonexistent and we can only presume that if any count was taken on these objects it was primarily as a matter of curiosity and no record was made."[40]

The flagrant deception in this response became glaringly clear in the 1980s, when "hidden files" from the Kline case were accidentally discovered in a University of Tennessee archive by researcher Clifford Honicker.[41] Included in these files was a document recording the "relative intensities" of radiation exposure of all eight men in the room, based on measurements from blood serum, film badges, coins, and so on, the collection of which Bradbury explicitly discussed in the memo cited earlier. In a memo to General Groves, written six days after the accident, Colonel C. W. Betts similarly acknowledged the collection and analysis of these materials: "All members of the party of eight were immediately hospitalized and placed under observation. Other experts spent the following night checking the radioactivity of metal articles in the possession of the victims of the accident and taking blood and urine radioactivity counts."[42] The data, which were withheld from Kline, make clear that, after Slotin and Graves, Kline received the highest dosage of radiation from the accident, one well over the maximum permissible dose, even by 1946 standards.[43]

Why were these medical data kept from Kline? It appears that Los Alamos doctors were explicitly directed not to cooperate with Kline because of concerns about litigation. In response to a request by the Chicago-based doctor J. J. Nickson to hospitalize Kline "for further medical study," Hempelmann wrote a revealing letter on December 10, 1946, nearly seven months after the accident. He acknowledged that the "case was being handled in a most unusual manner" and that he had been instructed "not to contact Kline directly nor to commit the project in any way." As for the reasons behind this lack of cooperation, Hempelmann admitted that "the prospect of a lawsuit seems to have caused a most remarkable case of jitters."[44]

Later that month, prompted by the Kline case, Warren recommended introducing policy measures that would protect the AEC from future legal cases. Again, the explicit motivation for this policy "clarification" was to "save possible embarrassment of the Government by medical legal suits."[45] Part of the issue for Warren and Hempelmann was that Kline refused to participate in any further medical examinations by Manhattan Project or AEC doctors. Kline objected because he justifiably felt he was being scientifically examined rather than medically treated. Warren's proposed policy was, in essence, to better facilitate examinations of workers following similar accidents in order to prevent future lawsuits. Again, Warren was evidently motivated not by concerns for Kline's health but by a desire to maintain "good public relations," an issue he mentioned three times in the policy proposal.[46]

The Omega Site accidents, and the Kline case in particular, provide another example of the pattern of caution, co-optation, and complicity we have observed in the doctors' involvements in various episodes of the dawn of the nuclear age. Doctors offered warnings about the critical assembly experiments. These warnings were disregarded or not taken seriously. When accidents did occur, the doctors were used to procure scientific data and then became complicit in hiding evidence, motivated, once again, out of fear of litigation. These cases also demonstrate the inadequacy of quick assessments and the lack of concern about potential long-term consequences. When Hempelmann conducted the follow-up study in 1979, he demonstrated that the Omega Site accidents had outcomes that extended well beyond the unfortunate deaths of Daghlian and Slotin. Hempelmann had conducted an earlier follow-up study in 1952 in which six of the eight survivors agreed to participate. Two, both from the Slotin accident, did not participate: Kline, for reasons that should be clear, and Cleary, because he was away fighting in the Korean War, where he would die in combat at the age of twenty-seven.

Kline's lack of participation in the 1952 study clearly frustrated Hempelmann, a response that reveals the manner in which a scientific mind-set superseded a medical one. At the same time that Kline was trying to retrieve his medical records and reach some kind of settlement with the AEC, Hempelmann and others were insisting that Kline first participate in another examination, for the purpose of completing the 1952 study, which Hempelmann and others were working on at the time. In a December 1949 letter, for example, Hempelmann wrote, "My interest in the Kline case is not limited to a desire for a speedy and fair settlement. I also want Kline to submit to an examination and to permit us to include his case in our study of radiation illness."[47] Kline, of course, refused, and "Case 5" is conspicuously missing in both the 1952 and the 1979 follow-up studies. During a 1980 interview, Hempelmann tried to explain Kline's absence from the studies, stating that Kline "was so disturbed by this experience that he . . . became a lawyer and then sued I think the AEC or something like that. I think we settled out of court or something like that and he would not cooperate with the follow-up."[48]

In the 1979 study, four of the six who had been reexamined in the 1952 study were now dead. Two (including Hemmerly) died from leukemia and two (including Graves) from heart conditions, all of which could plausibly be traced to the radiation exposure they received. As Hempelmann conceded, albeit with qualification, in 1979, "It seems likely that the two leukemic deaths represent late effects of the radiation exposure. . . . The other two deaths could conceivably have been related to the exposure."[49] Again, as was the case in Japan, early and quick assessments simply could not capture the full extent of the radiation injuries from the Omega Site accidents.

Further Studies of the Effects of Radiation in Japan

More long-term studies in Japan would similarly reveal the inadequacies of the Manhattan Project team's spot check and would demonstrate that Warren's findings, not to mention Groves's testimony, were themselves, at best, misleading. When Warren testified before the same Senate committee a few months after Groves had, he claimed that only 5 to 7 percent of the overall casualties in Japan could be attributed to radiation effects. He also stated that when his team departed from Nagasaki in early October, "the cases in the hospitals averaged 20 cases of fire burns to one of gamma-ray injury."[50] This assertion does not comport with information reported by General James B. Newman Jr., on October 5, of a ratio of "about three burns to one gamma ray injury case" in Nagasaki.[51] Nor does it square with the findings of John Flick, of Ashley W. Oughterson's team, who observed of patients in one of the largest hospitals (five wards of about fifty beds each) in the Nagasaki area (likely Omura), at around the same time, that "nearly all [were] irradiation cases."[52]

Also challenging Warren's estimate was the US government's Strategic Bombing Survey, one component of which investigated the biological effects of the atom bombs in Hiroshima and Nagasaki. This group of more than 110 men, who spent ten weeks in Japan between October and December 1945, cooperated with the elements of the Joint Commission that remained in Japan. In its June 1946 report, the Strategic Bombing Survey argued that Warren's estimate was "far too low." Instead, as stated in the report, "most medical investigators who spent some time in the areas . . . generally felt that no less than 15 to 20 percent of the deaths were from radiation."[53]

Shields Warren and Oughterson, the heads of the other two American teams forming the Joint Commission, published a comprehensive report of their findings in 1956, *Medical Effects of the Atomic Bomb in Japan.* Included in their analysis is a survey of the different types of injuries found among a sample of 9,292 casualties in Hiroshima and Nagasaki, all of whom were still alive twenty days after the explosions. Of this sample, 4,262, or 46 percent, were observed to have some kind of radiation injury, though sometimes in combination with blast or burn injuries.[54] Given these kinds of data, it is not surprising that Shields Warren and Naval Captain Rupert Draeger would conclude that, rather than constituting only a very small percentage of overall casualties, a "greater number of injuries was probably caused by ionizing radiation-blast effects, gamma rays, and neutrons than by any other type of injury resulting from the explosion of the bombs."[55]

Regarding potential harm from residual radioactivity, rather than outright denying its presence, as did Farrell and Groves, Shields Warren and Draeger allowed that it was a real possibility: "Residual radioactivity due to contamination of the area by fission products of the bomb is a conceivable happening."[56] In fact, a classified report written by Nello Pace and Robert Smith, two members of the Joint Commission's navy contingent, found measurable residual radiation, both near the points of detonation and downwind from the explosions in Hiroshima and Nagasaki. With respect to induced radiation, more significant than gamma rays, Pace and Smith reported, was the induced radioactivity at the epicenters caused by neutron penetration. Pace and Smith even observed that isotope production by neutrons was "several orders of magnitude" greater than isotope production by gamma rays.[57] Recall that all that was reported on in Stafford Warren's preliminary report supplied to Groves for his Senate testimony was the impact of gamma rays.

The navy doctors also found downwind radiological fallout from both bombs, most significantly from the plutonium bomb, where an easterly-northeasterly wind blew fallout over Nishiyama, a small village about two miles east of Nagasaki. This finding was in keeping with the observations of Nagasaki Medical School doctor Raisuke Shirabe, as discussed with Barnett and measured by Collins, considered in Chapter 5. According to Pace and Smith, Nishiyama villagers received radioactive fallout that approached "the magnitude of the maximal tolerance dose." The navy medical officers estimated the roentgen dosage absorbed by villagers to be about fifty-six roentgens, a level of radiation "capable of producing measurable physiological change."[58]

Japanese scientists, studying the same region, similarly found measurable fallout in Nishiyama. A team of researchers from Kyushu Imperial University discovered, in 1947, an increase in the number of leukocytes in over half of the villagers and cases of hyperchromic anemia (reduction in red blood cells) in about a third. As late as 1975, researchers reported higher concentrations of the radioisotope cesium 137 among Nishiyama residents than in the nonaffected population.[59] This is the same radioactive isotope, as we will see in Chapter 7, that would eventually prevent Bikini Islanders from returning to their atoll after postwar testing of nuclear weapons in the Marshall Islands.

Regarding residual radiation at the hypocenters in Hiroshima and Nagasaki, a number of accounts suggest that both Japanese rescuers and American servicemen who entered one or both cities in the early weeks and months after the explosions were found to have a range of radiation sickness symptoms, including diarrhea, nausea, high fevers, and hair loss. Even more severe illnesses—including various cancers, infertility, cataracts, and liver disorder—have been attributed to secondary radiation exposure.[60] Some of these more serious cases resulted in death.

Kiyoshi Tanimoto, for example, one of John Hersey's interlocutors, directly observed a number of instances in Hiroshima in which "people, who had not been in the city at the time of the explosion but had entered later, had died." As recorded in the September 10, 1945, entry of his diary, "Mrs. K. Okinishi, from Furuichi ten kilometers away, had come to pick up the bones of her daughter who had died in her home located near the Buddhist temples in Tera-machi, a kilometer from the explosion." As a consequence, Tanimoto wrote, she "died a few days later." In another instance, a man named I. Nishimoto visited Hiroshima after the bombing in search of his daughter's home in Mikawa-machi, which was also about "one kilometer from the explosion." Nishimoto's daughter was only recently married and was running a fish shop in Mikawa-machi. After visiting the ruins of his deceased daughter's home, he likewise "died a few days later." Another woman, "Mrs. Oguro's mother," had been living in Otake, about twenty miles away, at the time of the explosion. After visiting Hiroshima several times in search of "Jun's bones," she eventually contracted "the atomic disease," which included "a high fever" and "finally died." According to Tanimoto, "There had been many cases like that."[61]

Accounts from US military personnel who were part of the occupying forces in Japan after the war also suggest serious effects from residual radiation. Bill Griffin, for example, a marine who entered Nagasaki on November 1, reported that he lost teeth, his hair fell out, and his skin flaked off as a result of radiation exposure in Nagasaki.[62] Another marine stationed in Nagasaki, Sam Scione, was never told "anything about radiation or the effects it might have," though he and other US occupation troops went to ground zero many times. After a year in Japan and upon his return to the United States, Scione's "hair began to fall out and he was covered with sores." He suffered a number of radiation-related ailments for years.[63]

Another marine, David C. Milam, who was stationed in Nagasaki during the occupation period, likewise noted the effects of radiation on himself and his fellow servicemen. Among the first signs of radiation he witnessed while in Nagasaki was hair loss among some of the men. "It came out in clumps," Milam remembers. Next came the loosening of teeth, severe headaches, and even leukemia. One of his friends began to experience fatigue and then, after finally reporting to the sick bay, died a few weeks later. Others experienced what Milam referred to as "cancer of the blood," and Milam himself discovered years after the war that the residual radiation in Nagasaki had made him sterile.[64] Some recent studies indicate "significant exposure" for those who entered the bombed-out cities within a week of the explosions.[65] These findings are in keeping with what the radiologist Takashi Nagai and other Japanese doctors observed of residual radiation in Hiroshima and Nagasaki during their efforts to treat patients in the first weeks after the bombs.

Such outcomes should not have been surprising to Groves, given Warren's warnings about the potentially significant hazards troops might face when entering an area following a nuclear explosion.[66] However, Groves treated these data in the same way he treated Warren's preliminary report for his Senate testimony. That is, he fully misrepresented and distorted the information when communicating it to others. Just a few days after receiving Warren's warnings in late July 1945, Groves sent a memo to

George C. Marshall, army chief of staff, stating, "No damaging effects are anticipated on the ground from radioactive materials. . . . We think we could move troops through the area immediately preferably by motor but on foot if desired."[67] Historian Sean Malloy finds Groves's willingness to disregard warnings that directly affected the safety of American troops as "one of the most shocking aspects of the entire story" and evidence that Groves may have internalized his own compartmentalization policy, resulting in a delusional sort of "self-compartmentalization."[68]

The dynamics of the complicated relationship between Groves and Warren, represented in these communications, continued even after the war. In April 1957, for example, when Warren was dean of the University of California, Los Angeles, Medical School, the *New York Daily News* printed an article debunking stories about radiation-induced two-headed salmon, likely in reference to the contamination of waters around the Hanford plant in Washington. The article dismissed the genetic effects of radiation, as such, as communist propaganda aimed at discouraging the continuation of nuclear testing in the Marshall Islands. The article cited the "respected Dr. Stafford Warren" as an authority to discount these stories. Warren was quoted in the article as having stated that "there is no conclusive evidence . . . that radiation has any effect on reproductive processes or results." He was even reported to have said, "Nobody in any test area has suffered any damage from radioactive fall-out during the tests."[69]

When Groves read the article, he was delighted. Evidently still trying to manage the radiation narrative twelve years after the end of the war, he wrote Warren asking him to send any papers related to his refutation of the genetic effects of radiation exposure on salmon. In this letter, he also wrote disparagingly of those who continued to make claims about radiation injuries. "I am sure that you will agree that, like many others, I have had experience with a few, more or less queer people, all of them born before July 15, 1945 [the day before the Trinity test]. Their queerness cannot logically be blamed on radiation from atomic bombs."[70]

In an effort to diplomatically respond to Groves but also to set the record straight, Warren sent Groves a cover letter and accompanying paper. "We, too, have our share of odd-ball people," Warren offered in the cover letter, "some probably born that way; others who assume the role to attract attention." However, in the attached paper, though Warren defended the ongoing testing of nuclear weapons in the Pacific, he also acknowledged that "there is no doubt . . . that radiation can cause genetic mutations," most of which "are harmful in some degree." It's clear from the paper that he saw statements attributed to him in the *Daily News* article as having been taken out of context and misrepresenting his views as well as the scientific data on the topic. This exchange between Groves and Warren is indicative of previous efforts on Groves's part to appropriate Warren's expertise and on Warren's part to maintain a modicum of intellectual integrity while also trying to appease his boss.[71] In this instance, given the substance of his paper, it's hard to see how Warren's response would aid Groves's efforts, though one could plausibly say the same of previous memos sent from the colonel to the general.

While the United States still maintains the position that the residual radiation near the epicenters of Hiroshima and Nagasaki was negligible and thus not harmful, to officials in Japan the evidence of injuries from secondary radiation has been convincing enough that the Japanese government eventually increased health care coverage for those who entered within 1.25 miles of ground zero in either city within two weeks of the bombings.[72]

While the effects of residual radiation are still debated and difficult to document scientifically, the long-term effects of initial radiation are indisputable. Summary reports by the Radiation Effects Research Foundation, for example, show that survivors who were within 1.5 miles of the hypocenter at the time of the explosions were twice as likely as the unexposed population to die from leukemia, and those within 0.75 miles were six times as likely.[73] The younger the individuals, moreover, the greater the likelihood that they would one day contract leukemia. Children under ten, for example, who were within a mile of the hypocenter were diagnosed with leukemia at a rate eighteen times that of the general population. In addition to leukemia, studies show higher rates of stomach, lung, colon, and breast cancer among survivors. Interestingly, while deaths from leukemia among survivors peaked in the first five to ten years after the bombs, it took approximately twenty years for the long-term effects of other types of cancer to peak.

Long-term studies also show higher rates among survivors of such noncancer diseases and abnormalities as heart disease, stroke, kidney disease, benign thyroid tumors, liver disease, and cataracts.[74] Radiation-induced cataracts, for example, did not appear until between three months and ten years after exposure.[75] Studies also reveal that those exposed in utero were "adversely affected by radiation exposure." For example, exposure within eight to fifteen weeks of conception "led to severe intellectual impairment, decreased academic performance and intelligence quotient (IQ) scores, and increased epileptic seizures."[76] In utero exposure also resulted in children born with microcephaly, or markedly reduced head size, which was relatively frequent among those exposed within sixteen weeks of conception.[77] In her recent book on Nagasaki, in which she follows the lives of several *hibakusha,* Susan Southard also demonstrates the considerable social consequences and psychological strains endured by survivors. Because of their disfigured bodies and fears that radiation injuries could be passed on to children, *hibakusha* sometimes were shunned, were embarrassed to be seen in public, and experienced difficulties finding marriage partners.[78]

Thus, regardless of how careful and accurate the Manhattan Project doctors had been in their five weeks of observing the damages in Hiroshima and Nagasaki, a spot check, as such, could never have been adequate. The full consequences of this destructive new technology could only be understood on a longer-term basis, a reality that was not always lost on the doctors, who more than once recommended the sort of long-term studies that would be performed in research conducted by the ABCC and the Radiation Effects Research Foundation.

Plutonium Injections

Efforts by the doctors to understand the long-term consequences of radiation exposure took a rather dark turn following one of the earliest accidents in Los Alamos. This accident occurred on August 1, 1944, in Building D of the main Los Alamos lab, almost a year before the first critical assembly accident in the Pajarito Canyon. At the time, only very miniscule amounts of plutonium had been delivered to Site Y. So valuable were the microscopic plutonium samples that a special group was assigned for the sole purpose of recovering any plutonium that had been somehow misplaced, whether absorbed into rags or dropped on the floor, even to the point that "they were prepared to tear up the floor and extract the plutonium, if necessary." According to Hempelmann, the "Recovery Group" would even "dissolve a bicycle. . . . They went to great extremes to recover everything."[79]

On the morning of August 1, Don Mastick, a twenty-three-year-old chemist from Berkeley who had been recruited by Oppenheimer to join the secret project on the mesa, was working in Building D with a small glass vial containing ten milligrams of plutonium. When the neck of the vial accidentally snapped off, the liquid spilled out, some of which ricocheted off the wall in front of Mastick and splattered back into his mouth. Mastick carefully returned the broken vial to its wooden holder and then made his way to Hempelmann's office to report the accident. After numerous mouth rinsings, using concoctions recommended by Stafford Warren, Hempelmann then pumped Mastick's stomach. Demonstrating just how valuable were these small samples of plutonium at the time, after pumping Mastick's stomach, Hempelmann handed to the young chemist the four-liter container of his vomit and instructed him to chemically extract the plutonium from it.[80]

The accident, as well as the toxic effects of plutonium in the lab more generally, caused considerable anxiety among the workers. Two weeks after the accident, Hempelmann sent a memo to Oppenheimer describing these worries and urging him to initiate research that would deepen understandings of the effects of radioactive materials on the human body.[81] Hempelmann and the Health Group doctors simply didn't know how Mastick's body would handle the plutonium to which it had been inadvertently exposed. How much of the plutonium, for example, would be excreted from his body, and how quickly? How much would remain in his system, and what harm, if any, might it cause? Scientists had conducted some tests on rats in the Berkeley lab in an effort to answer these questions, but the extrapolation of their findings to humans remained uncertain.

In response to Hempelmann's memo, Oppenheimer authorized "the development of methods of detection of plutonium in the excreta," recognizing that these methods might involve "even human experimentation."[82] Two weeks later, Hempelmann confirmed plans to pursue, among other tests, "tracer experiments on humans to determine the percentage of plutonium excreted daily."[83] Oppenheimer fully supported and signed off on the program, though, for reasons that are not entirely clear, he wanted the tests conducted at sites other than Los Alamos. Then, in March 1945, representatives from the Chemistry Division and the Health Group met with, among others, Hymer Friedell and Stafford Warren to discuss implementation of this new program, after which Hempelmann issued a memo suggesting that "a hospital patient at either Rochester or Chicago be chosen for injection of from one to ten micrograms of material and that the excreta be sent to this [Los Alamos] laboratory."[84]

A few days later, a candidate was discovered who was viewed as suitable for the first plutonium injection, though he was in Oak Ridge, rather than Rochester or Chicago. The first "patient" selected for this test was a fifty-three-year-old "colored male" named Ebb Cade. Cade, a cement worker at the Oak Ridge Site, had been involved in an automobile accident while on his way to work in the early morning of March 24, 1945. The accident resulted in multiple injuries, including a broken leg and arm, the former of which required surgery. Cade, who was in otherwise generally good health, was assigned the code name HP-12 (Human Product 12) and was injected on April 10 with 4.7 micrograms of plutonium, nearly five times what was accepted at the time to be the maximum body burden for ingested plutonium. It was not enough plutonium to cause acute symptoms, though it was understood, even at the time, to be sufficient to eventually cause cancer.

Joe Howland—who would be heading to Nagasaki as part of the Joint Commission in about four months—was instructed to make the injection. At first he refused, demonstrating his unease with the experiments. According to Howland, he only acquiesced after his boss, Friedell, issued a written military order insisting that he make the injection. Howland recalled that Cade neither consented to the procedure nor was told what substance was being injected into his body. The operation to reset his leg did not take place until April 15, five days after the injection and nearly three weeks after the accident. Delaying the surgery until after the injections enabled the doctors to measure levels of plutonium deposited in the bones. During the procedure, the doctors biopsied two bone specimens from Cade's leg. Additionally, doctors removed fifteen of Cade's teeth, which were also eventually sampled for plutonium. It is not clear whether his teeth were removed primarily for medical or scientific testing purposes, though the doctors at the Oak Ridge Hospital noted that Cade had considerable "tooth decay and gum inflammation."[85] On the day after the operation, Friedell shipped a box "containing 21 urine and stool specimens, 2 bone specimens and one blood sample" to Los Alamos "for analysis by Dr. Wright Langham."[86]

After his reset bones healed, Cade discharged himself from the hospital and eventually moved to Greensboro, North Carolina. The doctors were unable to locate him for follow-up studies. Eight years after the injection, at the age of sixty-three, Cade died of a heart attack. Eileen Welsome points out that Cade came from a family with longevity in their genes, including a sister who lived to be over one hundred.[87] Cade was the first of eighteen patients who would secretly be injected with plutonium by Manhattan Project doctors, though he was the only one injected at Oak Ridge. Three patients were injected at the University of Chicago, three at the University of California, and eleven at the University of Rochester. At least two of the three Chicago patients were injected at the Billings Hospital, the same hospital where Allan Kline had been "treated" before he stopped cooperating with Manhattan Project and AEC doctors.

One of the California patients was a four-year-old Australian boy with a rare disease, who had been flown from Australia to the University of California hospital for special treatment. The ideal was to inject patients who were terminally ill, so that the potential long-term consequences of the injections would never be realized. However, not all patients were terminally ill, as was the case with Cade, and some who were thought to be seriously ill had been misdiagnosed. A forty-nine-year-old woman in Rochester, for example, had been misdiagnosed with a terminal illness. Doctors admitted, after the injection, that this woman "may have a greater life expectancy than originally anticipated due to an error in the provisional diagnosis."[88] In addition to the plutonium injections, six patients were injected with uranium and five with polonium. The latter types all took place at Rochester. In the case of the uranium injections, it was even understood that there could be possible acute effects from the injections. Of all the patients, only one apparently gave consent, though, even in this case, the doctors did not make clear to him what they were putting into his body. None of the patients were told that they were being injected with radioactive material; they were not told the reasons for the injections; and there were no anticipated therapeutic benefits. Indeed, it was understood that these injections could cause harm.

When Shields Warren assumed leadership of the Biology and Medicine Division of the newly created AEC in the fall of 1947, he soon learned of the existence of this secret program and was not pleased with what he discovered. He subsequently introduced policies that would prohibit such practices in the future, requiring that there be informed consent and that there be a therapeutic benefit for any such procedure. However, it appears that these new standards did not stop follow-up work on those previously injected (including the exhumation and reexamination of dead bodies) and that, at least in California, new experiments continued. Even in the follow-up studies, patients were not informed as to the real purposes for their "medical" examinations.

As late as 1949 and 1950, Robert Stone and General James Cooney were pushing for new total-body irradiation tests on prisoners with life sentences.

Stone, for example, proposed experiments in which healthy prisoners, on a voluntary basis, be exposed to 25, 50, and even up to 150 roentgens of full-body radiation, to better understand the effects of nuclear radiation on the human body. At the time, the military was interested in the development of nuclear-propelled aircraft; and then, starting in 1950, the military feared that nuclear weapons would be used in the Korean War. Military officials wanted to understand what this might mean for American troops entering into bombed-out areas. This time, however, some of the doctors, including Shields Warren and Joseph Hamilton, expressed strong reservations.

With the full impact of the Nuremberg trials still fresh in the public memory, Hamilton feared that such total-body irradiation tests "would have a little bit of the Buchenwald touch."[89] Hamilton had participated in the plutonium injections of the California patients and would himself die from leukemia before his fiftieth birthday, likely because of his extensive work with nuclear materials in the Rad Lab. Shields Warren's comparison to the Nazis was even more explicit. "It is not very long since we got through trying Germans for doing exactly that thing," he asserted. Warren, who had been part of the Joint Commission, also argued that, given all the data they had collected in Japan, further experiments were unnecessary. "Actually, we have got the results of an enormous experiment. We have the experiment involving over 200,000 people in the Nagasaki and Hiroshima areas, and I think that those results are real. I was there, and I saw the people when they got sick."[90] The *hibakusha* who complained of feeling like guinea pigs at the hands of Joint Commission and ABCC doctors would likely agree with Warren's characterization of the bombs and the studies that followed as an "enormous experiment."

Despite his reservations, even after learning about the plutonium injections, Shields Warren determined that data on the tests should remain classified. Once again, concerns about public relations and potential lawsuits were the motivating factors that kept the experiments secret. As the Advisory Committee on Human Radiation Experiments (ACHRE) concluded, "It appears that this decision [to keep the experiments secret] was based on concerns about legal liability and adverse public reaction, not national security."[91] It was not until the 1990s, largely because of the investigative work of the Pulitzer Prize–winning journalist Eileen Welsome, that the plutonium experiments became public. Welsome's reporting sparked a government investigation into the tests, directed by Secretary of Energy Hazel O'Leary, during the Bill Clinton administration.

On October 3, 1995, after a comprehensive and detailed investigation by the ACHRE, Clinton and O'Leary held a press conference at which they publicly released their findings. At the press conference, Clinton noted that some of the experiments conducted by doctors during the early years of the nuclear age "were unethical, not only by today's standards, but by the standards of the time in which they were conducted." In this context, he made explicit reference to the eighteen plutonium injections. He acknowledged further that these experiments were "carried out on precisely those citizens who count most on the government for its help—the destitute and gravely ill. . . . Informed consent was withheld. Americans were kept in the dark about the effects of what was being done to them. . . . These experiments were kept secret."[92]

The ACHRE's final report provides a thorough accounting of these and related human radiation experiments that were conducted between 1944 and 1974. A few years after release of the ACHRE report, Welsome published her book *The Plutonium Files,* which provides in more narrative form the disturbing development, execution, and cover-up of these tests. That the troubling findings of the ACHRE did not create a greater public stir, Welsome argues, may be due, in part, to the timing of the report's release—on October 3, 1995, the same day as the announcement of the verdict in the O. J. Simpson trial. The wall-to-wall press coverage of the "trial of the century" verdict arguably prevented a fuller public recognition of the significance of the ACHRE's findings.[93]

Obscuring the Medical Paradigm

As the unfolding of the dawn of the nuclear age makes clear, the plutonium experiments were really only the most extreme manifestation of a more general pattern that one finds at a number of critical moments in which the Manhattan Project doctors were involved—for example, the Trinity test, the Los Alamos accidents, and the postwar investigative work in Japan. With what little knowledge the doctors did have about the dangers of radiation, they offered warnings. These warnings were often ignored, dismissed, or misrepresented. When some of the outcomes of their warnings were subsequently realized, doctors were then put in a position of having to cover for the military, often out of concerns about litigation and public relations.

The military prerogatives of security, secrecy, and speed superseded the medical prerogatives of health, healing, and patient care. The cover-up and secrecy of the Los Alamos accidents and the plutonium injections suggest that overriding military concerns caused doctors to, in essence, violate one of the central tenets of the Hippocratic ideal: "First, do no harm." Indeed, in the case of the plutonium injections, though the doctors were motivated by a desire to establish proper safety measures for those working with radioactive materials, they were the ones who actually initiated and implemented the experiments, albeit with the clear support and direction of Oppenheimer, and operating within a program determined by military objectives.

In this instance, the doctors allowed a scientific paradigm of experimentation and the quest for knowledge to obscure a more purely medical paradigm, which resulted in doctors treating sick people as objects or products rather than as human patients. While the circumstances of the moment (a war mentality) and the structure of the situation (a hierarchical military bureaucracy) shaped decisions and determined certain behaviors, this is not to deny the place of human agency. For example, it appears that Nolan and Hempelmann may have had different perspectives on the acceptability of the plutonium injections and may have, as a consequence, participated differently as a result.

Nolan seems to have had little, if any, involvement in the experiments, though he was certainly aware of them, and I have found no evidence that he publicly objected to them. In fact, the first specimens sent from Oak Ridge were addressed to Nolan—who was head of the hospital at the time—though with instructions that they be given to Wright Langham for analysis. Nolan is not mentioned once in the ACHRE report, nor is he implicated in Welsome's study. In the Atomic Heritage Foundation's description of the plutonium injections, he is not listed among the eight Manhattan Project doctors who participated in the experiments. He was not present at the 1944 and 1945 meetings that launched the program. Why was he not more deeply involved, as were Warren and Hempelmann, with whom he so often collaborated at this time? One explanation may be that, when the programs were first imagined and initiated, he was still the post surgeon and overwhelmed with running the hospital in Los Alamos. In other words, he was occupied with his work as a doctor and thus simply not available.

It's possible, however, that his lack of participation was more than circumstantial. That is, unlike Hempelmann, he may have, on principle, preferred his role as a doctor and been uneasy with what could be viewed as a clear departure from the physician's vocation. His daughter, Lynne, remembers that he actually saw himself as different from Hempelmann on this score. He would jokingly refer to himself as a "practitioner" and to Hempelmann, neologistically, as a "theoreticer." That is, Hempelmann was more "the archetype of the crazy scientist . . . a pure scientist." She also recalls her father saying of his good friend that he "never treated people." Moreover, in reference to the plutonium experiments, Lynne understands that it was because of practices such as these that "Dad wanted out of that whole thing, of this whole business of the disposability of people."[94]

My father similarly recalled that his dad saw himself primarily as a doctor: "He was first and foremost a physician whose No. 1 concern was the welfare of his patients." Lawry recollected a clear sense that, given some of the tensions and pressures Nolan faced at Los Alamos, his parents wanted to leave the place: "My parents were anxious for us to return to their home town, St Louis, where my father could resume his career as a physician and medical school professor. They could not wait to leave the Hill."[95]

The use and perceived disposability of people was an issue at the heart of the ACHRE's moral critique of the experiments. As pointed out in the committee's final report, "In the conduct of these experiments, two basic moral principles were violated—that one ought not to use people as a mere means to the ends of others and that one ought not to deceive others—in the absence of any morally acceptable justification for such conduct."[96] A common image invoked for making sense of how humans were used in these experiments is that of a guinea pig. For example, this is how Joe Speed described what had happened to his friend Elmer Allen (or CAL-3), the eighteenth and final patient injected with plutonium and the third of the California patients involved in the tests. Allen was thought to have terminal bone cancer in his leg. Three days after the injection, his leg was amputated. Speed recalls Allen's understanding of what had happened to him: "He told me they put a germ cancer in his leg. They guinea-pigged him. They didn't care about him getting well. He told me he would never get well."[97]

Many Japanese have used similar imagery to describe their experience in postwar Japan. In coverage of the Joint Commission's work in Hiroshima in early September 1945, for example, a Japanese newspaper article began, "At last, natural science entered the new century called the atomic era. Unfortunately, our country was cruelly made the guinea pig of a bomb that was used without consideration of whether it was reasonable to do so."[98]

Critics of the ABCC in Japan have likewise referred to *hibakusha* as guinea pigs, especially in light of its no-treatment policy. Recall also that Allan Kline used the same terminology in objecting to the treatment he was offered by Manhattan Project and AEC doctors following the May 21, 1946, accident at the Omega Site. Likewise, Tina Cordova has invoked this image to describe the plight of the Trinity downwinders.[99]

As we turn to the next chapter of the dawn of the nuclear age, in which the Manhattan Project doctors again played a central role, we find that actual guinea pigs—sixty of them, to be precise, as well as two hundred mice—were used to study the biological effects of the fourth and fifth atomic bombs detonated in human history. At one point during their debate about total-body irradiation tests and animal experimentation, General Cooney noted that one of his generals, who was evidently worried about the potential effects of nuclear radiation on his troops, had asked him, "What are we—mice or men?" As we venture again to the Pacific, we will be given another opportunity to reflect on this prescient question, as both mice and men (and guinea pigs) would be exposed to high levels of nuclear radiation and doctors would once again be put in the difficult position of trying to understand and manage this exposure.

The ACHRE recognized the tensions that the Manhattan Project doctors faced in their conflicting roles "that linked the arts of healing and war in ways that had little precedent," where doctors "at one and the same time . . . counseled the military about the radiation risk to troops . . . and debated the need for rules to govern atomic warfare-related experimentation."[100] In such a context, with competing vocational interests and pressures, did the doctors still bear moral responsibility for their actions? At least with respect to the plutonium experiments, the ACHRE concluded without much qualification that "the medical professionals responsible for the injections are accountable for the moral wrongs that were done."[101]

7

Bikini and Enewetak

> The Bikinese . . . are not the first, nor will they be the last, to be left homeless and impoverished by the inexorable Bomb. They have no choice in the matter, and very little understanding of it. But in this perhaps they are not so different from us all.
>
> —David Bradley, *No Place to Hide*

> The Enewetak people became further casualties of the Atomic Age and Cold War; helpless victims of circumstances beyond their control, and of forces beyond their understanding.
>
> —Jack Adair Tobin, "The Resettlement of the Enewetak People"

On February 10, 1946, the Bikini Islanders had just completed their Sunday-morning church service when a seaplane arrived from Kwajalein Atoll carrying US commodore Ben H. Wyatt. At the time, Wyatt was serving as the military governor of the Marshall Islands, a region that had come under American control after Japan's defeat in World War II. Having determined that it would continue testing nuclear weapons, the US military selected the Bikini Atoll—one of twenty-nine atolls and five islands that compose the Marshall Islands—as the ideal location. Wyatt was given the unenviable task of "asking" the Bikinians to evacuate their homeland for this purpose.

Using language that resonated with the Bikinians' Christian faith, Wyatt, by his own account, told the islanders that they were like "the children of Israel whom the Lord saved from their enemy and led into the Promised Land." The Americans, Wyatt explained further, wanted to test nuclear weapons "for the good of mankind and to end all world wars."[1] The Bikinians considered this request and, after some deliberation, agreed to move off their island. Their chief, whom the American press referred to as King Juda, reportedly said to Wyatt, "If the United States government and scientists of the world want to use our island and atoll for furthering development, which with God's blessing will result in kindness and benefit to all mankind, my people will be pleased to go elsewhere."[2] It's questionable whether this statement represents a full and accurate rendering of the Bikinians' sentiments at the time. However, it is clear that the Bikinians were left with the understanding that the Americans would take care of them during their exile and that their relocation would only be temporary.

On March 7, less than a month after their meeting with Wyatt, the last of the 167 Bikinians then living on the island boarded a navy LST for transport to Rongerik Atoll, another circle of islands some 125 miles southeast of Bikini. With sadness and uncertainly about the future, they left behind the idyllic and largely self-sufficient life they enjoyed on their beloved atoll. It was a life characterized by a harmonious, intelligent, and cooperative coexistence with their surrounding natural environment. Through use of large handcrafted outriggers, as well as smaller individual canoes, Bikinians were skilled sailors and fishermen, and the Bikini lagoon offered an ample stock of fish to feed their community. The atoll also contained a plentiful

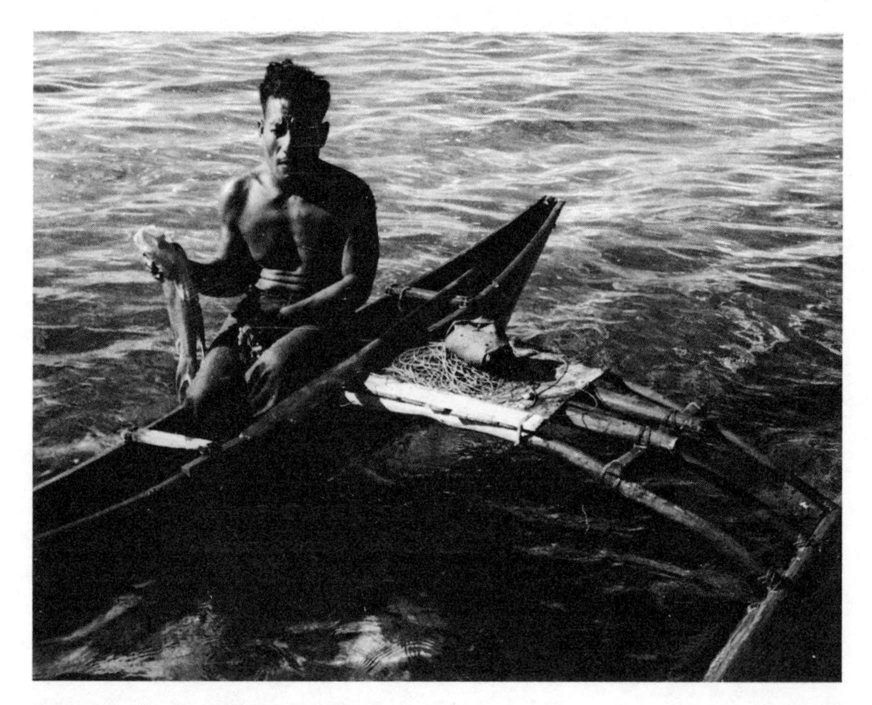

Bikini Islander fishing in small individual canoe.

supply of coconut, pandanus, and breadfruit trees; Bikinians raised pigs, ducks, and chickens as additional food sources.[3]

Operation Crossroads

Such a life would be significantly and irreparably disrupted with the American initiation of Operation Crossroads, a military effort to test nuclear weapons in the Marshall Islands in 1946. What was the purpose of Operation Crossroads? The war was over. The US military had obliterated two Japanese cities and fully demonstrated the destructive force of the atom bomb. Why was it necessary to test more nuclear weapons? The answer to this question is complicated. To begin with, not all supported Operation Crossroads. Robert Oppenheimer, for one, saw the tests as completely unnecessary. In a frank letter to President Harry S. Truman dated May 3, 1946, he carefully articulated his opposition and argued that his misgivings were shared widely within the scientific community. He questioned the wisdom of engaging in these tests while the United States and other countries were beginning efforts to establish international controls over the development of nuclear weapons. He argued further that the estimated costs (approximately $100 million) made the tests indefensible, and that the desired results could be attained more cheaply and accurately through laboratory experiments.

Finally, he questioned the usefulness of testing the effects of an atom bomb on naval vessels. "If an atomic bomb comes close enough to a ship," he stated, "it will sink it." Elaborating on this point, Oppenheimer added, "I do not think that naval applications are the important ones to test, nor that the test as it will be carried out will in fact be a good measure of naval applications, nor that the measurements which are to be made are the right measurements to make."[4] Truman forwarded the letter to Dean Acheson, acting secretary of state, along with a note dismissing Oppenheimer as that "cry baby scientist" who, six months earlier, had visited his office "ringing his hands and telling me they had blood on them because of the discovery of atomic energy."[5]

Oppenheimer's discussion of "naval applications" points to an important justification that was driving the operation—that is, an interagency contest between the army and the navy. The navy was concerned that the discovery and use of atomic weaponry would make naval ships obsolete. During congressional hearings in December 1945, for example, Senator

Edwin Johnson said to navy admiral William H. P. Blandy, "It does seem to me that atomic energy has driven ships off the surface of the sea. I don't see how a ship can resist the atomic bomb."[6] At the time, the air force was not a separate branch of the military but rather a part of the army. Both the army and the navy were threatened by and thus vying for control of air operations. Moreover, the navy wanted to demonstrate that, far from being outdated, its vessels—including, importantly, aircraft carriers—could withstand a nuclear attack.

Lewis L. Strauss, Oppenheimer's nemesis and future head of the Atomic Energy Committee (AEC), had earlier written to James Forrestal, secretary of the navy, arguing for the necessity of the tests to dispel the sort of views articulated by Johnson. "If such tests are not made," he wrote, "there will be loose talk to the effect that the fleet is obsolete in the face of this new weapon," thus jeopardizing future appropriations to the navy.[7] This rationale was precisely what others in the scientific community saw as the real motive for the tests. Albert S. Cahn, a physicist at the University of Chicago, for example, argued at the time, "This isn't a test of atomic power. This is a demonstration for power by the Navy. They are staging it for Congress so that the Navy will look pretty good and they can get bigger appropriations and a bigger Navy."[8] Though he hesitated, and even delayed the start of Operation Crossroads, Truman eventually approved the tests, as did Congress. It would ultimately be commissioned as a joint military effort (Joint Task Force One), under the leadership of the navy's Admiral Blandy. The joint nature of the task force did little to hide or mitigate interagency tensions.

The plan was to use ships captured from Germany and Japan, as well as older American navy vessels, to test the effects of nuclear attacks. In total, ninety-four target ships were used, including five battleships, two aircraft carriers, eight submarines, and twelve destroyers (one of which was the *Ralph Talbot,* a destroyer that participated in the rescue of the 316 survivors of the ill-fated USS *Indianapolis*). The original plan was to subject the ships, distributed at various points throughout the 243-square-mile lagoon, to three nuclear tests: an aerial drop, a bomb detonated ninety feet below water in the lagoon, and a deep-water explosion. The weapons, similar in design to the Nagasaki plutonium bomb, were given the military code names Able, Baker, and Charlie. In addition to the ships, Joint Task Force One would measure the effects of the bomb and nuclear radiation on a variety of animals—including five thousand rats, 204 goats, two hundred pigs, two hundred mice, and sixty guinea pigs—distributed on the vessels scattered across the Bikini lagoon.[9]

Radsafe

Among the groups making up Joint Task Force One was the radiation safety (or radsafe) section, led by Stafford Warren. Warren faced a daunting task in recruiting the necessary number of radiation monitors, as Operation Crossroads would ultimately involve forty-two thousand military and civilian personnel, as well as press, members of Congress, and invited dignitaries from around the world, including representatives from the Soviet Union. Less than a year after the end of World War II, qualified military and civilian personnel were not inclined to travel away from home again. As Warren recalled, "This was the time when the families of the men had decided to have their first vacation after the war."[10] His recruiting efforts were made more difficult when Truman decided, for a variety of reasons, to delay the operation by six weeks.

Nolan was one of the first men Warren recruited for the mission, though, having left the military, Nolan would participate in a civilian capacity. Fearful that the delay might affect Nolan's earlier commitment to the project, Warren sent him a rather urgent letter on April 19, 1946. "As you no doubt have read in the newspapers," he wrote, "postponement of operations CROSSROADS was ordered by the President some weeks ago. Accordingly, schedules are having to be changed." After discussing the new timeline, he pleaded with Nolan, "Your participation as a monitor is urgently needed. It is hoped you can rearrange your plans to meet some part of the above schedule; particularly, that concerning the first test. Can I count on you for one or both tests?"[11]

Nolan agreed to participate and served with the radsafe section of Operation Crossroads for the first two tests, though he would depart just a few days after the Baker test. On May 25, only four days after the Slotin accident, Nolan received his instructions to travel from Santa Fe to San Francisco and report to the commanding officer of the USS *Haven* by May 29. He departed from Los Alamos two days later, arriving in San Francisco on May 27. He then checked into the Durant Hotel in Berkeley, California, where Warren and his family had been staying since early May. The next day Nolan boarded the *Haven,* a hospital ship that had been specially retrofitted to serve the operation's medical, testing, and safety purposes.

It had been less than a year since Nolan boarded another naval ship in the same harbor, a vessel that would, less than three weeks later, end up on the bottom of the Philippine Sea. This time Nolan was among some 130 other safety monitors aboard the *Haven* destined for the Bikini Atoll. Because of his responsibilities with the Slotin accident, Louis Hempelmann remained at Los Alamos. He and additional radsafe monitors would travel by plane to the Marshall Islands later. By the time of the Able test, there were more than 300 radsafe personnel at Bikini.

During the two-week journey across the Pacific on the *Haven,* radsafe monitors were lectured on a wide range of radiation-related topics, including on what Warren, Nolan, and others had seen firsthand in Hiroshima and Nagasaki, radiation sickness, the differences between varying types of radiation (that is, alpha particles, beta particles, gamma rays, and neutrons), ionization and quantum concepts, the fission process, and the uses of Geiger counters and other monitoring devices.[12] As Warren recalled, "We had classes about twelve hours a day and the boys worked like mad to get themselves indoctrinated."[13] On the *Haven,* Warren faced what he and others on the radsafe team had encountered before and would continue to experience once they got to the Marshall Islands—namely, skepticism and lack of cooperation from the military officers, some of whom scoffed at Warren's warnings about the bomb's power and the dangers of radiation exposure. Warren described the attitude of two officers in particular: "The two of them were, of course, professionals, and I was just a country doctor. They wouldn't believe me."[14]

After a brief stopover in Hawaii, the *Haven* reached Bikini Island on June 12. For the remainder of the month the military prepared for the nuclear tests. The Able test took place on July 1 and the Baker test on July 25. As the test dates approached, there was considerable anticipation both among those participating in the tests in the Pacific and among those waiting for news of the blasts back in the United States. In a radio broadcast on the day of the Able test, a news correspondent aboard the USS *Mount McKinley* observed that Admiral Blandy was pacing his ship "like an expectant father." Upon hearing this description, a woman listening to the broadcast on Long Island objected. "Expectant father," she muttered. "Of all the lousy metaphors. . . . This is a death watch, not a maternity ward."[15]

As we have seen, this was not the first time the detonation of an atom bomb had been likened to the delivery of a newborn. In spite of the hype and expectation, the Able bomb was, at least initially, seen as less spectacular and destructive than anticipated. However, the blast did sink five ships, including two destroyers, and immobilize six others. Moreover, fires broke out on another twenty-three target ships.[16] The Baker explosion, ignited ninety feet below water, however, resulted in what Jonathan Weisgall refers to as our "first nuclear accident."[17] The blast lifted two million tons of water more than one mile into the air. The mushroom cloud of radioactive material extended nearly three miles wide and then rained down on the entire fleet of target ships. The explosion sank nine ships and seriously damaged dozens of others.[18]

In spite of warnings from the radsafe team, military officers were eager to see the effects of the bombs on their ships. Before the tests, Warren had explicitly warned the military that the radiation hazards from the Baker test

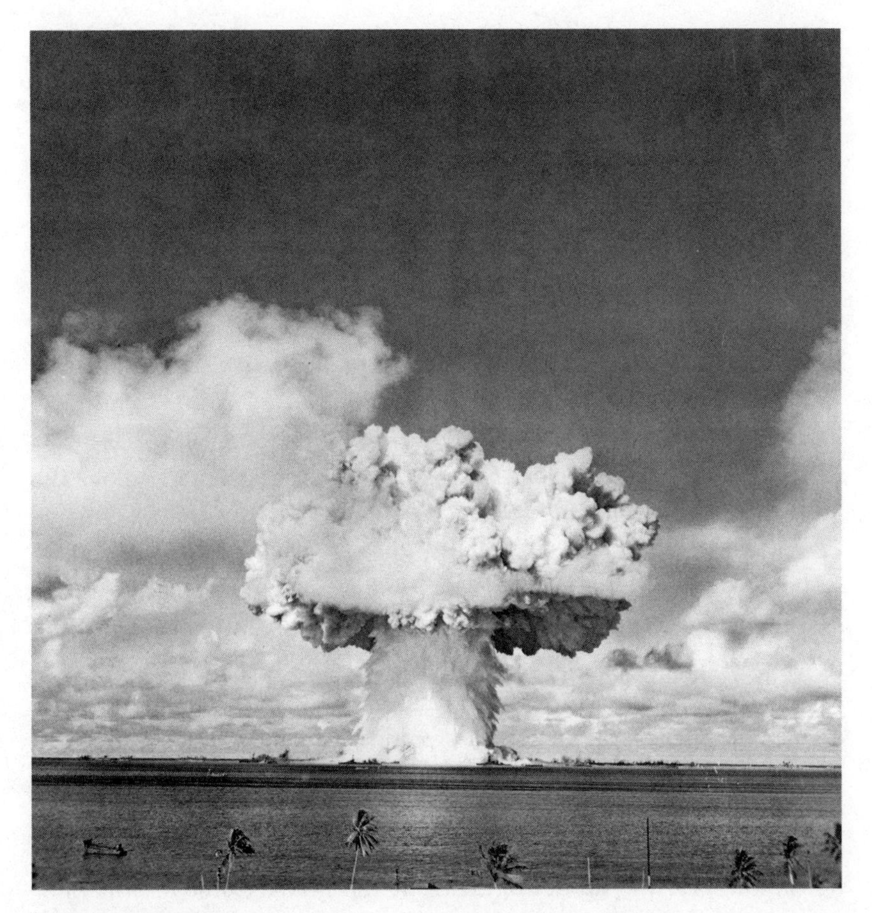

The July 25, 1946, Baker test.

would be very serious and that the spread of radioactive materials would be much greater than during the Able test, "possibly as much as 100 times as great."[19] The military was warned further that if the "column" over the lagoon following the blast rose to less than ten thousand feet, as in fact happened, "the water contained in the plume, and in the spray arising from it, and in the spray and splashes it produces as it falls back into the lagoon, will be heavily contaminated with radioactive fission products." As a result, Warren advised, the contaminated target ships would "remain dangerous for an indeterminable time thereafter."[20] These cautionary words were ignored.[21] After both tests, military personnel were keen to investigate their ships, and the overworked radsafe monitors had difficulty holding them back.

The *Skate*

Among the first vessels examined after the July 1 Able bomb was the naval submarine the *Skate.* Given the navy's preoccupation with proving its own relevance, Blandy and others were eager to demonstrate that navy ships could withstand a nuclear explosion. At the time, Blandy boasted that "modern submarines were capable of withstanding terrific pressures because the hulls necessarily are thicker than those of any surface craft." Such an attitude provides context for what happened to Nolan when he was directed to test radiation levels following the Able test. Nolan traveled with Blandy and Forrestal on the navy's flagship, the USS *Mount McKinley,* which entered the lagoon on July 2. Nolan was sent out on a small picket boat, equipped with monitoring devices, to assess levels of radiation. Among the first boats he tested was the *Skate.*

As reported in the *New York Times* on July 3, "James Nolan of St. Louis, radiologist at Los Alamos, N.M., atomic bomb laboratory, carried a Geiger counter that registered radioactivity on its dial and by earphones. After the picket boat had circled the Skate and was lying alongside, he reported radiation so intense that the counter was 'off the scale,' meaning there was more radioactivity than the sensitive instrument could register."[22] Blandy's response was indicative of the general attitude of the navy. Determined to demonstrate the invincibility of its fleet, Blandy was disposed to underemphasize the nature and extent of the damage. Thus, the high level of radiation found near the surface of the *Skate* was not welcome information. Blandy tried to downplay Nolan's findings. Turning to Forrestal, he ex-

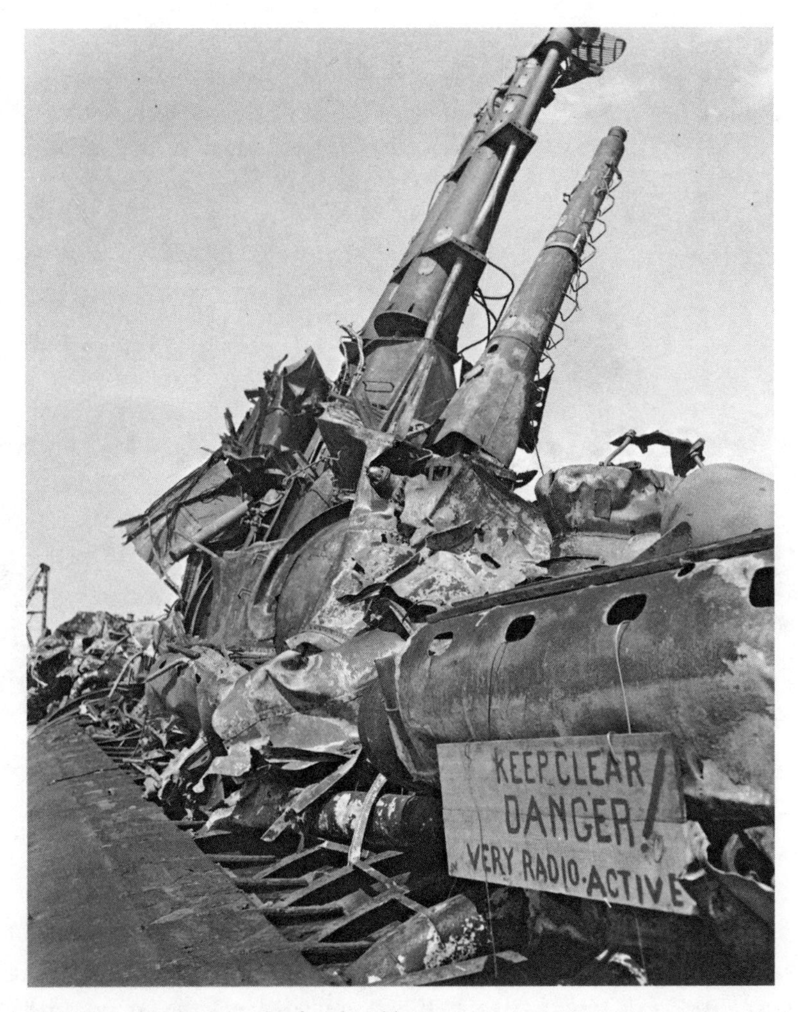

The *Skate* submarine shortly after the Able test.

plained with a laugh that "Nolan's counter was so delicate that 'my luminous watch dial will make it go off the scale.'"[23]

In spite of the warnings from the monitors (and the placement of a sign on the submarine's deck that read KEEP CLEAR, DANGER! VERY RADIOACTIVE), the *Skate*'s entire crew boarded the battered vessel only three days after the Able test and proudly saluted Blandy when his flagship passed by. Robert Henderson, a member of the Los Alamos assembly team, recalled, "That submarine was hotter than hell . . . but here is the Navy, all gung-ho lining up sailors and showing that it was invincible."[24]

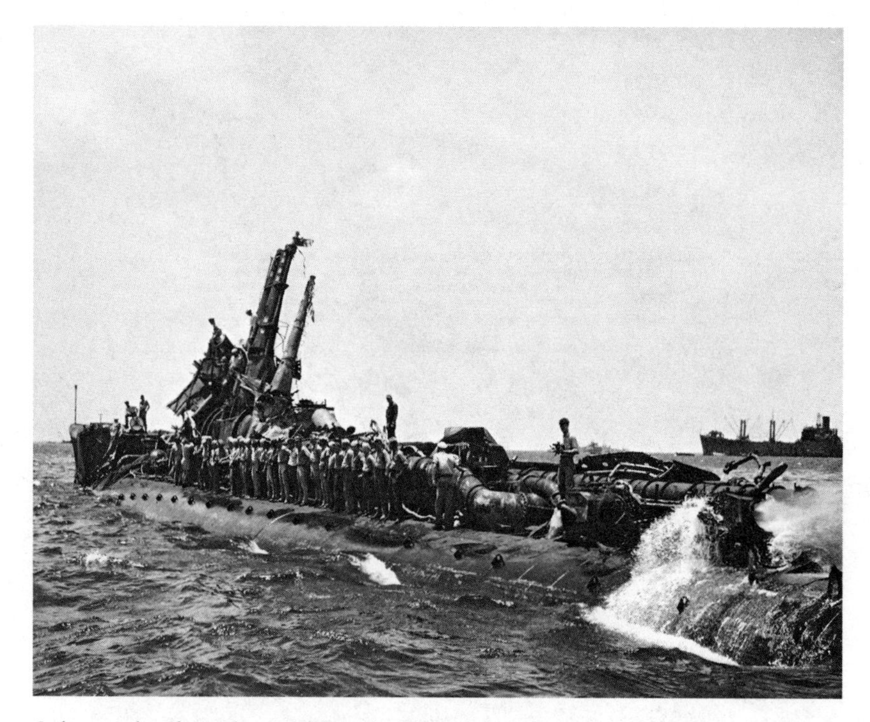

Sailors on the *Skate* submarine three days after the Able test.

USS *New York*

The story of the USS *New York* is also emblematic of the larger drama surrounding Operation Crossroads. On the day before the Able blast, the captain of the *New York,* Lowe H. Bibby, pulled down the American flag hanging off the stern of his ship and bid farewell to his now empty vessel. Bespeaking the triumphalist (and defensive) attitude of the navy, Bibby then scrawled on a gun turret with chalk, "Old Sailors Never Die." On the day after the Able test, Nolan was among the first to board the USS *New York* in order to assess levels of radiation. Though the ship had suffered visible damage, it was deemed radiologically safe.

Forrestal, Blandy, and other military officers then boarded the *New York* and even posed for a picture under Bibby's inscribed message concerning the immortality of aged sailors. Blandy seized the opportunity to hold forth again about the navy's strength. He even pointed out that "while Army material exposed on her decks was damaged, 'the heavy [that is, navy] parts of the ship itself were undamaged.'" He reminded Forrestal that "the Navy had promised Governor Dewey that his State would receive the old *New York* as a shrine if she survived the tests," and anticipated that "the *New York* could sail back under her own power," though he acknowledged the vessel had yet to face the Baker test.[25]

The *New York,* as was the case with nearly all of the remaining target ships anchored in the Bikini lagoon, would not fare so well from the Baker explosion. In fact, both the *New York* and the *Skate* would ultimately be deemed unsalvageable and were sunk in the deep waters of the Pacific. In the aftermath of the Baker bomb, the *New York* was the first of the irradiated ships that the navy would fruitlessly attempt to decontaminate. Sailors first tried hosing the ship off with salt water. Then they tried scrubbing the surface of the ship with soap, detergent, lye, cornstarch, charcoal, alkali, even coffee grounds. Nothing worked. The ship, or at least parts it, remained dangerously contaminated.

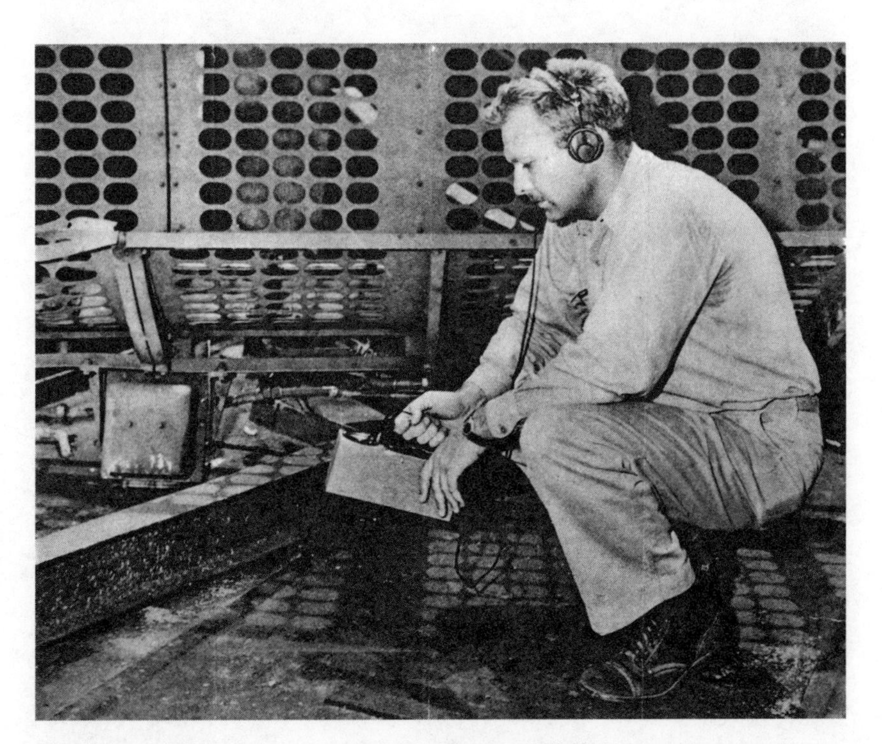

Nolan aboard the battleship USS *New York,* July 2, 1946, before an inspection party boarded the ship.

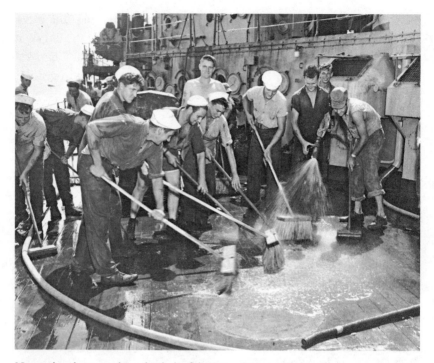

Navy enlisted men washing the deck of the *Prinz Eugen* in a futile effort to remove radiation.

More than two weeks after the Baker test, Nolan's fellow radsafe monitor David Bradley examined the ship again. Running a Geiger counter over various parts of the vessel, Bradley discovered wide variation in levels of radiation. He found fission products to be particularly potent in porous wood, rust, tar, rope, and caulk. Captain Bibby and his crew refused to believe that radiation was still a problem. According to Bradley, the captain was "completely bewildered." The deck looked clean enough to eat off, so "what was all this goddam radioactivity?"[26]

Regardless of pushback from the military, the radsafe team became increasingly worried about radioactivity, which was being detected on the nontarget ships as well, including the *Haven*. Radiation monitors tried to limit access to ships in the lagoon. But because Operation Crossroads personnel could not smell, feel, or taste the radiation, military officers resisted the warnings of the radsafe team. Another member of the safety team, George M. Lyon, for example, complained of one officer "who insists on a 'hairy-chested' approach to the matter with a disdain for the unseen hazard, an attitude which is contagious to the younger officers and detrimental to the radiological safety program."[27]

Solberg versus Radsafe

Because of his responsibilities handling the fallout from the Slotin accident back in Los Alamos, Hempelmann arrived late to Bikini. When he finally reached the atoll, he was assigned to Rear Admiral Thorvald A. Solberg's tugboat. Solberg was in charge of the salvage and repair of damaged vessels. Hempelmann's time with Solberg was characterized by notable friction. After the Able test, for example, Solberg was desperate to move quickly in toward the target ships. However, a system had been set up whereby Joint Task Force boats were not meant to approach the target ships until given specific instructions from Stafford Warren. After repeatedly sending requests to Warren and not receiving any word back, Solberg "couldn't stand it anymore" and decided he would approach the target ships anyway.[28]

At this point he turned to Hempelmann and said, "Louis, if we go in there, will you keep us safe?" Dumbfounded, Hempelmann responded, "Admiral Solberg, I can't give you permission to go in there." Solberg then clarified his statement, "I'm not asking for your permission, all I'm asking is for you to keep us safe." So, without approval, Solberg's tugboat moved forward, sailing in and around the target ships. Following this unauthorized tour, Solberg motored his tugboat straight to the USS *Mount McKinley,* where a large dinner for officers was taking place. At the dinner, Solberg gave a full account of all that he had seen and bragged of how little damage was done to the navy ships. Periodically, he would turn to his embarrassed radiation monitor to back up his account, "Isn't that true, Louis?" For his part, Hempelmann, knowing that Solberg's journey had not been approved, "was trying to shrink into the woodwork." He remembered the awkward occasion as "honest to God . . . one of the low points of my life."[29]

After the Baker test, Solberg again could not contain himself. He noticed one of the naval ships, the *Saratoga,* listing to one side, and thought that if he could get close enough to cut the ship's anchor, the *Saratoga* might be salvaged. Peering through his binoculars, Warren was alarmed to see Solberg's "tug going like mad with a big bow wave toward the Saratoga." Hempelmann was standing at the front of Solberg's vessel with a Geiger counter, which quickly recorded dangerously high levels of radioactivity. This time Solberg listened to Hempelmann's warnings. Warren watched through his glasses as Solberg's boat "all of a sudden . . . slowed down, stopped, and then backed up furiously."[30]

Warren likewise encountered resistance from the navy in a tense meeting with a group of over one thousand officers and petty officers on one of the barracks ships. "You could just feel a kind of wall of hate when I walked in," Warren remembered of the encounter. "The tension was just terrific." Blandy handed Warren a microphone and made him explain to the officers present why he was restricting access to their ships. In an exhausting effort, Warren tried to explain the nature and extent of the radiation hazards. "Well, I had it hot and heavy for an hour. I was nice and wringing wet when I got through." While the interchange did little to alleviate tension, Blandy ultimately acquiesced to Warren's position. "I guess that is all gentlemen," he stated, "and we will go on as before."[31]

However, Warren and the radsafe team finally determined that they could not even go on as before, but should abort the mission altogether and scrap the Charlie test. Solberg remained one of Warren's most forceful adversaries and maintained that the damaged ships could be decontaminated and restored. What finally persuaded Blandy, interestingly, was the evidence of an irradiated fish from the Bikini lagoon. Because the lagoon was so thoroughly contaminated, the fish were consuming algae and other organic material that was toxic. Radsafe personnel, working in the makeshift labs in the *Haven,* began testing fish using x-ray film. Photographic plates would pick up the alpha particles emitted from the fish and, remarkably, leave a clear imprint on the film. The pictures revealed not only the radiation distributed throughout the whole body of the fish but the particularly contaminated material in the fish's stomach.[32]

Accompanied by Deak Parsons, Warren went to Blandy with one of the films, which finally convinced Blandy of the dangers they faced. "If that is it," the admiral said, "then we call it all to a halt." A relieved Warren wrote home to his wife, "A self x-ray of a fish . . . did the trick."[33] Warren would worry for years about the Crossroads accident. Having seen firsthand the consequences of radiation exposure in Hiroshima and Nagasaki, he had nightmares about the potential harm done to American servicemen at Bikini. As Crossroads participant Anthony Guarisco testified before a Senate committee in 1985, Warren "spent countless nights, sleepless nights . . . haunted by the knowledge that atomic veterans of Crossroads were suffering and dying from their involvement in these nuclear explosions."[34]

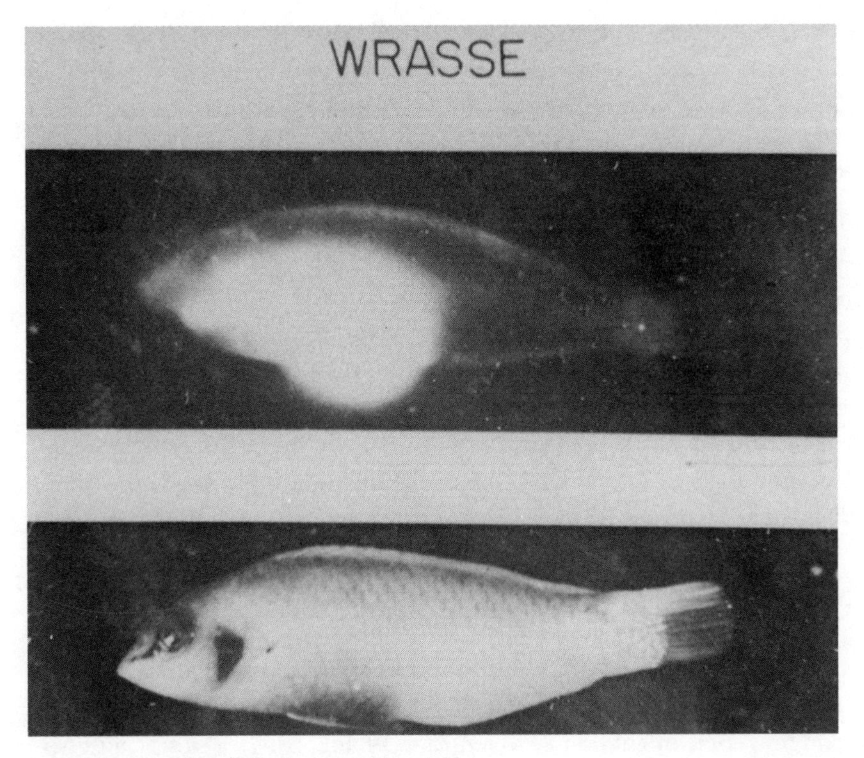

X-ray film of irradiated fish from the Bikini lagoon.

The Bikinians on Rongerik

While Nolan and others on the radsafe team returned to the United States shortly after the Baker test, others stayed on to aid the military with the attempted decontamination and relocation of the damaged target ships. Bradley was among those who remained in the Marshall Islands for another eight weeks. When the navy finally acknowledged the futility of decontaminating its fleet, Bradley and four other radsafe monitors were granted reprieve to go on a little fishing excursion. They joined Captain George Clancy's crew on his one-hundred-foot mine sweeper boat for a brief expedition, the ostensible purpose of which was to test radiation levels of fish in nearby atolls. Two days into the trip, the group decided to try the waters off the coast of the Rongerik Atoll. Passing near the shore of a small island, they noticed several people waving them ashore. Clancy maneuvered the boat close to the main island and, with some of the crew, went onto dry land, only to discover that the invitation came from the relocated Bikinians.

Six months after their resettlement, the Bikinians, whom Bradley found to be a "mild and friendly people," were not faring well. The visit evolved into a sort of conference between Clancy and King Juda. A man named Phillip, who spoke some English, served as a translator, while many from the native community observed the interchange. The message from the Bikinians was clear and straightforward. "We . . . are very hungry," said Phillip. "We . . . have nothing to eat . . . yes. Now I shall tell you something about this island. This is . . . a very poor island. We . . . have not enough coconuts . . . no. For many days now we eat nothing but fish."[35] With a landmass about one-quarter the size of the Bikini Atoll, the supply of coconuts and pandanus on Rongerik was not nearly as plentiful as advertised or anticipated. Moreover, many of the fish caught in the Rongerik lagoon—which was about one-fifth the size of the Bikini lagoon—made the Bikinians sick. Sympathetic to their plight, Clancy ordered supplies brought ashore from his ship. The Bikinians were delighted with the load of flour, sugar, cigarettes, and fishhooks given to them, and offered a number of handcrafted items to the Americans in return.

Before leaving, Clancy and his men were asked one final question. Translating for King Juda, Phillip said, "King Juda would like to know when he and his people might be able to return to Bikini." This was a difficult question and Clancy did not try to sugarcoat his answer. He explained that the village and many of the trees on the island had been destroyed and that water and food from the atoll and lagoon were unsafe and might remain so for months if not years to come. Bradley recalls Phillip's sad and respectful response: "Oh. We very sorry to hear this."[36]

Today, more than seven decades after their removal, the Bikinians still cannot live on their homeland, which remains too toxic for habitation. High levels of the induced radioisotope cesium 137 are traceable in the soil, thus contaminating some of the fruit and wildlife on the atoll. The plight of the Bikinians is a sad story indeed. Difficulties securing enough food on the Rongerik Atoll only intensified after the visit from Clancy and his radsafe fishing party. To compound their problems, in 1947 a fire burned nearly one-third of Rongerik's coconut and pandanus trees, which even before this misfortune had yielded less than the trees on the Bikinians' home atoll had. When Leonard Mason, an anthropologist from the University of Hawaii, visited Rongerik in early 1948, he found the Bikinians near starvation. Alarmed by their situation, he quickly summoned food supplies and medical care and encouraged another relocation. Nearly two years after their

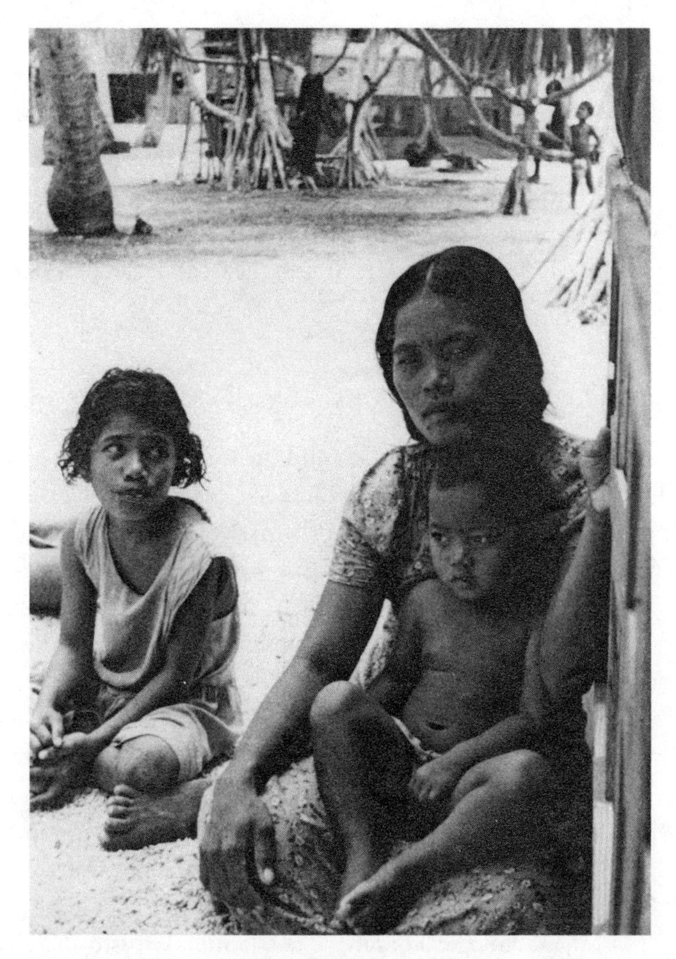

Bikinians on Rongerik Island, September 1946.

forced migration to Rongerik, the Bikinians were moved again, this time to Kwajalein Atoll, the location of a US military base. The Bikinians were set up in tents along the military airstrip, where they remained for almost eight months before another location could be determined.

It was finally decided, after some deliberation and several visits to alternative sites, to move the Bikinians to Kili Island, a small island in the southern part of the Marshall Islands, about 425 miles south of the Bikini Atoll. Because Kili is an island, not an atoll, the absence of a lagoon made impracticable their traditional methods of fishing. Thus, the Bikinians became dependent on imported food supplies, resulting over time in what has been called a "dole psychology" among the relocated islanders.[37] After the move, the Americans also provided the Bikinians with a converted forty-foot whaleboat, which had both sails and an engine, to enable easier travel to other communities in the Marshall Islands. In a painfully ironic gesture, the boat was named *Crossroads,* the same name as the military operation that required the Bikinians to relocate in the first place. The Bikinians had no experience with motored vessels and had trouble operating *Crossroads.* In less than a year of use, the boat crashed on Kili's reef and was abandoned.[38]

Medicolegal Board

As occurred with both the Trinity test and the nuclear accidents at Los Alamos, during Operation Crossroads the doctors set up radiation record-keeping procedures in order to protect themselves against potential future litigation. Toward this end, they went so far as to establish a medicolegal board. One of the main purposes of the board, as Jonathan Weisgall explains, was to "provide a paper trail designed to lay the groundwork for future denial of legal claims that might be brought against the U.S. government arising from Operation Crossroads."[39] Several weeks after the Baker test, Robert Newell, the chair of the medicolegal board, which initially included Nolan and Hempelmann as members, admitted that the board was established in order to "reassure Col. Warren that the safety measures adopted by RadSafe were such as to attract no justifiable criticism, and to give what assurance was possible that no successful suits could be brought on account of the radiological hazards of Operation Crossroads."[40]

Thus, the pattern of caution, co-optation, and complicity was repeated. The doctors offered multiple warnings about harmful radiation at Crossroads. These warnings were in many instances ignored by the military. To protect themselves from any "accusations of laxity" should anticipated radiation injuries occur, Warren established a hand-picked medicolegal board to provide cover. Admiral Solberg's instructions to Hempelmann capture well the complexity of the situation. Solberg didn't want to follow radsafe instructions; he just wanted Hempelmann to keep him safe. This incident is emblematic of the nearly impossible position in which the doctors were placed and of the manner in which they were co-opted. Arguably, here as elsewhere, the doctors ultimately became complicit in the manner in which they downplayed the harmful effects of radiation on Joint Task Force One personnel.

Newell implausibly concluded in his summary report of the medicolegal board, "The Operation Crossroads, Tests Able and Baker, were carried through without irradiation injuries to any persons."[41] As with the early "spot check" reports from Japan, time would reveal that such a conclusion was premature. Over time, a number of Joint Task Force personnel would attribute illnesses, including cancer, to the exposure they received while at Bikini.[42] Among these was John Smitherman, a navy sailor who had helped put out fires on target ships following the Able test. Several weeks after the Baker test, Smitherman discovered red marks on his legs and feet. As was apparently typical (see the photo earlier in this chapter), he had labored in the Bikini lagoon wearing little more than shorts, tennis shoes, and a T-shirt. He was diagnosed with "malignant lymphoma," and, over time, his legs began to balloon in size. Eventually both legs and an arm had to be amputated. He died in 1983 at the age of fifty-four. He never received any compensation for his injuries or any acknowledgment from the government that radiation from the Bikini tests caused his ailments.[43]

Enewetak

The Able and Baker tests would not be the end of nuclear testing in the Marshall Islands—far from it. Less than two years after Operation Crossroads, the United States initiated further experiments with the new atom bomb, this time on the Enewetak Atoll, approximately 220 miles west of Bikini. As was the case with Bikini, an indigenous community lived on Enewetak; in fact, two communities, the Enewetak and the Enjebi peoples, occupied two separate halves of the atoll. Enewetak had been under Japanese control since the beginning of the twentieth century, though until the start of World War II the atoll and the communities living on it had largely been left alone. The Enewetak people lived a similar sort of self-sufficient existence as had the Bikinians.

During the war, given its northwestern location in the Pacific, the Japanese came to regard the atoll as an important strategic site and built a military base with a large airfield on one of the islands, Engebi. By the end of 1943, however, having already conquered the relatively larger Kwajalein and Majuro Atolls in the Marshall Islands, the American military set its eyes on Enewetak in its island-hopping march toward the Japanese mainland. A fierce five-day battle with the Japanese ensued on Enewetak in February 1944, resulting in the loss of 3,400 Japanese troops and 348 American

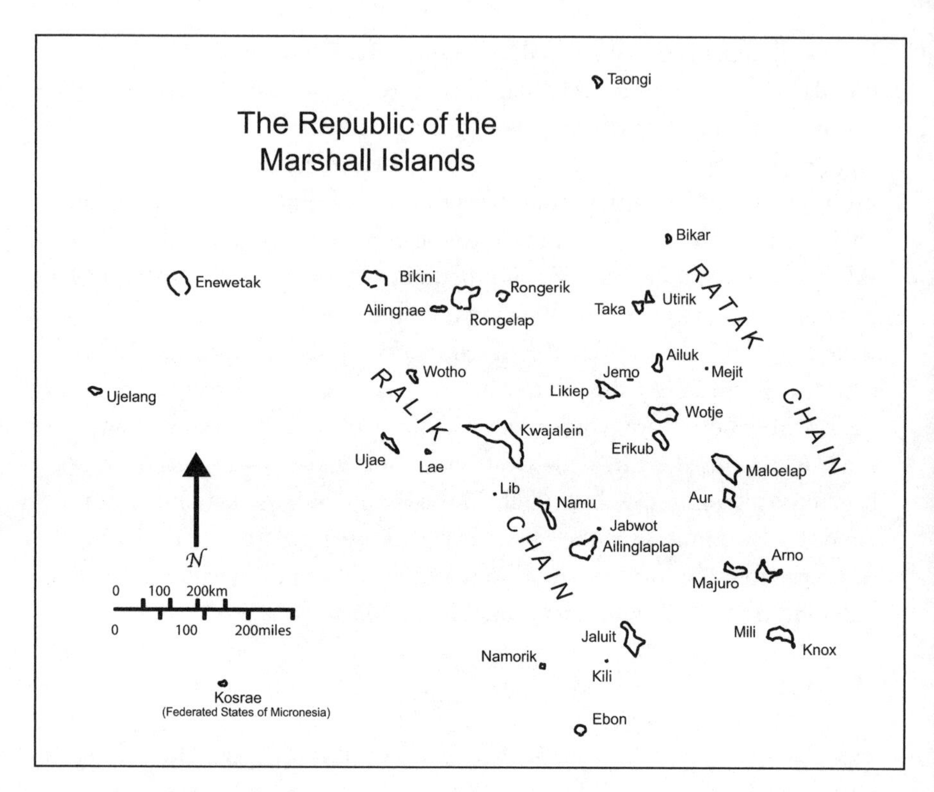

Republic of the Marshall Islands.

troops.[44] After securing the atoll, the American military allowed Marshallese laborers from other atolls—who had been imported to work on the Japanese base—to return to their home atolls. A number of Marshallese had been killed during the fighting, and the US military helped to feed and house the Enewetak community after taking control of the atoll. Utilizing some of the infrastructure left from the Japanese occupation, the American military then established an important advance base for its ongoing war in the Pacific.

With an airfield and base already in place, Enewetak became an attractive option for ongoing nuclear testing after the end of the war. The remote northwestern location was also an appealing feature, in that prevailing easterly trade winds would presumably carry radioactive material over the open sea to the west, rather than toward the populated atolls and islands to the east and southeast. Moreover, the military determined that the geography of the Enewetak Atoll afforded enough space for three separate land-based nuclear detonations.[45] As was the case with Bikini, Enewetak was inhabited, and the 142 Enewetak and Enjebi peoples would be forced to relocate.

It was determined that the Ujelang Atoll, approximately 120 miles southwest of Enewetak, would be an ideal new home for the Enewetak and Enjebi peoples. For a short time, Ujelang had also been considered as a potential new home for the Bikinians. While the dislocated Bikinians were struggling to survive on Rongerik Atoll in late 1947, construction on Ujelang had commenced for this purpose. However, in December 1947, once it was determined that Enewetak would become the permanent proving ground for further nuclear testing, the US military decided to give the uninhabited atoll to the Enewetak peoples instead.

For several reasons, the relocation of the Enewetak community was a more successful resettlement than was the unfortunate odyssey and final placement of the Bikinians. For one, the Ujelang Atoll *is* an atoll, not an isolated island like Kili. Moreover, Ujelang's climate and ecology are similar to Enewetak's, and the inhabitants (and former inhabitants) of the two atolls shared some ancestral ties. In fact, some members of the Enewetak community had actually lived for a time on Ujelang, when a previous community had occupied the atoll, and were thus familiar with the geography and natural resources of the place.

Nevertheless, the Enewetak people were leaving their homeland, and the adjustment to the new atoll was not easy. Like the Bikinians, they missed their home atoll and wanted someday to return to it. As occurred in the Bikinians' initial transfer to Rongerik, the Enewetak people were transferred to a much smaller atoll. The move constituted a reduction in landmass from 2.26 to 0.67 square miles and a decrease in lagoon size from 387 to 25.4 square miles.[46] The availability of natural resources was thus significantly reduced. As a consequence, like the Bikinians, though to a lesser extent, the displaced community became more dependent on externally imported supplies.[47] While acknowledging positive aspects of life in Ujelang and the comparatively more successful relocation process than occurred with the Bikinians, anthropologist Jack Tobin, in his comprehensive study of their resettlement, concludes that the forced migrants from the Enewetak Atoll "became further casualties of the Atomic Age and Cold War; helpless victims of circumstances beyond their control, and of forces beyond their understanding."[48]

Operation Sandstone

The military operation that necessitated the relocation of the peoples of the Enewetak Atoll was called Operation Sandstone. After a political battle in the United States between the military and the scientists, atomic matters were placed under civilian control with the establishment of the AEC in January 1947. Therefore, Operation Sandstone was a civilian-run operation (Joint Task Force Seven), with the military playing a supporting role. As had been originally planned for Operation Crossroads, there would be three tests at Enewetak, code-named X-Ray, Yoke, and Zebra, and scheduled for detonations on April 15, May 1, and May 15, 1948. As with Trinity, the test bombs would be blasted from towers, this time two hundred feet high, built on three different islands on the Enewetak Atoll (Enjebi, Aomon, and Runit). Whereas Crossroads was a military operation testing the effects of nuclear weapons on navy ships, Sandstone would be a scientific experiment testing or proving the effectiveness of new nuclear weapons designs—thus the name for these ongoing tests, the Pacific Proving Ground.

Sandstone was different from Crossroads in other respects. It was smaller (about ten thousand instead of forty-two thousand personnel), more controlled, and much less of a media spectacle. Because Sandstone was testing new bomb designs, this operation returned to the normal modus operandi characteristic of the Manhattan Project—that is, a high level of secrecy, an orientation that would again have interesting consequences. Some lessons from the Crossroads disaster were taken to heart, including giving radsafe a more central and prominent place in the operation. Colonel James Cooney would lead the radsafe group; like Stafford Warren before him, Cooney was a radiologist and military doctor. Warren was not available for Joint Task Force Seven, as he had by this time assumed his new duties as the dean of the University of California, Los Angeles, medical school. As with Crossroads, however, there was pushback against radsafe; only this time it was more from scientific than military personnel.

Once again, it was acknowledged that 0.1 roentgens constituted the maximum permissible daily dose. However, as occurred at Trinity, the scientists were able to negotiate the acceptability of a higher dose in some instances—specifically, "a maximum exposure of 3 R for certain approved specific missions."[49] As head of radsafe, Cooney was concerned with "insuring that the safety of personnel would not be subordinated to the urgency of recovery of scientific data."[50] In the end, the scientists and the radsafe team reached something of a compromise whereby "under unusual circumstances, the Scientific Director and the Radsafe Officer may authorize a total exposure up to three (3) roentgens." Cooney worried that the so-called unusual circumstances represented a loophole through which the scientists could "obtain test results at any costs."[51]

Nolan and Hempelmann would both be involved in Operation Sandstone. However, as in the delivery of the Hiroshima bomb and the Joint Commission in Japan, Nolan was given the overseas assignment, while Hempelmann stayed at home to handle matters at Los Alamos. For Operation Sandstone, Nolan was made the civilian head of a three-person advisory unit, which also included Harry Whipple, another doctor who had worked with the Health Group at Los Alamos and had traveled with Nolan to Japan.[52] The purpose of the advisory unit was to "furnish radiological and safety and medical legal advice to Colonel Cooney."[53]

Once again, then, the doctors were mindful of potential legal consequences. In fact, they anticipated "possible long range effects of minor radiation and . . . possible future legal complications involving the Government or the AEC." Following a game plan similarly employed at Crossroads and at Trinity, it was determined that documentation of radiation exposure levels would be a necessary precaution. Thus, the radsafe group "decided to forward a permanent record of all exposed civilian personnel to the AEC and of all military personnel to the respective Suregon's General [*sic*]."[54]

In his capacity as head of the advisory unit, Nolan participated in a series of three meetings before the tests with Cooney and other medical officers, discussing issues related to radiation. During these meetings, the doctors showed slides of the injuries of *hibakusha* in Japan, which garnered "particular interest" from those in attendance.[55] Available military records indicate that in addition to his advisory role, Nolan may also have participated in some of the actual monitoring exercises, including going to Engebi Island after the X-Ray test and before the Yoke test to "supervise radiological safety operations" on the island.[56] In the main, though, it appears that he was mostly stationed at the RadSafe Center on the USS *Mount McKinley* or the USS *Bairoko* advising Cooney and other officers on radiation safety matters.[57] After Crossroads, navy commander Frank Winant commended Nolan for his "advisory" role, which "proved invaluable in the task of rendering decisions which could well involve the life and health of those for whom we were responsible."[58]

Because greater care was given to safety measures at Sandstone, some of the more dangerous consequences of Crossroads were avoided. Nevertheless, secondary fallout resulted in "widespread, but low-level exposure" not only on Enewetak but as far away as the Kwajalein Atoll.[59] Additionally, there were some unexpected and more acute radiation injuries to American military personnel. At Sandstone, drone planes flew through the mushroom clouds following the detonation of each test. After they landed, members of the radiochemistry group would quickly recover filters from the drone planes, which were then placed in a container for shipment back to the Los Alamos lab for analysis. Members of the team were meant to use tongs to recover the filters before placing them in the containers, but because of the wind on the island and the need for a quick recovery effort, they used only their glove-covered hands instead.

One radiochemistry group member after the Yoke test and three others after the Zebra test received serious beta burns on their hands while recovering the contaminated filters. It was only after several weeks that severe blistering from the beta burns became acute. In the case of the Zebra test, the three group members had registered exposures of 3.8, 5.6, and 17.0 roentgens, respectively, all exceeding the allowable dosages, even for "unusual circumstances."[60] All four of those exposed eventually found their way back to Los Alamos, as did the data samples from the filters.

The radiochemistry team member exposed during the Yoke test was initially misdiagnosed as having only a bruise on his hand. As a consequence, this "resulted in the forward area's not being advised, before the Zebra Test, of the excessive dosages possible in the procedures used at Eniwetok."[61] In a letter to Robert Stone dated June 28, 1948, Hempelmann conveyed, in notably scientific terms, the outcome of his examination of these victims. His language calls to mind the same sort of posture that was evident in the "treatment" of Allan Kline and the other victims of nuclear accidents in the Omega lab. That is, the accidents provided the doctors with an excellent opportunity to study the effects of radiation on the human body. As Hempelmann wrote to Stone concerning the Sandstone cases, "I would like very much to give you a preview of our excellent series of colored photographs. I learned several things from following the cases. The most interesting is that beta ray burns can look a lot like a bruise. The first one was completely mis-diagnosed by us because it was located in a place where we did not think radiation burns could occur. It was interesting to correlate changes in blood count with the visible day-by-day progress of lesions."[62]

As occurred with the Omega Site accidents, Hempelmann and Shields Warren were interested in publishing an article on the biological effects from the Sandstone injuries. "Shields Warren was here recently," Hempelmann wrote to Stone, "and he wants us to publish the cases after a six-month's follow up."[63]

A full follow-up would require more than six months. The injured men would remain in the Los Alamos Hospital for months before finally being transferred to St. Louis to receive skin grafts on their hands. All three men from the Zebra test received grafts, the last of which was not finally completed until a decade later.[64]

The Legacy of Bikini and Enewetak

The Able, Baker, X-Ray, Yoke, and Zebra bombs would not be the last weapons tested on Bikini or Enewetak. In fact, between 1946 and 1958 a total of sixty-seven atom bombs were tested in the Marshall Islands, twenty-three at Bikini and forty-four at Enewetak, yielding the total equivalent of 108 megatons of TNT, more than seven thousand times the force of the Little Boy bomb.[65] The largest bomb exploded during this testing period was Castle Bravo, a hydrogen or thermonuclear bomb detonated at Bikini on March 1, 1954. Castle Bravo alone yielded a force of 15 megatons, nearly double the force that was anticipated. The bomb, one thousand times more powerful than Little Boy, vaporized three of Bikini's islands and left a crater that was 6,500 feet in diameter and 250 feet deep.

Bravo also blew radioactive fallout at a distance of more than 125 miles, not to the north, as expected, but to the east, dropping contaminated coral dust on the atolls of Rongelap, Utirik, and Ailinginae. Though the islands were exposed to dangerously high levels of radioactivity, the inhabitants of Rongelap and Utirik, and the eighteen Marshallese camping on Ailinginae (a total of 239 islanders), were not fully evacuated until three days after the detonation. Like the Bikinians, the Rongelapese to this day cannot live on their home atoll. Following Bravo, Marshall Islanders, particularly the sixty-four inhabitants of Rongelap, which was the most contaminated of the affected atolls, suffered both acute radiation sickness and other symptoms, some of which, including multiple thyroid tumors, were not recognized until years later.[66]

Castle Bravo also dropped radioactive ash on a Japanese fishing boat, misnamed the *Lucky Dragon.* All twenty-three members of the *Lucky*

Dragon were affected by the fallout. One died shortly after the accident, and others suffered for years with various symptoms of radiation sickness. The accident stirred renewed resentment from the Japanese and generated a wave of antinuclear activism both in the United States and internationally. One of the Japanese physicians who examined the injured crew members was Masao Tsuzuki, the same Japanese surgeon who had worked with Nolan and Stafford Warren during the Joint Commission in 1945.

In the late 1970s, the US government plowed 3.1 million cubic feet of radioactive waste into a section of Runit Island on the Enewetak Atoll, the location of the Zebra test bomb from Operation Sandstone. Over the pile was placed a concrete dome (eighteen inches thick and 328 feet wide) to contain the radioactive material. It was meant to be temporary but has remained untouched for more than four decades. With rising sea levels, there are growing concerns that the so-called Runit Dome, where cracks are already visible, will be compromised further, thus threatening to leak large quantities of radioactive waste into the surrounding environment.[67] In addition to the damage done to the Enewetak Atoll from forty-four atomic bomb tests, it was recently revealed that in 1958 the United States, unbeknownst to the Marshallese, had shipped 130 tons of sand from the Nevada Test Site to Enewetak and, a decade later, had tested biological weapons on the atoll—"bombs and missiles filled with bacteria designed to fell enemy troops."[68]

While the indigenous people and the natural ecology of the Marshall Islands have suffered for decades as a consequence of the nuclear age, what of the legacy of Enewetak and Bikini elsewhere? During the summer of Operation Crossroads, the French clothing designer Louis Réard had crafted a new bathing suit scheduled to be unveiled in Paris on July 5, 1946. The Able test, which took place four days earlier, was front-page international news. Capitalizing on the story, Réard named his new design after the island where the bomb had been dropped. Produced from only thirty square inches of fabric, the new bikini bathing suit was advertised as "smaller than the smallest bathing suit in the world." It was so skimpy that Réard could not find a professional model willing to wear it in public. He finally had to hire a Paris stripper named Micheline Bernardini, who modeled the new bikini at the Piscine Molitor pool in Paris. The design, though controversial at the time (several European countries initially outlawed it), eventually became an international success.

As for Admiral Blandy, after Operation Crossroads, he returned to Washington, DC, and on November 1, 1946, officially dissolved Joint Task Force One. The event was celebrated on November 7 in the Officers' Club of the Army War College in Washington, DC, at the same time that the Bikinians living on Rongerik were struggling to provide enough food for their survival. At the center of the gathering was a cake, the base of which read OPERATION CROSSROADS. On top of the cake was the mushroom cloud of a nuclear explosion, and Blandy's wife wore a hat that appeared to match it. A photograph of the event was taken and published in the society pages of the *Washington Post* the next day. The photograph became widely published, including in Russia, and understandably engendered much commentary.

Such an image, of course, says a lot about military attitudes regarding the bomb and the dawn of the nuclear age. It also conveys much about the relative indifference to the plight of the Marshallese, some of whom were

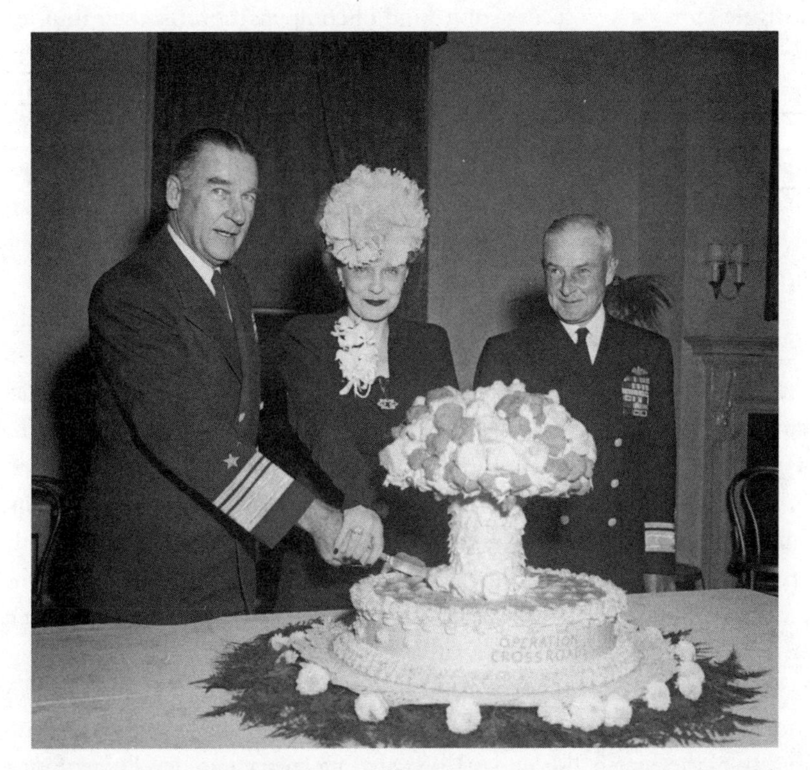

Left to right: Admiral William H. P. Blandy, his wife, and Rear Admiral George M. Lowry at the Army War College in Washington, DC, November 7, 1946, celebrating the end of Operation Crossroads.

exiled from their homelands and whose culture and way of life were irreversibly altered by the bomb. With assistance from people like Jonathan Weisgall and Jack Niedenthal, the former Trust Liaison for the Bikinians, the Marshallese eventually secured monetary compensation for their sufferings. However, such reparations, though appreciated, could not give the islanders—especially the Bikinians and the Rongelapese—what they wanted most, a return to their beloved homelands. The sort of indifference exhibited for years by the United States toward these indigenous people might best be summarized by the words of Henry Kissinger, offered during a 1969 discussion with Interior Secretary Walter Hickel. Hickel had recently returned from a trip to Micronesia and was concerned about US policy in the region and the plight of the people living there. "There are only 90,000 people who live out there," Kissinger responded. "Who gives a damn?"[69]

The Marshallese were not the only humans affected by the nuclear tests in the Pacific Proving Ground. Like John Smitherman, many US servicemen struggled for years to secure some kind of compensation for their injuries. For decades the Department of Veterans Affairs denied claims for compensation on the grounds that the servicemen could not prove that their cancers and other medical troubles were caused by exposure to radiation during the tests. What documented evidence was available did not provide proof that the nuclear tests were the source of their illnesses. Arguably, then, Warren's medicolegal board succeeded in its intended purpose of preventing future legal claims.

As late as 1985, radsafe monitor David Bradley, in testimony before the Senate Veterans' Affairs Committee, forcefully questioned the fairness of these denials. He made several important points in this regard. First, he acknowledged that it was because of Warren's repeated warnings about the dangerous effects of radiation that the "tough intelligent military leaders" finally, sixteen days after Baker, acquiesced and agreed to "abandon the ships and the test."[70] Bradley also argued that the ships in the lagoon, especially after the Baker test, were heavily irradiated. As happened in Japan, the radiation-measuring instruments, according to Bradley, were limited in their effectiveness. They could not really measure alpha or beta particles; some of the film badges only registered up to two roentgens; and instruments measuring gamma rays were often made dysfunctional by the heat and humidity of the Marshall Islands. Thus, proving an accurate level of exposure for an individual serviceman, especially since many did not even wear film badges, was impossible.

Bradley also argued that the accuracy of blood tests was "meaningless" and "futile" and measurements of urinalysis tests "meaningless or worse."[71] Part of the problem with the urinalysis tests, according to Bradley, was that radsafe monitors were not given enough information to meaningfully analyze the samples. After Nolan and others had returned home following the Baker test, Bradley stayed on to perform a range of tasks, including making sense of three thousand buckets of urine samples stored in the *Haven*'s survey laboratory. After being given this assignment, Bradley asked for "a book giving some guidelines or some standards" in order to organize and interpret the urine samples. He was told that he could not see the book because "it is secret. It is classified."[72]

Recall that during the Joint Commission in Japan, when some of the non–Manhattan Project doctors asked for greater insight into the nature of the nuclear explosions—the effects of which they were ostensibly studying—they were likewise denied this information on the grounds of secrecy. Thus, as it concerns Crossroads, the sum total of the lab's library was the random notes on urine samples that Bradley scribbled in his notebook. "That," Bradley stated with stinging irony, "is how good, how scientific we were." It is no wonder that he described data from urine samples as "meaningless or worse."[73]

As far as Nolan was concerned, Operation Sandstone represented the end of his direct involvement with the production and testing of nuclear weapons. He was keen to return to his work as a medical doctor. While he was critical of the ongoing testing of nuclear weapons that would follow Sandstone, he was nevertheless eager to use new radiation technologies in the treatment of his gynecological patients.

8

Dr. Nolan and the Quandary of Technique

> We should have learned a lesson from the making of the first atomic bomb and the resulting arms race. We didn't do well then, and the parallels to our current situation are troubling.
>
> —Bill Joy, "Why the Future Doesn't Need Us"

In the summer of 1946, after Operation Crossroads, James F. Nolan had returned with his family to St. Louis to take a position as assistant professor of obstetrics and gynecology at Washington University. During this short stint as a full-time teaching faculty member, Nolan began to explore the use of other radioisotopes, in addition to radium, to treat cancer. For example, he proposed using an isotope of cobalt (cobalt-60) as a cheaper alternative to radium, and he received a $9,800 Atomic Energy Committee grant to test whether a radioisotope of gold (gold-198) would be an effective treatment against cancerous tumors. Shortly after the completion of Operation Sandstone, however, on July 1, 1948, Nolan resigned from his post at Washington University to take a position at the Los Angeles Tumor Institute. A year later, he also joined a team of four other gynecological oncologists at the Southern California Cancer Center, a division of the California Hospital Medical Center, and became a clinical professor of gynecology and obstetrics at the University of Southern California. In 1972, he became director of the Cancer Center.

The reason for the move to California seems to have been twofold. First, after the war he had been offered use of a rare cobalt machine by the military to treat cancer patients. Washington University's Barnes Hospital apparently wanted 40 percent overhead for use of the unit, while the Los Angeles Tumor Institute offered to house the equipment without an overhead charge.[1] That members of Ann Nolan's family were living in the Los Angeles area was likely an additional motivating factor for the move to California. Ann's father, Rolla Lawry; brother, Bill Lawry; and sister, Jane Reynolds—with whom she and her kids had lived during Nolan's time overseas—were in the Los Angeles area. In 1948, then, after Nolan resigned from his position at Washington University, he, his wife, and their two children, Lawry (now ten years old) and Lynne (now five years old), moved permanently to Los Angeles.

Nolan was keen to get away from the military aspect of nuclear technology and to use radiation for helpful medical purposes. This is how his daughter, Lynne, remembers his attitude in the postwar years. The sense she got from her father was that the faster "he could get away from the military aspect of the whole thing, the better." Instead he wanted to see "peaceful uses for the whole business, not only in energy but in the treating of disease."[2] Nolan's son, Lawry, remembered his father's disposition in a similar way. In a lecture he gave at the College of the Holy Cross in January 2006, Lawry recollected that his dad could not wait to get away from the military and to a place where he could use nuclear technology for positive ends, especially in the realm of medicine. "He was convinced that great good" would "flow from the peaceful use of radiation, particularly in the field of medicine." Lawry added that his father "spent the rest of his professional life discovering, designing, and employing life-saving radioactive isotopes to locate and kill cancer cells" and also designed and built devices to "send rays to destroy cancer."[3]

Concerning the continued testing of nuclear weapons in the Marshall Islands and in Nevada, Nolan was privately critical. Lynne remembers her father reading about the atmospheric and underground testing of weapons in the Nevada Proving Grounds with disapproval. "Dad used to shake his head and say, 'They have no idea what they're doing.'" This is a man who had witnessed firsthand the ongoing suffering and deaths of *hibakusha* in Hiroshima and Nagasaki in the weeks after those detonations. One can only imagine what he thought of military testing efforts that required marines to march directly toward ground zero moments after a nuclear explosion in the Nevada desert—what the military in one report euphemistically called a "coordinated air-ground maneuver against the attack objective."[4] Not surprisingly, as with the military personnel and the native inhabitants in the Marshall Islands, soldiers serving in the Nevada Proving Grounds would suffer for years from a variety of radiation-related injuries and illnesses.[5]

Dr. Nolan and the Instrumentalist Perspective

With no direct involvement in the ongoing military aspects of the nuclear age, in Los Angeles Nolan gave himself fully to his work as a medical practitioner and cancer researcher, using radiation technology to treat cancer patients. In other words, he lived out his view that nuclear technology could be used for beneficial purposes in the area of medicine. Such a perspective is a fitting illustration of what philosopher Albert Borgmann refers to as the instrumentalist view of technology. In his discussion of technology as a cultural force, Borgmann identifies the instrumentalist view as the official or most commonly held perspective on the role of technology in modern society, a view that posits that technology "is neither good nor bad. . . . It depends on us and our values whether it is used well or ill."[6]

While Borgmann sees important limitations to the instrumentalist view, he acknowledges that "there is obviously some merit" to this perspective and that it "is undoubtedly correct at its avowed level of observation."[7] As to the observable good Nolan achieved with radiation therapy, it was considerable. For the next thirty-plus years as a medical researcher and practitioner, he did admirable work in his field. He trained medical students in obstetric and gynecological care, and he developed new treatments for several forms of gynecological cancer, using a variety of radioisotopes, most commonly radium. As noted in Lawry Nolan's Holy Cross lecture, he also developed devices for performing biopsies and for applying radiation therapy to cancer patients. One innovative tandem apparatus he devised, used for the application of radium to patients with cervical cancer, came to be known in the field as the Nolan applicator.[8]

Nolan's medical papers, published over a period of four decades, demonstrate a keen and practical eye for developing radiation treatments aimed at more effectively killing cancer cells (carcinoma) but avoiding harm to surrounding healthy tissues. Consideration of various treatment strategies were generally aimed at determining the proper dosage—in terms of quantity, duration, and type—that would best serve patients with different types of gynecological cancer.

Treatment methods considered in Nolan's medical papers include external and intravaginal x-ray therapy, the implantation of radium seeds strategically placed next to cancerous tumors, the application of multiple radium capsules for irregularly shaped uteri, and the use of radiogold in colloidal form (that is, gel) to treat "carcinoma of the uterus." The papers

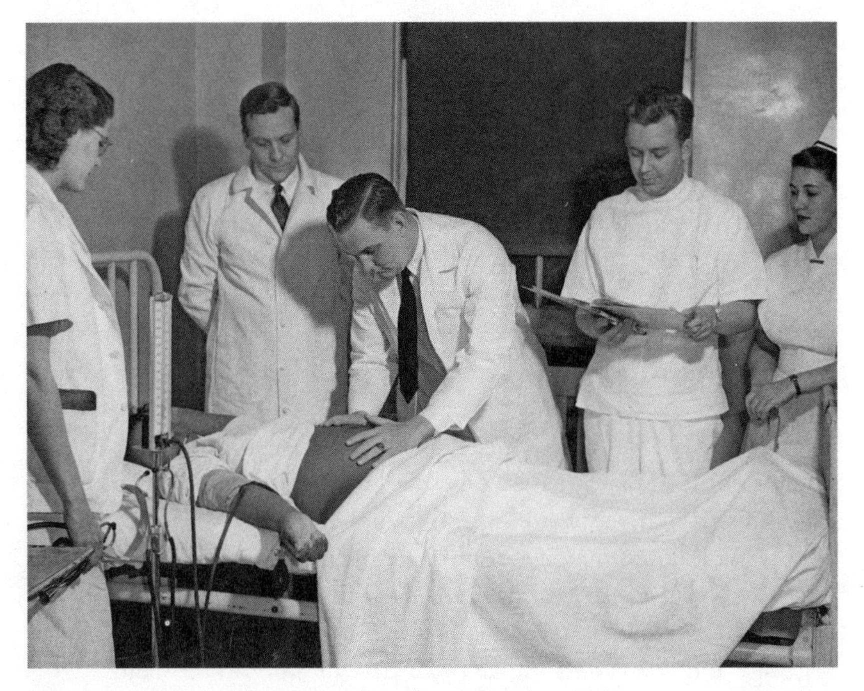

Nolan supervising the examination of an obstetrical patient, 1948.

also offer analyses of the flexible application of combined treatments, the innovative use of new devices for taking biopsies and applying radiation therapy, and the effectiveness of specific surgical procedures for excising different types of cancerous lesions.[9] The papers reflect a vocational perspective—evident also in Takashi Nagai's postwar work in Nagasaki—that seamlessly integrated scientific research with patient care.

In 1971, Nolan was elected president of the American Radium Society, one of four medical societies for which he served as president or chairman during his medical career. In March of that year, he gave the presidential address at the society's annual meeting, which took place in Mexico City, Mexico. His words offered in this context provide a rare window into his thinking, as he reflected on the radiation hazards to which he and other doctors had been exposed during decades of work in the field. The address was offered in an intentionally ironic style, in keeping with the distinctive quality of Nolan's unique sense of humor. Departing from the more academic and data-driven style of previous addresses, Nolan instead offered himself as the subject for his lecture, a more personalized focus, he explained, "which cannot be subjected to the usual restraints of the scientific approach."[10]

At the start to the talk, Nolan recollected the first American Radium Society meeting he attended, in Atlantic City in 1942, the year before he moved his family to Los Alamos. He recalled the missing fingers he saw on the hands of many participants, pioneers in the field who had delivered their new medical product with heroic self-sacrifice. Turning to the radiation risks to which he had been exposed, Nolan focused on his almost twenty-five years of providing medical care in the years after the war. Consistent with the ideal of secrecy with which he had been so thoroughly indoctrinated during his military service, he only made oblique reference to his wartime experience and claimed that, during those years, "personal radiation exposure was minimal and largely theoretical."[11]

In the nearly twenty-five years of clinical practice that followed, in contrast, he observed that radiation exposure "must be considered appreciable." He estimated that between 1950 and 1970, he had been exposed to 2,029 radium applications, ranging from 80 to 150 applications a year, or an average of about 100 per year. He calculated that he had received approximately "50 rem total body irradiation . . . during those 20 years or 2.5 rem per year" and about four to five times that amount on his hands.[12] It is highly likely that, as with his wartime work, he significantly downplayed the amount of exposure he had received in these years of medical practice.[13] As to the physiological effects of this exposure, he claimed that none could be found at the time.[14]

However, he acknowledged that his red blood cell count had been "consistently higher than the normal range." A pathologist diagnosing "the subject" concluded that this condition might have been caused by a "physiologic compensatory mechanism" and noted that "a common chronic respiratory irritant [was] producing bronchiolar spasm and strongly recommended the discontinuation of its use."[15] Translation: my grandfather was a heavy smoker (unfiltered Camel cigarettes), and the pathologist advised him to give up the habit—advice that he did not heed.

Nolan also implicitly acknowledged that he may have become infertile as a consequence of radiation exposure. In addition to offering himself as the experimental subject, he employed a colleague—of the same age and experience but without radiation exposure—as the control subject. Given Nolan's age (he would have been fifty-six at the time), they decided not to test for infertility. As Nolan explained in the lecture, "Testicular biopsies were not performed as the control subject considered the possible information to be gained to be irrelevant. Actually the F_1 generation for the experimental subject was launched before any significant exposure was accumulated, and the F_2 generation is well on its way."[16] In other words, Nolan had two children, both conceived before moving to Los Alamos; and by 1971, he already had five grandchildren (the author of this text included). Thus, he regarded knowing whether he was infertile as irrelevant.

However, it was the case that he and my grandmother were not able to conceive after the war. They had hoped to have as many as four children. He used to jokingly say that he had "two only children."[17] Just as in Hiroshima, when he and Stafford Warren attributed their diarrhea (a common feature of radiation sickness) to Japanese food, he speculated that his infertility was less attributable to radiation exposure than it was to his use of "adult mood modifying substances," a euphemistic reference to his consumption of alcohol.[18] Both Lynne and his daughter-in-law, Karen Nolan, remember Nolan commenting on how much radiation exposure he had received and how remarkable it was that he had lived as long as he had without apparent effects.

In the 1971 lecture, Nolan also identified other risks, unrelated to radiation exposure, that represented potential hazards to medical doctors. Interestingly, lawyers and the fear of litigation were among these additional hazards. Nolan identified "exposure" to the malpractice suit, for example, as "one type of hazard that can be very distressful." He lamented that "as long as it is profitable, one can depend on the contingency fee, res ipsa loquitur, and the theory of informed consent to promote this type of exposure."[19] Given the Manhattan Project doctors' involvement in the plutonium injections, Nolan's seemingly dismissive reference to the "theory" of informed consent is unsettling. His more general identification of physicians' worries about lawsuits should be no surprise given the Manhattan Project doctors' consistent preoccupation with legal matters and efforts to protect themselves from lawsuits during the early years of the nuclear age. As to the effects of these lawyerly hazards on this subject, "electrocardiographic studies have so far shown no significant defects."[20]

In the last part of the lecture, Nolan reflected on physicians' reasons for being willing to take on the risks of radiation exposure. He first identified, then debunked, several possible motives. Could it be the monetary rewards? "Extra hazardous duty pay has never been associated with radium applications. . . . This type of reward is of insignificant consequence." Perhaps it was for all the expressions of gratitude doctors received from their patients. "Almost 2,000 years ago," Nolan observed, "10 lepers were cleansed and told to return to the temple to give thanks, but only one did. The proposition of present day patients responding in a similar manner remains about the same."[21] Could it be the heroism associated with innovative medical care? "There is no bravado involved." What about the attitude, "Someone has to do it"? "There never has been a dearth of practitioners in the field to make such a necessity."[22]

If not these motivating factors, then what? Nolan was quite clear on this point. Doctors took on the risks because of a superseding "interest in patient welfare." In pursuing this end, he identified a number of developments in the field, including the use of new, more effective, and safer medical technologies. Though he was offering himself as the subject for his "farcical" and "editorialized" analysis, he argued that new developments in the field, though safer for the practitioner, were not aimed at "achieving greater protection for the physician." Rather, they were "directed toward more effective patient care."[23]

Doctors in the field—like the early pioneers who had lost their fingers applying radiation treatment—had accepted these risks because of their overriding interest in "delivering quality health care." Nolan's student, and then colleague, Robert Futoran, who for years worked closely with my grandfather in Los Angeles, remembers that both were fully aware of the significant amount of radiation to which they were regularly exposed, but they simply "did not want to stop doing what [they] were doing." Futoran was later diagnosed with lymphoma; and though it was successfully treated, he attributes having contracted the disease to radiation exposure.[24]

Shifting back to the subject of his talk, Nolan offered a final and rather ominous long-term assessment and prognosis of his own condition: "Data in reference to possible shortening of the life span or the nature of the terminal event are, as yet, unavailable."[25]

Optimistic Technological Determinism

In addition to the instrumentalist perspective, for which Nolan's exemplary medical career offers a useful illustration, Borgmann also identifies the determinist view as another notable, though less common, way of making sense of technology as a cultural force. The determinist perspective comes in two varieties, the optimistic and the pessimistic. The optimistic determinist views the development and application of new technologies as inevitable and as a net good for society. "If you are an optimistic determinist," says Borgmann, "you welcome the problems and the blessings of technology, and you will warn critics and opponents that you can't stop technology."[26]

The views of *New York Times* journalist William L. Laurence represent a classic example of optimistic technological determinism. As discussed in Chapter 5, Laurence displayed an almost religious commitment to the bomb and to the advent of the nuclear age. A fundamentally determinist perspective allowed him to rationalize any misgivings he might have had about the destructive effects of nuclear weaponry. "As you look back at it," said Laurence in an interview, "you rationalize a thing like that. You are in it. You say it's one of the inevitables of history; there is nothing you can do about it to change it; it would happen anyway; there are forces in history that are set in motion, that somehow human beings become like automatons—they play the part but nevertheless it's a part written for them by some external force, which they are just playing out."[27] Later in the same interview, Laurence acknowledged that he was able to resist any feelings of compassion toward the Japanese victims of the bomb by reminding himself, "You had nothing to do with it. This determination, this destiny, has been decided on long ago by forces much greater than any human decision can make or influence."[28]

Optimistic determinists do not disregard the problems associated with technological innovations, but they see technological progress as, in the main, for the good. Any negative outcomes can be remedied by even newer technological solutions, the so-called technological fix. Most significantly, though, optimistic determinists view technological advancements as inevitable. Any resistance will ultimately be futile.

tech fix

While Laurence is an example of an optimistic determinist from the early nuclear age, Ray Kurzweil, Google's director of engineering, is a more contemporary example. Kurzweil is convinced that technology is on an accelerating self-determining path, such that by 2045 (exactly a century after Hiroshima and Nagasaki) we will reach the tipping point of singularity—that is, a point in our evolutionary process when artificial intelligence (AI) will surpass human intelligence. As an "optimistic futurist," he views this coming AI world not with fear and trepidation but as something to enthusiastically celebrate. According to Kurzweil, AI will perform great wonders and solve all of our problems, environmental, medical, and otherwise.

The accelerating development of this brave new world, according to Kurzweil, is not limited to the expanding intelligence of computers or robots. In addition, the new superintelligent machine will merge with the human, thus enabling humans to transcend the limits of our biological bodies and brains, to become transhuman, better than human. By merging with the machine, the argument goes, humans will benefit from the much-improved capacities of new information and genetic technologies. For example, the introduction of billions of microscopic nanobots in the human brain will "vastly extend human intelligence."[29] These nanobots, introduced into the capillaries of our brains, will enable the brain to connect to the cloud, which not only will make humans smarter, says Kurzweil; "We're going to be funnier, we're going to be better at music. We're going to be sexier."[30]

According to Kurzweil and other optimistic determinists, the synthesis of the virtual and the real will also open up new avenues for human self-expression and creativity. As more experiences "take place in virtual environments," humans will be less able to distinguish virtual reality from "real reality." As such, individuals will be offered a range of new opportunities for creative self-expression. For example, people will be able to choose "to be a different person both physically and emotionally," with such benefits as allowing your romantic partner "to select a different body for you than you might select for yourself (and vice versa)."[31]

Communications theorist Neil Postman once posed that for every new technology, we should ask the question, "What is the problem to which this technology is the solution?"[32] This provocative question is meant to underscore the extent to which so-called problems are often "discovered" only after a technology has been invented. Concerning the atom bomb, the original problem for the physicists who initiated the Manhattan Project was a fear that the Germans might get the bomb first. When that problem disappeared, the physicists—carried forward by the momentum of the project—continued to build. Only then did Japan, an anticipated costly land invasion, and the need to end the war quickly come into focus as the problems for which atomic technology was the solution.

Following Postman, we can ask, What are the problems to which new advances in bioengineering, nanotechnology, more intelligent computers, and robotics are the solutions? In reading Kurzweil, one gets the distinct impression that the fundamental problem is humanity itself. The human mind, body, emotions, and even spirituality are too slow, limited, constrained, and lacking in creativity and imagination. The measures against which Kurzweil and other optimistic determinists judge the limitations of humanity are themselves based on the values and criteria dictated by technique, by a distinctively technical world view and morality. It is only by operating within such a paradigm—along with the availability of these new technologies—that humanity comes to be viewed as a problem.

Pessimistic Technological Determinism

Like the optimistic determinist, the pessimistic determinist understands technology as "an encompassing and irresistible force." However, the pessimistic determinist, writes Borgmann, has a "darker view of technology," which he or she views as "a culturally and environmentally destructive force." Pessimistic determinists "reveal grave problems" about technology, but these are "usually swept under the rug."[33] The views expressed by physicists Robert Wilson and Frank Oppenheimer represent this type of determinism. That is, in looking back at the fervor with which the scientists continued to build the bomb in the spring of 1945, even after Germany had surrendered, Wilson and Oppenheimer could not quite comprehend why they so willingly and unquestioningly continued to move forward with the project. Using language similar to Laurence's, they claimed they saw themselves compelled as if by a force outside themselves, like mindless and ethically indifferent automatons.[34]

Robert Oppenheimer likewise spoke of a kind of technological determinism in an even broader cultural sense. He expressed this, most notably, in a remarkable letter to Haakon Chevalier, Oppie's close friend and associate from his Berkeley days, with whom he had a complicated and fraught relationship because of their shared communist entanglements. His relationship and conversations with Chevalier would become a central focus of Oppenheimer's devastating 1954 tribunal. On the day after the Hiroshima bomb, Chevalier wrote a warm letter to Oppie in which he noted Oppenheimer's "love of men" and thus imagined the possible regrets his friend was experiencing in having participated in such "a diabolical act in destroying them."[35]

On August 27, 1945, only eighteen days after the Nagasaki bomb, Oppenheimer wrote back to Chevalier and, though "heavy with misgivings," attempted to explain why he had participated in such an act. "This thing had to be done, Haakon," Oppenheimer pleaded. "It had to be brought to an open public fruition at a time when all over the world men craved peace as never before, were committed as never before both to technology as a way of life and thought and to the idea that no man is an island."[36] Oppenheimer's sociological insight offered here—that humans, at that moment in history, "were committed as never before . . . to technology as a way of life and thought"—represents a trenchant and pithy articulation of what the French sociologist Jacques Ellul refers to as technique in his important critique of the role of technology in modern society.

Ellulian Technique

In keeping with the reflections offered by Wilson and the Oppenheimers, Ellul writes of the deterministic quality of technology. That is, technology, once set in motion, becomes self-augmenting and difficult to resist. "Technique," according to Ellul, "has become the new and specific *milieu* in which man is required to exist." A defining feature of technique, then, is that it is "self-determinative" and acts "independently of all human intervention."[37] In Frankenstein-like fashion, it takes on a life of its own.

Importantly, part of the difficulty in saying no to technology rests in the social ubiquity of a technological mind-set. Technique is not limited to the machine, gadget, or device. It is an all-encompassing habitus, an "all-embracing consciousness."[38] Technique advances a world view that permeates society in such a way that the collective conscience is infused with, if not defined by, a technological ontology.[39] As Ellul puts it, "Modern man's state of mind is completely dominated by technical values." In keeping with Laurence's "nuclearism," Ellul sees modern humans approaching technology as "something possessing sacred character." As such, technique "is not solely an ensemble of material elements, but that which gives meaning and value to life."[40]

Ellul also directly and forcefully questions the instrumentalist view, even while acknowledging how common it has become for people to think about technology in such terms. "It is also held that technique could be directed toward that which is positive, constructive, enriching," writes Ellul, "omitting that which is negative, destructive, and impoverishing." Humans think that they can use technologies "in the direction of good and not of evil."[41] Ellul holds that such a view is naive and misguided. The good and bad of a technological innovation and its concomitant applications cannot be demarcated or compartmentalized as such.

He specifically highlights nuclear technology as a way to illustrate this point. Indeed, he identifies 1945 as the watershed year when technique became fully triumphant.[42] Nuclear technology, says Ellul, is received as a whole package. The military, medical, and energy-producing applications of atomic technology and all of their consequences—intended and unintended—are of a whole. They cannot be distinguished and separately applied. One cannot, for example, separate the benefits of nuclear energy from Chernobyl, Fukushima, and Three Mile Island, nor from the perennial difficulties of storing the thousands of tons of hazardous nuclear waste generated each year. Such distinctions, writes Ellul, "are completely invalid and show only that he who makes them has understood nothing of the technical phenomenon. Its parts are ontologically tied together; in it, use is inseparable from being."[43]

On this latter point, recall Oppenheimer's observation that the decision to use the bomb "was implicit in the project."[44] Or as Furman communicated to Samuel Goudsmit during the Alsos Project, "You understand, Sam, if we have such a weapon, we are going to use it."[45] That the bomb existed meant that it would be used. Ellul elaborates on this point: "Finding himself with so powerful an instrument, [the possessor] is led to use it. Why? Because everything which is technique is necessarily used as soon as it is available, without distinction of good or evil. This is the principle law of our age. We may quote here Jacques Soustelle's well-known remark of May 1960, in reference to the atomic bomb. It expresses the deep feeling of us all: 'Since it was possible, it was necessary.' Really a master phrase for all technical evolution."[46]

Concerning what Ellul refers to as "monism" (the inseparability of technology's beneficial and destructive features), when Nolan sought to use nuclear technology for the good of providing better medical care, on one level, he was successful. Or as Borgmann puts it, there is "obviously some merit" to this perspective. However, the good achieved, as such, cannot be understood as independent from the larger technological phenomenon, nor from the other uses made of nuclear technology. Indeed, at the end of his Mexico City lecture, Nolan took a parting shot at what he presciently anticipated to be emerging trends in the field of medicine. He warned against the move toward a more rationalized and scientifically informed method of collecting and statistically assessing medical data for the purposes of recommending methods of patient care. He worried that this development—clearly constitutive of a technological ontology—would problematically alter the nature, scope, and financing of medical treatment.

Nolan worried that this "more effective system" of "socio-economic innovations" would "de-humanize the future of individual vendors of the product," which would ultimately move toward "stereotypy and lack of latitude" and would "stifle" doctors' "zest and enthusiasm for their calling."[47] With the subsequent movement in the next several decades toward more managed care, increasingly influential actuarial interventions and oversight, and the introduction of a range of new medical technologies, Nolan's concerns about these additional "risks and hazards thereof" have surely been realized and have indeed resulted in the kind of dehumanizing consequences—for both doctors and patients—that he warned against. The important point here is that the very mind-set and corresponding processes to which Nolan objected were part and parcel of the larger systemic and cultural dominance of technique, a development to which the medical profession was not immune.

In a later work, Ellul writes of the important role of technological systems—that is, the large-scale institutions that assume a distinctively technological character and work in a coordinated fashion to advance technique. Thomas Hughes, a prominent historian of technology, emphasizes a similar theme in his book *American Genesis.* Hughes points to the considerable influence of coordinated bureaucratic systems of industry, military, government, and universities working together to develop massive technological projects that then take on a determinative force or momentum, which becomes virtually irresistible. Hughes identifies the Manhattan Project as the prototype of a large-scale "military-industrial-university" complex that built and established an enormous and expensive system, which moved forward, even against those inclined to resist it, with a forceful "technological momentum."[48]

Princeton physicist Freeman Dyson identifies this feature of the Manhattan Project as the reason that military and scientific personnel continued to build and then ultimately use the bomb, in spite of the reservations and objections of some of the physicists on the project. Dyson writes, "Why did the bomb get dropped on the people at Hiroshima? I would say that it's almost inevitable that it would have happened, simply because all of the bureaucratic apparatus existed by that time to do it. The Air Force was ready and waiting at that time. They had prepared big airfields at Tinian and in the Pacific from which you could operate. The whole machinery was ready. The President would have to have been a man of iron will to put a stop to it."[49] Thus, Dyson acknowledges the determinative power of technique and identifies the role that a large, coordinated, forceful system played in moving the project forward. Also in keeping with Ellul's understanding of technique, Dyson recognizes the dominance of a technological ontology, which influenced human thinking, resulting in a sort of "technical arrogance that overcomes people when they see what they can do with their minds."[50]

In the Shadow of Manhattan

For both Ellul and Hughes, the Manhattan Project is only one example of a broader social phenomenon. However, it is so significant an example that it represents an archetype for which to think about the development and application of new and emerging technologies more generally. Bill Joy makes just this point in his much-discussed 2000 *Wired* article "Why the Future Doesn't Need Us." Joy, one of the cofounders of Sun Microsystems and an early pioneer in computer technology (thus, no Luddite), became alarmed by what he saw emerging on the horizon with the ever-expanding and ever-accelerating advancements in nanotechnology, genetic engineering, and robotics.

Like the Manhattan Project physicists, Joy acknowledges the excitement and intoxicating effect of scientific exploration and experimentation and realizes that, while scientists are absorbed in the discovery process, the potential dangers of their discoveries rarely enter into the calculus. Recall Oppenheimer's statement offered during his 1954 security tribunal, "When you see something that is technically sweet, you go ahead and do it and you argue about what to do about it only after you have had your technical success."[51] Joy sees this as a common and dangerous attitude among scientists and technologists; caught up "in the rapture of discovery and innovation," technological innovators often fail "to understand the consequences of our inventions."[52]

Dyson similarly observes the process by which scientists, captivated by the thrill of discovery, rarely take the time to consider what might be the harmful outcomes of their innovations. "When something is technically sweet it is like climbing a mountain. It beckons you and you climb it just because it's there. And you only think about the consequences afterward." Dyson also, in essence, points to the Ellulian understanding of "self-augmentation"—that is, once discovered, technology assumes "a self-generating process" in which "technique generates itself."[53] While pursuing their technically sweet discoveries, says Dyson, scientists fail to "notice that the progress to newer and more powerful technologies can take on a life of its own."[54]

Joy notes that the Manhattan Project continued to progress even "after the initial impetus had been removed." Why? In keeping with explanations offered by Ellul, Hughes, and Dyson, Joy points to the "momentum that had built up" as the "likely reason the project continued."[55] With advancements in genetic engineering, nanotechnology, and robotics, Joy sees the same sort of momentum and the same basic technological arrogance among scientists and technologists today. Technological innovators are still pursuing with great enthusiasm the "technically sweet," and they still don't stop to consider what might be the long-term consequences of the development and use of these new technologies. Only this time, there is not a long and costly world war to justify such developments. Rather, writes Joy, "we are driven, instead, by our habits, our desires, our economic system, and our competitive need to know."[56]

Concerning the relationship between nuclear technology and the many technological innovations that have developed since, not only do we find a similar mind-set among scientists and technologists, but many of the technologies that permeate society today are themselves a direct outgrowth of the discovery and use of the atom bomb. The internet, GPS, drones, laser technology, and even the American interstate system all stem at least in part from efforts to develop, monitor, and test nuclear bombs and to prepare for a possible nuclear conflict.[57] Moreover, the large, coordinated systems of the military, corporate industry, and universities, discussed by Ellul and Hughes, continue to work together to advance and promulgate applications of these technologies. Anthropologist Joseph Masco does not overstate matters when he says, "America in the twenty-first century remains a society built around, and to a large extent, through the bomb."[58]

The application and the dramatic social consequences of these and other new technologies illustrate Ellul's important challenge to the instrumentalist view. Indeed, one sees in the discovery and use of nuclear-engendered technologies many of the insights offered by Ellul. For example, recent history reveals that once new devices are discovered, they are necessarily put to use. Once put to use, the technologies take on a life of their own, often fostering the development of even newer technologies, which result in new problems. "Every technique implies unforeseeable effects," says Ellul.[59] In response to these unforeseeable effects, we look to new technologies for a solution, and so it goes. Again, the proliferation of technique cannot be understood as neutral. That is, the ostensibly positive applications cannot be disaggregated from their ill effects. In Ellul's words, "Pernicious effects are inseparable from favorable effects."[60]

The smartphone, the internet, and social media applications may connect more people, give faster access to more information, and allow for the dissemination of a greater variety of world views and perspectives, but they also have been found to increase loneliness and to decrease capacities to remember, pay attention, reason, be patient, read deeply, and write well.[61] Moreover, rather than exposing people to a range of different perspectives, widespread use of communication technologies has been found to discourage "bridging social capital" and to encourage the reinforcement of already entrenched views, what some have referred to as "cyberbalkanization" or the "echo chamber" effect.[62]

Social media was once celebrated for the positive role it played in fostering such ostensibly democratic movements as the Arab Spring. Yet the same tools have also been used in the consequential manipulation of the American electoral system by a foreign entity and, more generally, have made it increasingly difficult for citizens to accurately discern what is real and what is "fake news," the same process of mixing the virtual with the real that Kurzweil celebrates. Moreover, the long-term success of achieving peace and democratic governance in the Middle East, as aided by social media communications, can now be viewed as questionable at best.

In light of some of these troubling outcomes, Tim Berners-Lee, the inventor of the World Wide Web, now has serious regrets about what he helped set in motion more than thirty years ago—an invention, incidentally, that was originally aimed at helping nuclear scientists share data among themselves.[63] Berners-Lee is dismayed at the dysfunctions he sees in the current state of his communications innovation, problems that include "state-sponsored hacking[,] . . . the viral spread of misinformation," and the "outraged and polarized tone and quality of online discourse."[64] During a March 2019 meeting of the Web Foundation, he offered a summary assessment of the web that represents a trenchant illustration of Ellulian monism. "And while the web has created opportunity, given marginalized groups a voice, and made our daily lives easier," Berners-Lee stated, "it has also created opportunity for scammers, given voice to those who spread hatred, and made all kinds of crime easier to commit."[65]

In a 2018 interview he gave with *Vanity Fair,* the ominous shadow of the Manhattan Project was not far from view. During the interview,

Berners-Lee remorsefully reflected on the role of Russian hackers in influencing the 2016 elections, as well as the revelations about the monopolistic data-sharing and surveillance practices from which Google, Facebook, and Amazon have amassed enormous profits. Like Oppenheimer, and invoking his words, Berners-Lee now worries "that his invention could become . . . a destroyer of worlds." "I was devastated," said Berners-Lee. "The mushroom cloud was unfolding before his very eyes," observed *Vanity Fair* reporter Katrina Brooker.[66]

Just as, after the end of World War II, the Manhattan Project scientists sought to rein in the spread of their creation through the scientists' movement and through efforts to establish some kind of international controls, Berners-Lee is determined to do something about the problems he helped to unleash. In keeping with Ellul's characterization of technique, however, the proposed solutions to the problems themselves are wholly technological in quality. In terms of the disorders, Berners-Lee says, "we should see them as bugs: problems with existing code and software systems that have been created by people—and can be fixed by people." He proposes a new web-based platform called Solid that he hopes will decentralize, democratize, and offer greater privacy protections for users.[67] Should Solid, or something like it, be implemented, we can anticipate new problems for which further technological solutions will no doubt be proposed to fix them.

The same sort of monism is evident in the widespread use of another technology generated by the nuclear age. GPS may make elements of travel easier, but it has also resulted in a range of problems, including putting greater distance between humans and nature, making it more difficult to remember directions, and rendering travelers less capable of interpreting and gauging their physical surroundings. In addition to "shrinking our cognitive maps," reliance on GPS has encouraged a misguided trust in the wisdom of the device and has resulted in enough tragic outcomes that park rangers have invented a new phrase, "death by GPS."[68] Like other technologies, GPS helps to shape a certain kind of consciousness within a technological society, or, as Greg Milner puts it, GPS "may fundamentally change us as humans."[69]

New surveillance technologies have also come with both beneficial and pernicious effects. GPS, closed-circuit television cameras, facial recognition technology, drones, dash cams, and body cameras—not to mention the millions of megabytes of data people willingly pour into cyberspace each day through the use of Facebook, Instagram, LinkedIn, Twitter, and Snapchat—

give parents, teachers, and law enforcement officers unprecedented monitoring and security capacities. Police can now investigate criminal activity and solve difficult crimes in ways once viewed as inconceivable. Along with advances in, and widespread use of, information technology, such biological interventions as urine testing and DNA sampling have also aided law enforcement efforts. The use of GEDmatch to catch the Golden State Killer in California is just one example of the benefits of DNA technology in cracking long-unsolved crimes.

Yet the broad extension of surveillance and monitoring practices can make George Orwell's Big Brother society seem innocuous and traditional notions of privacy almost quaint. The sharing of data about individuals—often including information that people knowingly and uncritically themselves provide—has been used not only for security and law enforcement purposes but even more extensively for commercial and marketing ends. The degree to which users of these technologies are happy to forsake privacy for the convenience of using such sites as Amazon and Facebook clearly has limits, evident, for example, in the outcry that followed Cambridge Analytica's harvesting of data from Facebook during the 2016 elections. People are also bothered when they attend a private party and unflattering images show up in places like YouTube or Instagram or when individuals receive pop-up advertisements on their computer screens suspiciously related to their online purchases or searches. The widespread use of these new technologies seriously threatens traditional understandings of privacy.

In the area of biotechnology, the genetic modification (GM) of plants became widespread in the United States with virtually no public discussion of the practice, whereas in Europe there has been greater resistance. With more than 80 percent of corn and more than 90 percent of soybean crops genetically modified in the United States, it is practically impossible to resist consumption of these products, particularly with the success that agribusiness industries have achieved in preventing the labeling of GM foods. Proponents argue that GM products make food less expensive, easier to transport, better tasting, and available to a greater number of people. Critics point to the long-term consequences that resulted from other biotechnological innovations, such as the negative effects of DDT and the overuse (and subsequent ineffectiveness) of some antibiotics—which only became realized over time—as just one reason to be concerned about the extended effects of GM foods.

A further indicator of the relationship between the Manhattan Project and new bioengineering practices is that some of the same industrial actors who participated in the large-scale nuclear production systems, discussed by Ellul and Hughes, are also major players in the world of agribusiness—and, in both cases, these industries have collaborated with government and universities. Monsanto, for example, helped in the production of polonium for use in making both plutonium and uranium, and eventually took over the Clinton lab at Oak Ridge during the early nuclear age. Monsanto, of course, has also been a major player in the production, patenting, and global marketing of GM food products.

The genetic engineering of humans is of even greater consequence. As with the defenders of the genetic modification of crops, advocates for the bioengineering of humans argue that new forms of genetic editing are continuous with previous practices. The genetic modification of plants and animals, they argue, is really no different from previous selective breeding practices. So with humans, they say, genetic enhancements are really no different from the "hyperparenting" practices employed by parents to give their children a competitive edge in today's meritocracy. Moreover, it is argued further, a range of biomedical interventions—including human growth hormones, steroids, and psychotropic drugs—are now widely used not only to treat people with certain mental and physical deficiencies but also to enhance human performance.

A similar sort of continuity argument has been offered to justify use of the atom bombs in Japan. In defending the bombing of Hiroshima and Nagasaki, supporters of the dominant narrative observe that we were already engaged in a total war, such that the effects of firebombing places like Dresden and Tokyo (where more than one hundred thousand Japanese, mostly civilian, were killed) with conventional weapons were not substantively different from the destructive effects of the atom bombs. Stafford Warren, recall, offered this type of argument in defense of the Hiroshima and Nagasaki bombings, even going so far as to argue that the nuclear bombs were comparatively more merciful.

One could argue, however, that the similarities between these two forms of warfare, rather than justifying both, call into question the morality of total war itself, a point Father John Siemes strongly intimated in his discussion of Hiroshima, which was collected and translated by the Joint Commission. Michael Sandel suggests the same concerning the genetic enhancement of humans. Perhaps the ostensible continuity between recent child-rearing practices and new genetic enhancements, rather than justifying the latter, actually should lead us to question the validity of contemporary "hyperparenting" behaviors.[70]

Critics also worry that human genetic manipulations will result in a new eugenics, a new competitive arms race to improve the human mind and body, and a Frankenstein-like situation in which humans lose control of their genetically improved creations. Though there are strong voices of caution in the scientific and medical worlds concerning these practices, certain developments—including the successful implantation of a fiber-optic sensor in a man's brain to enable him to see colors and the announcement by Chinese scientist He Jiankui that he had edited the genes of two recently born twin girls—heighten the worries of some while they enliven and confirm the predictions and aspirations of Kurzweil and other optimistic determinists.[71]

As is reflected in the title of his article, Joy worries for the future. While the Manhattan Project provides helpful lessons about the dangers of technological momentum and its consequences, Joy fears that these lessons have gone unheeded. "We should have learned a lesson from the making of the first atomic bomb and the resulting arms race," says Joy. "We didn't do well then, and the parallels to our current situation are troubling." Indeed, Joy forebodingly anticipates that what lies ahead is a new arms race in the development of genetics, nanotechnology, and robotics.[72] Unlike nuclear technology, Joy adds, the new technologies are self-replicating and thus will be even more difficult to control.

A provocative fictional consideration of the connections between the Manhattan Project and new AI technology is found in Alex Garland's 2015 film, *Ex Machina.* In the film, an AI technologist named Nathan is in the process of developing sophisticated and high-functioning robots, which are on the threshold of achieving singularity. An unwitting programmer named Caleb is "randomly" selected by Nathan to interact with his most recent and advanced robotic creation, Ava, in a sort of Turing test. When Caleb finally realizes what Nathan is up to, he quietly quotes Oppenheimer's words uttered (or thought) in the moments after the Trinity test, "I have become death, the destroyer of worlds." Another indication of the perceived relevance of the Manhattan Project to new AI technologies comes from a 1980s song included in the film's soundtrack, "Enola Gay," by the British band

OMD (Orchestral Manoeuvres in the Dark). Among the song's lyrics are the following: "Enola Gay, is mother proud of little boy today? Oho, this kiss you give, it's never ever gonna fade away."

Freeman Dyson observes, concerning the development and use of the bomb, that in the face of the formidable technological momentum at play, "no one had the courage or the foresight to say no." Joy fears that the same lack of courage, failure to consider the consequences, and amnesia regarding lessons from the past persist today. In other words, the long shadow of the Manhattan Project, the salient metaphor of delivering Little Boy, is still with us. As in OMD's lyrics, the kiss it gives has yet to fade away.

Technique and the Competing Narratives

We have considered the competing narratives invoked to make sense of the bomb. Proponents of the dominant narrative generally hold that the bomb was necessary and that its use ended the war and saved thousands of American (and Japanese) lives. Defenders of the counternarrative argue that the bomb was not necessary, that Japan was prepared to surrender and would have done so sometime in the fall of 1945, without either a land invasion or the dropping of the bombs. Supporters of the counternarrative also contend that American officials were less concerned about ending World War II than they were with establishing an early advantageous position in the Cold War. That is, the bombs had more to do with the Soviet Union than with Japan.

How does the matter of technique, or even more specifically, "technological momentum," intersect with this ongoing debate? On one level, a deeper understanding of technique ascribes less human agency to the decision. Recall Leslie Groves's observation that Harry S. Truman did not really make a decision, that he was like "a little boy on a toboggan." Ferenc Szasz, in his excellent book on the Trinity test, notes that technological momentum essentially made the decision for Truman. Szasz goes so far as to argue, "Truman did not really make any 'decision.' Instead, the momentum of the Manhattan Project made the decision for him."[73]

While Truman claimed never to regret his "decision," a diary entry—which was not discovered until 1979—suggests that he had more misgivings than he was ever willing to admit publicly. On the night after learning about the success of the Trinity test, Truman entered into his diary, "I hope for some sort of peace—but I fear that machines are ahead of morals by some centuries and when morals catch up, perhaps there'll be no reason for any of it. I hope not. But we are only termites on a planet and maybe when we bore too deeply into the planet there'll [be] a reckoning—who knows?"[74] Szasz argues that too much attention has been given to the individual motives and decision-making powers of such actors as Truman, Groves, and Henry Stimson, thus overshadowing the explanatory significance of "technological momentum." Does this then suggest that human agency has no role? Is technological determinism so powerful as to deny any human resistance? Szasz proposes an interpretive paradigm that stands somewhere between "the heresy that man has no control over his destiny, on one hand, and that man has complete control on the other."[75] Though often portrayed as a pessimistic technological determinist, Ellul would agree with Szasz on this point and likewise argues for a more dialectical understanding of the relationship between human agency and deterministic forces.

Human Freedom and the Device Paradigm

Ellul denies being a determinist. Rather, he argues that recognizing the deterministic quality of technique is the first step toward realizing human freedom. Modern humans cannot act with freedom unless they first recognize and appreciate the extent to which they live in a technological milieu. If the very criteria we commonly employ to make decisions are themselves shaped and determined by technique, then we are not in a position to act with freedom. Sociologist Peter Berger makes a similar point. In his discussion of the sociological imagination, he compares humans to marionettes. Just as the puppeteer controls the actions of the puppet—through the artful manipulation of the attached strings—so society controls and determines human action, behavior, and thoughts.[76]

However, for Berger, as for Ellul, because we are humans and not marionettes, we can look up, see, measure, and understand the size, strength, and direction of the strings that guide us. Such recognition and understanding are the necessary first step toward acting with freedom against these determining forces. As long as we remain in ignorance of the determinative qualities of technique, says Ellul, genuine freedom is not possible. Rather, humans unwittingly "accept a condition of slavery." "It is only by making men conscious to what degree they have become slaves . . . that there is any hope of regaining liberty," and this "by asserting themselves, perhaps at the cost of much sacrifice, over the Technique which has come to dominate them."[77]

In Borgmann's final category for making sense of technology as a cultural force, he proposes an understanding that we live in a "device paradigm." According to Borgmann, the overarching presence and pressure of this paradigm must be recognized. Borgmann would agree with Ellul that presently the ubiquity and potency of this paradigm are not appreciated, certainly not in the realm of politics. Neither political party in the United States, says Borgmann, "has been willing to recognize and question technology as a cultural force."[78] Indeed, as sociologist Robert Wuthnow argues, political actors invoke America's technological prowess as a means of providing legitimacy to the modern state and are thus complicit in sustaining, if not advancing, technique.[79]

Borgmann recommends that, in response to a fuller acknowledgment of a life dominated by technique, we more fully engage with what he calls "focal things" and "focal practices," such as the shared, home-cooked family meal, the flow realized through a long walk in the woods, or playing a musical instrument, in order to act against the consequences of living in a technological society. A greater concentration on focal things and practices within what he calls "final communities" will result in the development of non–technologically determined life habits, the communal practice of which leads to the carving out of spaces that function in liberating contradistinction to the device paradigm.[80]

For both Ellul and Borgmann, the important first step, though, is less prescriptive than it is descriptive. Particularly for Ellul, his major intellectual contribution has been to describe well the overarching, penetrating, and ubiquitous quality of technique in modern society. Interestingly, Ellul self-consciously understands his diagnostic position, as such, to be like that of a physician or physicist who, like my grandfather in his 1971 lecture, "is describing a group situation in which he is himself involved," including being "exposed to radioactivity." In advancing such an analysis, "the mind may remain cold and lucid, and the method objective," but there is for Ellul, and one senses there was for Nolan as well, "a profound tension of the whole being."[81] Ellul elaborates on this sociologist-as-physician metaphor: "Before a remedy can be found, it is first necessary to make a detailed study of the disease and the patient, to do laboratory research, and to isolate the virus. It is necessary to establish criteria that will make it possible to recognize the disease when it occurs, and to describe the patient's symptoms at each stage of his illness. This preliminary work is indispensable for eventual discovery and application of a remedy."[82]

While Ellul himself does not offer a remedy to the condition he so thoroughly diagnoses, he does not deny the possibility of resistance, of human agency, of acting with freedom in light of a deeper understanding of the prevailing social condition. However, he underscores that a step toward freedom, as such, is only possible after one has become fully aware of the disorder. Such awareness, in other words, enables the possibility of freedom. "The very fact that man can see, measure, and analyze the determinisms that press on him," writes Ellul, "means that he can face them and, by so doing, act as a free man."[83] Berger, in his discussion of the puppet metaphor, says the same thing: "Unlike puppets we have the possibility of stopping in our movements, looking up and perceiving the machinery by which we have been moved. In this act lies the first step toward freedom."[84]

Ellul writes further that to deny the possibility of such resistance is actually to aid in the advancement of technological determinism: "If man does not pull himself together and assert himself . . . then things will go the way I describe"—that is, "determinants will be transformed into inevitabilities."[85] Borgmann recommends concentration on focal things and focal practices as one way of recognizing and resisting the technological milieu or the device paradigm. Ellul advises more broadly and abstractly that "each of us, in his own life, must seek ways of resisting and transcending technological determinants. Each man must make this effort in every area of life, in his profession and in his social, religious, and family relationships."[86]

In looking back at the early years of the nuclear age, one can imagine any number of instances when the course of history may have been very different had certain acts of resistance been pursued. What if officials had allowed Leo Szilard's petition to reach Truman in late July or early August 1945? What if Oppenheimer had been more open to the concerns expressed by Robert Wilson and other physicists after it was discovered that Germany did not have a bomb? What if Albert Einstein and Szilard's initial letter had never been written or had never reached Franklin D. Roosevelt? As illustrated in the life and actions of Joseph Rotblat, it was possible to say no, to walk away. When Manhattan Project personnel explored the possibility of using radiation as a weapon (that is, independent of a nuclear explosion), it was actually Groves who helped to table such an option.[87] Could he not have done the same with the bomb?

While the dominance of technique and the force of technological momentum must be more deeply appreciated, both Berger and Ellul recognize that technological determinants are only one part of the sociological equation. "We must not think of the problem in terms of a choice between being determined and being free," writes Ellul. "We must look at it dialectically, and say that man is indeed determined, but that it is open to him to overcome necessity, and that this *act* is freedom."[88]

In his sociologist-as-physician metaphor, Ellul sees himself as a diagnostician, offering a careful and full assessment of the technological society. However, unlike the sociologist, or at least a sociologist of an Ellulian ilk, a medical physician like Nolan does prescribe a treatment. Regardless of the efficacy of the treatment, the doctor is cognizant of a variety of contingencies, human vagaries, and outcomes. Reflecting on these possible outcomes, Ellul considers the manner in which the doctor "recognizes that God may work a miracle, that the patient may have an unexpected constitutional reaction, or that the patient . . . may die unexpectedly of a heart attack."[89] Ellul's last possibility mentioned here, as we will see, provides an interesting final connection between Ellul (the sociologist as physician) and Nolan (the physician as ironic keynote speaker), in that it curiously points to the "nature of the terminal event" for which, in Nolan's 1971 lecture, the data were "as yet, unavailable."[90]

9

1983

The most lionized of the alumni was former Captain James F. Nolan, M.D., the obstetrician who had delivered so many of the scientists' children on the mesa during the war.

—Peter Wyden, *Day One*

Nineteen eighty-three was an important year. The Cold War was at its zenith. In 1983, the United States had a stockpile of 23,305 nuclear weapons and the Soviet Union had 35,804. By this time, four other countries—the United Kingdom, France, China, and Israel—also possessed nuclear weapons. There existed more than 60,000 nuclear warheads worldwide.[1] Included in these arsenals were weapons, notably the hydrogen or thermonuclear bomb, that were as much as one thousand times more powerful than those dropped on Japan. Nineteen eighty-three was also the year in which President Ronald Reagan first used the term *evil empire* to describe the Soviet Union and in which he announced his plans for the new Strategic Defense Initiative (SDI), or the third wave of nuclear technology, a program sometimes disparagingly referred to as the Star Wars initiative.

It was also the year when the television movie *The Day After* was shown, a film that drew more than one hundred million viewers in 38.5 million households, becoming television's highest-rated movie in history. Set in Lawrence, Kansas, *The Day After* depicts a fictional full-scale nuclear war between the United States and the Soviet Union, giving particular and graphic attention to the effects of nuclear radiation. Reagan previewed the film in the month before its November 20 airing on ABC. He was moved by the film and, after watching it, entered into his diary, "It is powerfully done—all $7 million worth. It's very effective and left me greatly depressed."[2] Though he saw it as a validation of his administration's deterrence policy, the movie was reportedly one factor that led to the Intermediate-Range

Nuclear Forces Treaty signed by Reagan and Soviet president Mikhail Gorbachev in 1987. In a 1986 meeting leading up to the treaty, the Reagan administration sent a telegram to the film's director stating, "Don't think your film didn't have any part of this, because it did."[3]

Also in 1983, as though to offer a clear response to Father John Siemes's plea from 1945, "When will our moralists give us a clear answer to this question?" the US National Conference of Catholic Bishops issued a pastoral letter. In it they stated plainly that "it is never permitted" to direct weapons, nuclear or otherwise, to "the indiscriminate destruction of whole cities or vast areas with their populations" and that the "intentional killing of innocent civilians or non-combatants is always wrong." In light of this position, the US bishops viewed it as necessary "for our country to express profound sorrow over the atomic bombing of 1945." In the absence of such sorrow, the letter added, there would be "no possibility of finding a way to repudiate future use of nuclear weapons."[4]

Nineteenth eighty-three was also the year when the Marshall Islanders voted in favor of the Compact of Free Association, an important step toward full sovereignty, self-governance, and independence from the United States, but a move that also released the American government from responsibility for handling the long-term consequences of nuclear testing in the region. It was the year when John Smitherman, the navy enlisted man who had contracted multiple forms of cancer following Operation Crossroads, died. And it was the year when ninety thousand feet of colored film taken by a US military camera crew in Japan in early 1946, including graphic shots of *hibakusha* in Nagasaki and Hiroshima, finally became available for public viewing after decades of having been suppressed and hidden.[5]

The Fortieth-Anniversary Reunion

Nineteen eighty-three also marked the fortieth anniversary of the start of work at Los Alamos. As such, plans were set in motion for a reunion to be held in Los Alamos in April 1983. Those who had worked on the mesa beginning in the spring of 1943 were invited to participate, including James F. Nolan. More than one hundred Los Alamos alumni, including Nolan, traveled to Los Alamos for the reunion, which was covered in a CBS documentary by Bill Moyers. Interviews with the famous physicists in attendance conveyed a palpable sense of regret. On the drive up the winding

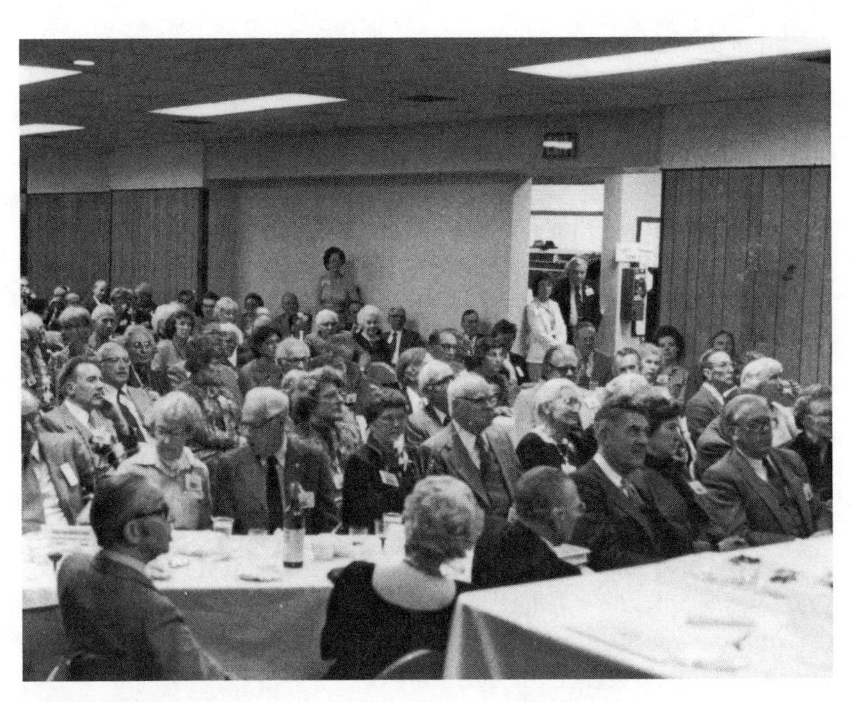

Nolan (standing in doorway under exit sign) attending the fortieth-anniversary reunion in April 1983 at Los Alamos.

road to the mesa, for example, Moyers asked Isidor Rabi how he felt about Los Alamos, returning to it after all these years. Rabi replied, "Sorrow that the place still exists." He added, as they approached the famous lab, which was still developing ever more powerful and sophisticated nuclear weapons at the time, "It's an abomination. . . . We should have put that thing to rest thirty years ago at least."[6]

During one of the gatherings at Fuller Lodge, the Nobel Prize–winning German physicist Hans Bethe stated that while he was happy to see his old friends, he had serious regrets about what had been done at the site. "We did a terrible job here. . . . What we produced is a great threat to the world."[7] In a retrospective article published two years later, he wrote of the "technological imperative" that had compelled the arms race forward. In terms strikingly Ellulian in character, Bethe wrote of the process by which each new innovation, from the hydrogen bomb, to intercontinental ballistic missiles, to antiballistic missiles, to multiple independently targetable reentry vehicles, to the new SDI or Star Wars initiative, was advanced by a perceived "technological imperative," which was "followed without regard for the consequences." He encouraged politicians to "show restraint" and to "not lightly follow the technological imperative."[8]

The Austrian-born theoretical physicist Victor Weisskopf gave a lecture at the reunion in which he, like Bethe, acknowledged the joy of seeing old friends and remembering the exciting years they had shared together on the Hill. Yet he also expressed profound disappointment that "the result of our work" had "developed into the greatest danger that humankind has ever faced," a danger that "threatens more and more to destroy everything on Earth that we consider worth living for." In terms of the ever-escalating arms race, Weisskopf anticipated that "future generations, if there are any, will regard this as a virulent case of collective mental disease." In keeping with the Ellulian critique of the "unforeseeable effects" of "technique," Weisskopf lamented, "Forty years ago we meant so well. At that time we did not foresee the consequences of our work."[9] Given all that had happened since 1943, Weisskopf acknowledged the "special duty" of the scientists to come to terms with the fact that their invention had resulted in "the unintended cause of the world's tragic predicament."[10]

In sympathy with Weisskopf's lament was a group of demonstrators who held a silent vigil outside the buildings where the reunion took place. Among the demonstrators was a scientist who had previously worked in the lab. During his lecture, Weisskopf advised his fellow scientists, "Do not condemn the demonstrators in front of our building. Some of their slogans may be simplistic, but they express the revulsion of the people against the nuclear arms race."[11] Another anti-nukes protest would take place two months later in Albuquerque. Included among the demonstrators at this event was Peter Oppenheimer, the son of the famous physicist who ran the Los Alamos lab during the war.[12]

The Olum Petition

Another physicist who attended the fortieth-anniversary reunion was Paul Olum. Recruited to Los Alamos when he was twenty-four years old, Olum had been a graduate student in physics and math at Princeton University. On the Hill, he worked with Weisskopf in the theoretical physics group. Olum had been a little nervous and unsure about attending the reunion. Like many of the other scientists, he felt badly about what had become of their innovation and was uncertain as to what they were meant to celebrate at the gathering. In reflecting on his time on the Hill, like both Robert Wilson and Frank Oppenheimer, Olum had difficulty making sense of why the scientists were carried forward with the project in the spring and summer of 1945 even after learning of Germany's defeat.

"When V.E. Day, victory in Europe, came in the spring of 1945," Olum observed, "we were quite certain the Japanese had no bomb. The Japanese had hardly gotten anywhere toward building a bomb, and there was no belief they possibly could have one. Why didn't we all stop and walk off the project then? We no longer needed what we had been trying so hard to achieve. We didn't have to worry about somebody else getting it first."[13] In an attempt to answer his own question, Olum—like other Manhattan Project scientists—acknowledged the intoxicating effect of scientific discovery and the technological momentum that carried the physicists forward. Olum recollected, "When you are involved in something like that . . . it just is hard to stop. You are totally caught up in it." He added, "I think very few of us stopped to think on V.E. Day that the justification we would have given for working on the bomb in the first place was no longer there."[14]

In addition to the remorse he felt about their work, Olum had also become a strong supporter of the nuclear freeze movement. Given this disposition, it is understandable why he was hesitant to attend the event. Therefore, before accepting his invitation, he contacted several of his physicist friends, including Bethe, Weisskopf, and Wilson, to discuss his concerns. They were in sympathy with his general sentiments and encouraged him to somehow address his apprehensions at the reunion. Subsequently, Olum drafted a petition letter calling for a "mutually agreed upon reduction of nuclear armaments" between the United States and the Soviet Union, and advocating for "the ultimate goal of the total elimination of such weapons."[15]

The letter acknowledged the Manhattan Project scientists' "special sense of responsibility" and asserted, "We are appalled at the present level of the nuclear armaments of the nations of the world and we are profoundly frightened for the future of humanity."[16] Olum carried the letter with him to the reunion, but the directors of the Los Alamos lab would not allow him to make an announcement about it from the podium. Instead, he and sympathetic friends personally handed the petition around during the course of the reunion and at the final banquet. It was eventually signed by seventy scientists, including five Nobel Prize winners—Bethe, Owen Chamberlain,

Richard Feynman, Ed McMillan, and Emilio Segrè—along with other such scientific luminaries as Wilson, Weisskopf, and Robert Serber.

The same number of scientists had signed Leo Szilard's petition back in 1945. Interestingly, there is not a single instance of a scientist having signed both petitions, which is not surprising given Oppenheimer's opposition to Szilard's petition when copies of it showed up in Los Alamos in 1945.[17] The seventy who signed the 1983 petition were an entirely new group of concerned scientists. Among those presented with the petition during the reunion's final banquet was Edward Teller. Not surprisingly, the father of the H-bomb, who was also on board with President Reagan's new SDI, refused to sign. When a signature was requested of Teller a second time, he banged the table and "warned that such a petition might mean war."[18] Isidor Rabi also didn't sign the petition, though not out of disagreement with the spirit of the letter, but because he found the language and purpose to be too vaguely stated. James F. Nolan was also among those who did not sign the petition.

Five Good Years Left

In the years leading up to the reunion, as the twilight of Nolan's medical career approached, he received a number of accolades for his impressive achievements in the field of gynecological oncology. In October 1976, for example, the Alumni Association of California Hospital threw a testimonial dinner for Nolan, which was attended by more than one hundred friends and associates, many of whom had trained under Nolan as residents or fellows at the Southern California Cancer Center. Several colleagues gave talks on different aspects of Nolan's illustrious career, including Louis Hempelmann, who spoke on the "war years." At the time, Hempelmann was the head of the Radiation Department at the University of Rochester.

Approximately eighteen months after the testimonial dinner, Ann Nolan died at the age of sixty-four from complications associated with her alcoholism. Karen Nolan remembers walking on the beach with her depressed father-in-law in the summer following my grandmother's death. Still mourning the loss of his wife, Nolan soberly and presciently stated that he thought he had about five good years left. A year later, he married Jane Davis Lamb, a woman with whom he and Ann had been friends since their St. Louis days. All three had attended the John Burroughs School together. In a September 1945 letter Ann Nolan sent to her husband while he was in

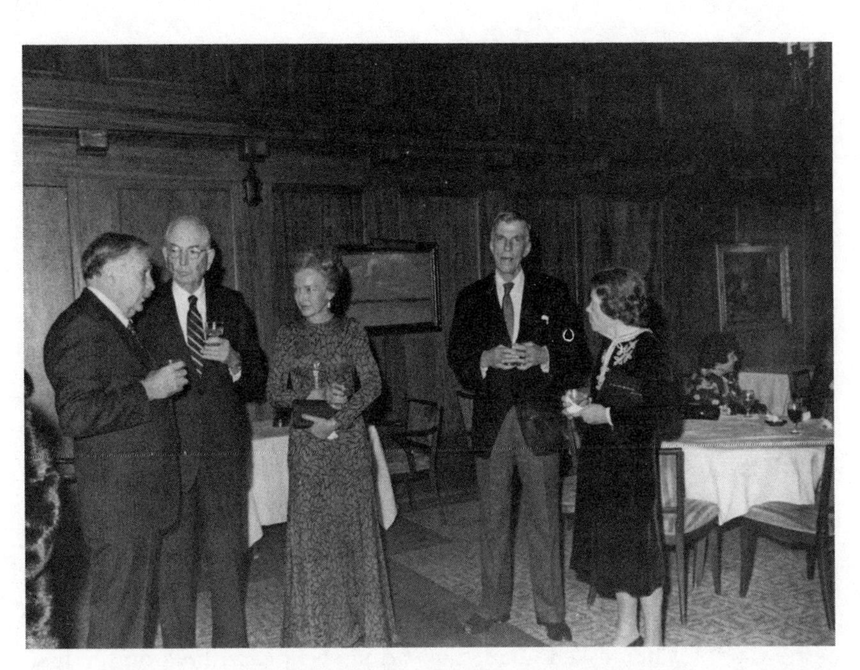

Left to right: James F. Nolan, Keith Russell, Elinor Hempelmann, Louis Hempelmann, and Ann Nolan at 1976 testimonial dinner, Los Angeles Athletic Club, October 30, 1976.

Japan, she had written with the news that Jane had left her husband "due to his drinking."[19] Jane wanted to visit Ann in Los Angeles, but Ann observed that space at the Reynoldses' home, where she was staying, was so crowded, "we couldn't squeeze in a widget." Nevertheless, in keeping with her reputation as a warm and hospitable host, Ann decided to rent a nearby hotel room and stay with Jane for a bit. She explained to her husband that, in the aftermath of the separation, Jane "sounded very low," and "for old times sake I felt I should make some sort of effort."[20] My grandfather would marry Jane in 1979, and he would attend the fortieth-anniversary reunion with her in 1983.

Another milestone came in 1981, when Nolan traveled with Jane and other members of his family to Dublin, Ireland. In Dublin, Nolan's contributions to the field of gynecological oncology were recognized through the establishment of the First James F. Nolan Conference on Gynecological Cancer at Trinity College, Dublin. Attended by leaders in the field from Europe and the United States, the conference was sponsored by the University of Southern California; Trinity College, Dublin; University College, Dublin; the Irish Cancer Society; and the Wimberley Society. While I have not found evidence that this conference continues today, a James F. Nolan Award is still given each year by the Western Association of Gynecologic Oncologists.

In 1982, Nolan retired from his position at the Southern California Cancer Center and moved with Jane to a retirement community in Laguna Hills, California, with the unfortunate name Leisure World. With his gallows humor, he would refer to the complex as "Seizure World," which he would say was populated by "the three C's: Cripples, Cardiacs, and Cadillacs." While living in the community, he gave his last interview about his life on the Manhattan Project. The phone conversation with Ferenc Szasz took place on May 24, 1983. The interview covered many aspects of his contributions to the dawn of the nuclear age, from his confrontation with Leslie Groves in Oak Ridge, to his responsibilities at Trinity, to his role escorting Little Boy and his time on Tinian Island, to his travels to Hiroshima, Nagasaki, Bikini, and Enewetak. He told Szasz that he was "now retired," and that he had been at Los Alamos for a total of "3 years, 3 months, and 3 days." When asked about the various people with whom he had worked during the war years, he referred to Groves as a "pretty hard cookie," Hempelmann as his "classmate" and one of his "best friends," Kenneth Bainbridge as a "real good guy," Jack Hubbard as "a lot of fun," and Stafford Warren as "full of it, but good."[21]

A couple of weeks later, he and Jane traveled up the California coast to attend my sister Kate's June 11 graduation from Santa Clara University. Kate was in sympathy with the nuclear freeze movement, which was popular at the time. At one point during the graduation events, she confronted her grandfather about his role in the creation and delivery of the bomb. "Was it really necessary to drop the bombs?" she asked. Family members remember the encounter as somewhat tense. Only two months earlier, Nolan had heard the regretful talks from Weisskopf and others in Los Alamos. Still, he responded in keeping with the official narrative, "It ended the war and saved American lives." Nolan had two brothers in the military during World War II, both of whom would have participated in the anticipated land invasion.

Kate looks back with regret on this exchange (though not on her views about nuclear weapons), as it was the last substantive conversation she had with her grandfather. Four days later, Nolan attended my sister Annie's high school graduation in Palos Verdes, California. He gave Annie a lapis lazuli ring as a graduation gift, made from a cufflink that was missing its matching pair, and told her it was because of their similar blue eyes. As he and Jane departed that day to return to their Laguna Hills condominium, there was talk of gathering again during the upcoming Father's Day. Nolan would not make it to Father's Day. The next day, June 17, 1983, we received a phone call from Lynne's husband, Tom Handy, who had been staying with his in-laws. I remember the moment well. I was in the kitchen area with my sister Annie and my parents. My dad answered the phone, and shortly into the brief conversation his body tightened up. "What?" I remember him asking. After a moment, he handed the phone to my mom and said, "Dad's dead." She took the phone as my grief-stricken dad disappeared upstairs.

My grandfather was sixty-eight years old when he died. In keeping with one of the three Cs he invoked to make fun of his retirement community, he died of a cardiac arrest. His death certificate lists as the cause "arteriosclerotic cardiovascular disease," a heart condition that has been associated with (or can be exacerbated by) radiation exposure. Given his consumptive habits (that is, use of "a common respiratory irritant" and "adult mood modifying substances"), it would be impossible to identify radiation as the sole or even the primary cause of his death. Moreover, given the degree to which he downplayed the amount of radiation he received during his military and medical careers, it's likely he would never have made such a claim himself, though he was certainly aware of the considerable level of radiation to which he had been exposed during his lifetime.

Though he had offered to my sister Kate the official narrative regarding the bomb, what did he really think about his unique role in the early years of the nuclear age? Was he troubled, for example, by what he saw in Japan, a topic he almost never discussed? When he did give talks on his wartime experience, he would mostly speak in a self-deprecating way about his awkward moments aboard the USS *Indianapolis* and the like. Or if asked about Los Alamos, he would respond, "I delivered the babies." However, family members suspected that the whole experience troubled him deeply. His nephew Bill Reynolds, for example, recalls several times asking Nolan about his service in Japan. Nolan would say that he couldn't really talk about it, though Reynolds remembers one occasion when his uncle soberly admitted of Japan that "it was utter devastation of the kind that is difficult to imagine."[22]

Reynolds believes Nolan was "fighting it in his head." It was "something he never fully came to terms with," and this private wrestling may have "pushed him to alcohol."[23] Nolan's colleague Robert Futoran also remembers that he did not like to talk about what he saw in Japan, but did once say of the devastation that it was "vast." His daughter, Lynne, agrees that he never talked about Japan. However, she also remembers that the memory of his wartime experience took a toll on him. She knew that it must have been difficult for him, as a man with compassion and faith who took joy in bringing life into the world. Lynne observes that "they saw stuff that they didn't ever want to talk about. The devastation must have been just horrifying because Dad never, ever talked about it." Nevertheless, she knew that it troubled him. "It's got to leave a mark," she remembers; "it did, and he would go through funks, he did. . . . I mean he walked in there right after the bomb went off and saw people dying. Not only the dead, but the dying."[24]

Others, including his daughter-in-law, Karen Nolan, remember these funks or dark moods. Among Nolan's favorite activities, in addition to golf and painting, was surf-fishing. While fishing, he would sit and stand for hours on the beach staring out into the ocean. Bill Reynolds once asked his uncle about his passion for fishing. Nolan told him that fishing allowed him "to be by himself and look out into the ocean." Or, as he put it in one newspaper interview, he liked to surf-fish "because it gave you a reason to

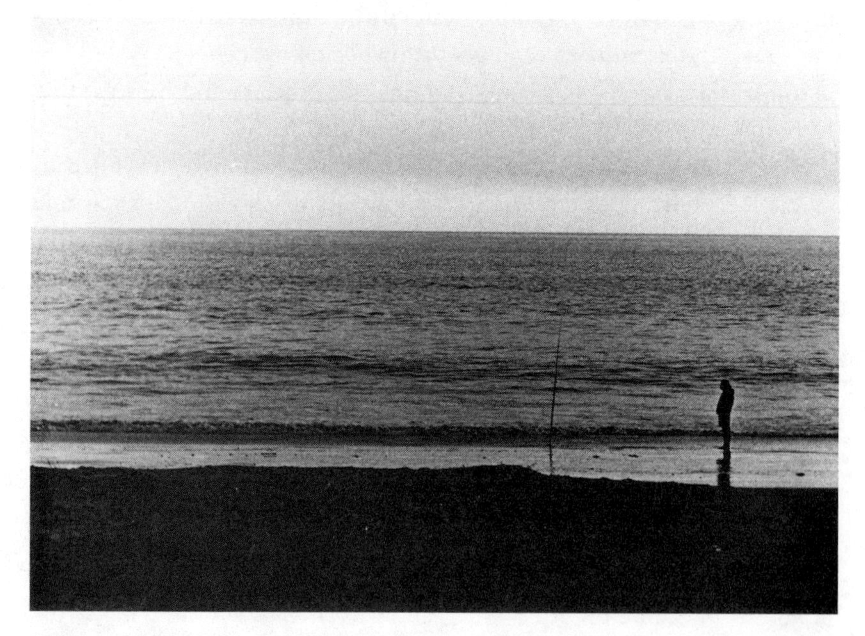

Nolan surf-fishing on the California coast.

sit there."[25] What did Nolan contemplate as he stared out into the ocean? What did he think about during his dark moods? Was it, as his daughter imagined, the dead and dying he saw in Hiroshima and Nagasaki? Did he consider the protesting type of questions asked of him by his young, idealistic granddaughter? Or was it the question scribbled by a friend on the newspaper clipping detailing Little Boy's journey through San Francisco: "Does this make you a hero or a villain?"

Delivering Little Boy: A Final Image

Given his reserve and his relative silence on the topic, one can only speculate regarding Nolan's inner thoughts about his journey through the early nuclear age. However, he certainly encountered questions about the ethical justification of the bombs at least as early as his time in Japan in the fall of 1945. Recall his late-night discussion with Japanese doctors while grounded near the Iwakuni Airport. Recall also Father Siemes's question put forth in the document collected and translated by the Joint Commission: "Does it not have material and spiritual evil as its consequences which far exceed whatever the good that might result? When will our moralists give us a clear answer to this question?"[26]

One moralist who did provide a recent answer of sorts to Siemes's question was Pope Francis, who issued in late December 2017 a card displaying the image of a young boy carrying his little brother to a crematorium in Nagasaki in the weeks following the detonation of the Fat Man bomb. The card was circulated at a time when the use of nuclear weapons was receiving renewed international attention as a result of the public statements exchanged between North Korea's Kim Jung Un and US president Donald Trump. Following North Korea's threat of taking "thousands-fold" revenge on the United States, Trump warned in August 2017 that North Korea "will be met with fire and fury the likes of which the world has never seen."[27]

Against the backdrop of these escalating threats, the pontiff circulated the card. This image of "delivering little boy," the final one considered here, was taken by Joe O'Donnell, a US Marine photographer who was in Nagasaki around the same time as were Nolan and the other members of the Joint Commission. O'Donnell walked into Nagasaki in September 1945. He would stay in Japan for more than six months taking photos, including ones of the victims in Nagasaki, Hiroshima, and other Japanese cities.

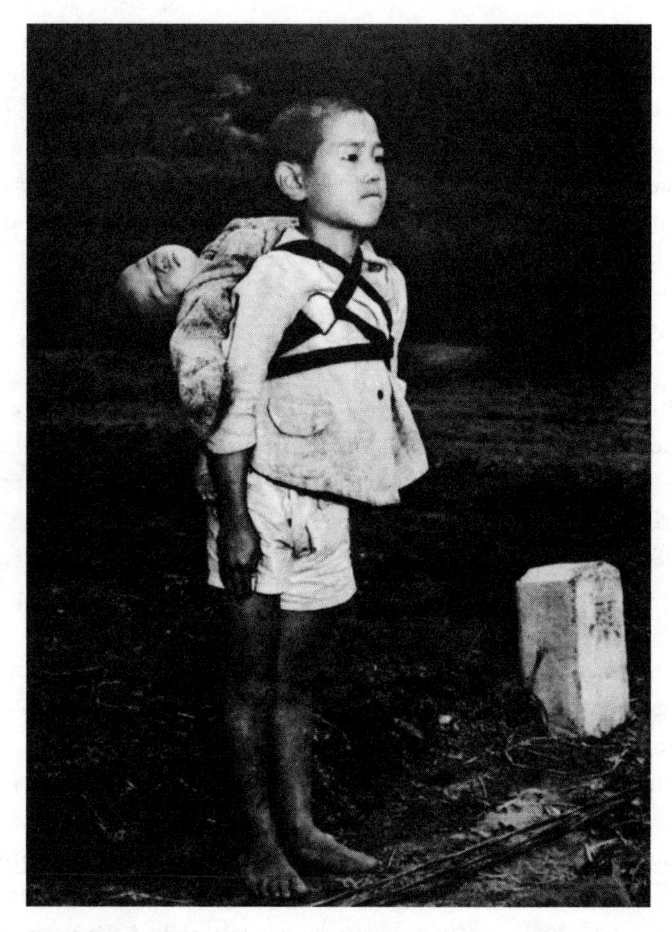

Boy delivering his baby brother to be cremated in Nagasaki.

O'Donnell carried with him two cameras; he would take two photos of each scene, one for the military and one clandestinely for himself. After returning to the United States, he put the negatives of his personal stash in a trunk, where they were stored untouched for decades in his attic. He reportedly found them too painful to view in the years immediately after the war. As time went on, however, he became haunted by what he had seen in Japan. "Years later, many years later, the nightmares began," O'Donnell recalled. "The voices of the children, the endless stretches of rubble and bone, the stench. Over and over again. The voices were always pitiful, always begging. Yet they were accusing, too."[28] Six years after Nolan's death and forty-three years after storing the photos in his attic, O'Donnell reopened the trunk and pulled them out. The pictures were published first in Japan in 1995 and then in the United States in 2005, under the title *Japan 1945: A U.S. Marine's Photographs from Ground Zero.*

Among the photos in the book is that of the boy carrying his little brother on his back to be cremated, a common practice in Nagasaki in the weeks after the bomb. Nolan, Warren, and other members of the Joint Commission witnessed images like this during their time in Japan. As Lynne Handy puts it, they saw "not only the dead but the dying."[29] One day, O'Donnell's son, returning from his summer job while in college, saw some of the recently unearthed photos spread out on his family's kitchen table. His attention was drawn to the picture of the boy carrying his little brother. He observed to his dad that the infant looked like he was sleeping. "No, son, he's not sleeping," O'Donnell said. "The little boy is dead."[30] In an interview with a Japanese journalist, O'Donnell recalled the scene: "The boy stood there for five or ten minutes. The men in white masks walked over to him and quietly began to take off the rope that was holding the baby. That is when I saw that the baby was already dead. The men held the body by the hands and feet and placed it on the fire. The boy stood there straight without moving, watching the flames. He was biting his lower lip so hard that it shone with blood. The flame burned low like the sun going down. The boy turned around and walked silently away."[31]

There had been plans to use some of O'Donnell's photos in the *Enola Gay* exhibit at the Smithsonian Institution scheduled for 1995, the fiftieth anniversary of the first and only combat uses of atomic weapons. The photos were jettisoned, however, following protests from *Enola Gay* pilot Paul Tibbets, *Bockscar* pilot Charles Sweeney, and other veterans, who regarded the story conveyed through the images as "revisionist history"—just one example of the continuing potency of the dominant narrative. O'Donnell, however, no longer shared this narrative. As he explained during an interview with National Public Radio, at the time of the controversy, based on what he had seen on the ground in Japan, he believed "Japan could have been defeated with conventional arms, and without the hundreds of thousands of American casualties that an invasion of the Japanese home islands had been expected to entail."[32]

After the war, O'Donnell became a White House photographer and covered a number of photo shoots with President Harry S. Truman over the years. Walking next to Truman on a Wake Island beach in the North Pacific in 1950, O'Donnell mustered the courage to ask Truman whether he ever had any regrets about dropping the atom bombs. "Hell yes," Truman responded, "I've had a lot of misgivings about it—and I inherited a lot more, too!" This somewhat cryptic response, though not in keeping with Truman's publicly stated confidence about commissioning the use of atomic weapons, does comport with his diary entry of mid-July 1945, when he expressed fears that "machines are ahead of morals by some centuries."[33]

O'Donnell died in 2007 at the age of eighty-five. He had suffered for years from medical issues that he and his family understood to be related to the radiation exposure he received during his months in Japan. The powerful image of the boy and his little brother taken by O'Donnell in 1945 and then reprinted and widely circulated by Pope Francis in late 2017 was accompanied in the latter case by the words "the fruit of war." As we have seen, the fruits of nuclear war, and of the nuclear industry more broadly, have been bountiful indeed. From the *hibakusha* suffering in Japan; to the relocated Bikinians who still cannot live on their beloved atoll; to the downwinders in Nevada and New Mexico; to the many other victims of radiation exposure; to the billions of dollars spent each year on nuclear weapons and on attempts to safeguard nuclear waste; to the many new technologies, and their multiple consequences, that were spawned by the atom bomb, it's safe to say, in the words of OMD's "Enola Gay," that the kiss given by Little Boy has yet to fade away. In other words, unlike the little boy in O'Donnell's potent image, the Little Boy delivered by Nolan and Robert Furman in the summer of 1945 is far from dead.

The image captured in O'Donnell's photo, however, is arguably deeply connected to and emblematic of the other meanings considered in the pages of this book: the literal delivery of the bomb to Tinian Island, the military code name used to communicate the success of the Trinity test, and the image of Truman riding a toboggan down the hill of technological determinism. The scientists at the fortieth-anniversary reunion could not celebrate any of these understandings of "delivering little boy." If not these meanings, then what could they commemorate at this event? Peter Wyden, who discusses the reunion in his book *Day One,* observes that, at the event, "the most lionized of the alumni was former Captain James F. Nolan, M.D., the obstetrician who had delivered so many of the scientists' children on the mesa during the war."[34]

Thus, while the scientists in 1983 could not celebrate their creation of a highly destructive and consequential technology—one that had (and continues to have) many "unforeseeable effects"—they could commend the work of the doctor among them who helped to usher life into the world.

Dorothy McKibbin, the cheerful and industrious gatekeeper of the Manhattan Project, also seems to have recognized this as Nolan's most significant contribution. In early 1952, she sent Nolan a clipping from the Santa Fe newspaper the *New Mexican* announcing the dedication of the new $2.5 million Los Alamos Medical Center. Fittingly, featured on the front page of the issue is a photograph of a woman holding her newborn, the "first baby to occupy the nursery at the new Medical Center." Scrawled at the top of the page commending Nolan's legacy is a handwritten note from McKibbin: "See what you started Jim!"[35] Bill Reynolds may well be right that the most fitting epitaph for Nolan, and the one that his uncle would have chosen for himself, would simply be, "I delivered the babies."

Notes

Introduction

1. James F. Nolan, interview by Lansing Lamont, 1965, Lansing Lamont Papers, Harry S. Truman Library, Independence, MO; James F. Nolan to Richard F. Newcomb, August 12, 1957, James F. Nolan papers, in the author's possession.

1. Life at Los Alamos

1. Nolan took twelve elective hours in radiology during his final year of medical school.

2. Louis Hempelmann, interview by Martin Sherwin, August 10, 1983, Voices of the Manhattan Project, Atomic Heritage Foundation.

3. Louis Hempelmann, interview by Paul Henriksen and Lillian Hoddeson, January 31, 1986, Los Alamos National Laboratory Archives (hereafter LANL), 3.

4. Hempelmann, interview by Sherwin.

5. In Oppenheimer's testimony before the House Un-American Activities Committee in 1949 and in his security clearance tribunal in 1954, he identified Bernard Peters as one among his former Berkeley associates who was a communist. At the time of the 1954 hearing, Bernard and Hannah were working at the University of Rochester, the latter in a lab adjacent to Hempelmann's. As a consequence of Oppenheimer's testimony—and the general hysteria of the McCarthy era—the Peterses left their jobs at Rochester and moved to India. Kai Bird and Martin Sherwin note that given Hannah Peters's communist affiliations, "the FBI concluded that she was a member of the CP [Communist Party]." Kai Bird and Martin Sherwin, *American Prometheus: The Triumph and Tragedy of J. Robert Oppenheimer* (New York: Vintage Books, 2005), 117.

6. Louis Hempelmann, interview by Barton Hacker, June 3–4, 1980, Department of Energy, Nuclear Testing Archive, Las Vegas (hereafter NTA).

7. Hempelmann, interview by Henriksen and Hoddeson, 3.

8. James F. Nolan to Richard F. Newcomb, August 12, 1957, James F. Nolan papers, in the author's possession (hereafter JFN papers).

9. Robert Oppenheimer to James Nolan, March 4, 1943, JFN papers.

10. The Washington University School of Nursing was represented during the war by the following: "Miss Harriet Peterson, Mrs. Sara Dawson Prestwood, Miss Amelia Komadina, Miss Helen Schneider, Mrs. Rosalyn Thomas Lindsay, Mrs. Jeanne Smoot Crumb, Mrs. Francis Foster Allen, Miss Loretta Ashby, and Miss Doris Allen." The doctors recruited from Washington University School of Medicine to Los Alamos during the war included James Nolan, Louis Hempelmann, Paul Hageman, Alfred Large, Jerry H. Allen, and Jack Brookes. Ann Perley, an instructor in biological chemistry in pediatrics, and technicians Annamae Dickie and Ann Earp were also recruited to Los Alamos from Washington University. "Medical School to Advise on Health Services, Research at Los Alamos," *Washington University Medical Alumni Quarterly* 10, no. 1 (October 1946): 14–15.

11. James Nolan to Robert Oppenheimer, March 6, 1943, JFN papers.

12. In a Western Union telegram sent from Hempelmann to Oppenheimer dated March 21, 1943, Hempelmann communicated, "NOLAN AND I WILL ARRIVE WEDNESDAY MARCH 24TH HAVE ARRANGE CLEARANCE FOR BOTH OF US WITH HILBERRY=LOUIS HEMPELMANN." JFN papers. William S. Loring writes, "Construction at Site Y reached a stage in March that the lab began receiving staff and among the first to arrive, on March 24, were medical doctors Louis Hempelmann and James Nolan." William S. Loring, *Birthplace of the Atomic Bomb: A Complete History of the Trinity Test Site* (Jefferson, NC: McFarland, 2019), 11.

13. Hempelmann, interview by Sherwin: "Although in the first year, I really didn't have too much to do in the laboratory. I mean, there weren't any radiation hazards yet. All the other occupational hazards were minimal. They were just more or less like they are in a university set-up like this. I would help Nolan with the practice. I would see the person who presented with medical problems."

14. Oppenheimer to Nolan, March 4, 1943, JFN papers.

15. Jonathan Weisgall, *Operation Crossroads: The Atomic Tests at Bikini Atoll* (Annapolis, MD: Naval Institute Press, 1994), 208.

16. Eileen Welsome, *The Plutonium Files: America's Secret Medical Experiment in the Cold War* (New York: Dial, 1999), 61.

17. Hymer Friedell, interview by Barton C. Hacker, June 12, 1979, NTA.

18. For a discussion of this clash between Warren and Stone, see Barton C. Hacker, *The Dragon's Tail: Radiation Safety in the Manhattan Project, 1942–1946* (Berkeley: University of California Press, 1987), 49–52.

19. Stafford Warren, interview by Barton C. Hacker, October 30, 1979, NTA.

20. Hempelmann, interview by Hacker.

21. James F. Nolan, interview by Ferenc Szasz, May 24, 1983, Ferenc M. Szasz Papers, Center for Southwest Research, University of New Mexico Library, Albuquerque. In a 1979 deposition, Hempelmann stated, "I met him [Warren] someplace, and I felt we need all the help we could get." Deposition of Louis H. Hempelmann, MD, December 20, 1979, 9, *Bernice Lasovick v. United States of America,* LANL.

22. Warren, interview by Hacker.

23. Stafford Warren, *An Exceptional Man for Exceptional Challenges,* oral history interview by Adelaide Tusler (Los Angeles: UCLA Oral History, 1983), 972.

24. According to Robert Norris, when the Manhattan Project commenced, "eight on the project had already won a Nobel Prize, and more than a dozen others would do so after the war." Robert S. Norris, *Racing for the Bomb: The True Story of General Leslie R. Groves, the Man behind the Birth of the Atomic Age* (New York: Skyhorse, 2002), 239.

25. Ferenc Morton Szasz, *The Day the Sun Rose Twice: The Story of the Trinity Site Nuclear Explosion, July 16, 1945* (Albuquerque: University of New Mexico Press, 1984), 22–23.

26. Quoted in Bird and Sherwin, *American Prometheus,* 230; Weisgall, *Operation Crossroads,* 82; Szasz, *Day the Sun Rose Twice,* 21.

27. Jane S. Wilson, "Not Quite Eden," in *Standing By and Making Do: Women of Wartime Los Alamos,* ed. Jane S. Wilson and Charlotte Serber (Los Alamos: Los Alamos Historical Society, 2008), 62.

28. Joseph O. Hirschfelder, "The Scientific and Technological Miracle at Los Alamos," in *Reminiscences of Los Alamos, 1943–1945,* ed. Lawrence Badash, Joseph O. Hirschfelder, and Herbert P. Boida (London: D. Reidel, 1980), 70.

29. Eleanor Jette, *Inside Box 1663* (Los Alamos: Los Alamos Historical Society, 1977), 87. Szasz similarly notes that "General Groves was frequently excoriated in absentia, and the people were so rude and ungracious to Lieutenant Colonel Whitney Ashbridge that he suffered a heart attack and had to be transferred." Szasz, *Day the Sun Rose Twice,* 22.

30. Nolan to Newcomb, August 12, 1957, JFN papers.

31. *Advisory Committee on Human Radiation Experiments: Final Report* (Washington, DC: US Government Printing Office, October 1995), 37.

32. Henry Barnett, interview by Joseph Dancis, 1996, Oral History Project, Pediatric History Center (Elk Grove Village, IL: American Academy of Pediatrics, 2000), 9.

33. Warren, *Exceptional Man,* 964.

34. Quoted in Shirley B. Barnett, "Operation Los Alamos," in Wilson and Serber, *Standing By,* 115.

35. Ibid., 115–116.

36. Lynne Handy, interview by author, September 4, 2015.

37. Nolan, interview by Szasz.

38. James L. Nolan, "Los Alamos and the Atom Bomb through the Eyes of a Young Boy" (lecture at College of the Holy Cross, Worcester, MA, January 24, 2006).

39. Nolan, interview by Szasz.

40. Hempelmann, interview by Hacker.

41. Welsome, *Plutonium Files,* 60.

42. Weisgall, *Operation Crossroads,* 208.

43. Paul Dodd, introduction to *Exceptional Man,* by Warren, xviii. Dodd himself did not concur with this particular assessment.

44. The main problem was that Warren "failed to supply full and correct titles and spellings." Ongoing editorial efforts were thus hampered by the "inconsistent or sometimes incorrect names supplied by Warren." Dodd, introduction, xxvi.

45. Quoted in Norris, *Racing for the Bomb,* 210.

46. J. F. Nolan's son (my father), James Lawry Nolan, often went by the name Lawry as a child and young man. However, as an adult most people called him Jim. In the pages of this book, I will refer to him as Lawry, both because that is what he was typically called as a child (the time period covered in this book) and in order to make clear when I am referring to James Findley Nolan rather than James Lawry Nolan.

47. Personnel Folder, April 10, 1943, JFN Personnel Files, LANL.

48. Quoted in Bird and Sherwin, *American Prometheus,* 81.

49. Quoted in ibid., 207.

50. Quoted in Jennet Conant, *109 East Palace: Robert Oppenheimer and the Secret City of Los Alamos* (New York: Simon and Schuster, 2005), 219.

51. Lynne Handy, interview by author, March 23, 2015. Lynne Nolan, daughter of Jim and Ann Nolan, would take the surname Handy, after marrying Tom Handy.

52. Quoted in ibid., 149.

53. Elsie McMillan, "Outside the Inner Fence," in Badash, Hirschfelder, and Boida, *Reminiscences of Los Alamos,* 43.

54. Hempelmann, interview by Sherwin.

55. Ibid.

56. Yearbook, Los Alamos, 1944, JFN papers. According to Barnett, "To a limited extent, the doctors took over the problem of pets. . . . The doctors . . . became their own and each other's veterinarians." Shirley B. Barnett, "Operation Los Alamos," 118.

57. Quoted in Conant, *109 East Palace,* 337.

58. Ruth Marshak, "Secret City," in Wilson and Serber, *Standing By,* 32.

59. Quoted in Peter Wyden, *Day One: Before Hiroshima and After* (New York: Simon and Schuster, 1984), 80–81.

60. Quoted in Bird and Sherwin, *American Prometheus,* 230.

61. Wilson, "Not Quite Eden," 60–61.

62. Lynne Handy, interview by author, March 23, 2015.

63. Ibid.

64. Jette, *Inside Box 1663,* 18; Shirley B. Barnett, "Operation Los Alamos," 109. Edith Truslow identifies the first three nurses as Sarah Dawson, Harriett Petersen, and Margaret Schoppe. Edith C. Truslow, *Manhattan District History: Nonscientific Aspects of Los Alamos Project Y, 1942 through 1964* (Los Alamos, NM: Los Alamos Historical Society, 1991), 85.

65. Shirley B. Barnett, "Operation Los Alamos," 111–112.

66. See Conant, *109 East Palace,* 127, on Hempelmann passing out during a delivery.

67. Hempelmann, interview by Sherwin.

68. Shirley B. Barnett, "Operation Los Alamos," 112.

69. This description is offered on a display at the small museum at the San Ildefonso Pueblo near Los Alamos in New Mexico.

70. Conant, *109 East Palace,* 143.

71. Ibid., 262–263; Bird and Sherwin, *American Prometheus,* 263; Bernice Brode, *Tales of Los Alamos: Life on the Mesa 1943–1945* (Los Alamos, NM: Los Alamos Historical Society, 2006), 5.

72. Szasz writes, "Nearly one thousand babies were born in that small community from 1943 to 1949; those 208 born during the war had birth certificates listing the place as simply Box 1663, Sandoval County, Rural." Szasz, *Day the Sun Rose Twice,* 18.

73. Marshak, "Secret City," 31.

74. Conant, *109 East Palace,* 214.

75. Hempelmann, interview by Hacker.

76. Marshak, "Secret City," 30.

77. Mr. and Mrs. Will Harrison to Lt. Col. Whitney Ashbridge, June 14, 1943, JFN papers.

78. Beverly Agnew, interview with Theresa Strottman, November 20, 1991, Los Alamos Historical Museum.

79. Henry Frisch, conversation with author, June 3, 2015.

80. McMillan, "Outside the Inner Fence," 43.

81. Jette, *Inside Box 1663,* 49.

82. Ibid., 50.

83. Among other references to this practice, Victor F. Weisskopf, leader of the Theoretical Physics Division at Los Alamos, remembers having to deal with this issue when he chaired the town council: "Prostitution raised its ugly head in Los Alamos supposedly by somebody who reported in the dormitories at some happenings there." Victor F. Weisskopf, interview by Ferenc M. Szasz, April 1981 interview, 15, Ferenc M. Szasz Papers, Center for Southwest Research, University of New Mexico Library, Albuquerque.

84. Hempelmann, interview by Sherwin.

85. Quoted in Truslow, *Manhattan District History,* 91.

86. Louis Hempelmann, "History of Health Group," March 1943–November 1945, 2–3, LANL. "During the first year there were very few radiation hazards," said Hempelmann. "The hazards there were just the same as in any college physics laboratory. So there really wasn't much for me to do the first year." Hempelmann, interview by Henriksen and Hoddeson.

87. Hempelmann, interview by Hacker.

88. Deposition of Louis H. Hempelmann, 19.

89. Hempelmann, "History of Health Group," 5; Hacker, *Dragon's Tail,* 78.

90. Hempelmann, "History of Health Group," 2.

91. Ibid., 14.

92. Deposition of Louis H. Hempelmann, 44.

93. Ibid., 61.

94. James Nolan, interview by Lansing Lamont, 1965, Harry S. Truman Library, Independence, MO.

95. Hempelmann, "History of Health Group," 5.

96. Groves's diary entry for Saturday, February 17, 1945, reads, "Col Warren called Gen. Groves from Knox . . . discussed need for additional hospital and warehouse facilities at Y. Gen asked about head doctor and Col. W. stated Cap. Barnett is now exec. In charge of hosp. which will release Nolan to help Hempelmann more." Entry for February 17, 1945, Groves Diary, Papers of Lt. Gen. Leslie R. Groves, National Archives, College Park, MD.

2. The Trinity Test

1. Samuel A. Goudsmit, *Alsos* (Los Angeles: Tomash, 1947), 70–71. The journalist William L. Laurence also stated that, by the end of 1944, the Americans had "definite evidence" that the Germans were not "anywhere near close to us, were way behind us." William L. Laurence, interview by Scott Bruns, March 28, 1964, 287, Columbia Oral History Archives, Columbia University.

2. Goudsmit, *Alsos,* 76.

3. Ibid.

4. Quoted in Kenneth Glazier, "The Decision to Use Atomic Weapons against Hiroshima and Nagasaki," *Public Policy* 18 (Winter 1969): 515.

5. Quoted in Jon Else, *The Day after Trinity: Robert Oppenheimer and the Atomic Bomb* (New York: Voyager, 1995), CD-ROM, supplemental files, 383–384.

6. Quoted in Jon Else, *The Day after Trinity,* supplemental files, 246–247.

7. Thomas P. Hughes, *American Genesis: A Century of Invention and Technological Enthusiasm, 1870–1970* (Chicago: University of Chicago Press, 1989).

8. Joseph Rotblat, "Leaving the Bomb Project," *Bulletin of the Atomic Scientists* 41, no. 7 (August 1985): 18.

9. Ibid.

10. US Atomic Energy Commission, *In the Matter of J. Robert Oppenheimer: Transcript of Hearing before the Personnel Security Board, April 13, 1954* (Washington, DC: US Government Printing Office, 1945), 2:266.

11. Groves's aide, Major Robert Furman, noted that even after it was learned that Germany had no bomb, Groves turned his attention to Japan and Russia. "So, the use of the bomb turned away from Germany quite quickly, in our favor, but I guess we still were ready to use it in case the Russians got out of control or something like that. It was hard for me to imagine those conditions that existed there at that end of the war. There was great fear that the Russians would just keep coming." Robert Furman, interview by Cindy Kelly, February 20, 2008, Voice of the Manhattan Project, Atomic Heritage Foundation. Though the extent to which concern about the Russians influenced the decision to use the bomb has been hotly debated, there is now considerable evidence that, as historian Gar Alperovitz puts it, "impressing the Russians was a consideration." Indeed, it would be "impossible to ignore the considerable range of evidence that now point in this direction." Gar Alperovitz, "Historians Reassess: Did We Need to Drop the Bomb?," in *Hiroshima's Shadow,* ed. Kai Bird and Lawrence Lifschultz (Stony Creek, CT: Pamphleteer's, 1998), 17.

12. James F. Nolan to Richard F. Newcomb, August 12, 1957, James F. Nolan papers, in the author's possession (hereafter JFN papers).

13. Louis Hempelmann, interview by Barton Hacker, June 3–4, 1980, Department of Energy, Nuclear Testing Archive, Las Vegas (hereafter NTA).

14. Nolan to Newcomb, August 12, 1957, JFN papers.

15. John Donne, *John Donne's Poetry: Authoritative Texts, Criticism,* ed. A. L. Clements (New York: W. W. Norton, 1966), 86.

16. Quoted in Else, *Day after Trinity.*

17. Sean L. Malloy, "'A Very Pleasant Way to Die': Radiation Effects and the Decision to Use the Atomic Bomb against Japan," *Diplomatic History* 36, no. 3 (June 2012): 537.

18. Stafford Warren, *An Exceptional Man for Exceptional Challenges,* oral history interview by Adelaide Tusler (Los Angeles: UCLA Oral History, 1983), 783.

19. Ibid., 798.

20. Hymer Friedell, interview by Barton C. Hacker, June 12, 1979, NTA.

21. Warren, *Exceptional Man,* 783–784.

22. Stafford Warren, interview by Barton C. Hacker, October 30, 1979, NTA.

23. Louis Hempelmann, "History of the Preparation of the Medical Group for Trinity Test II," June 13, 1947, LANL.

24. Ferenc Morton Szasz, *The Day the Sun Rose Twice: The Story of the Trinity Site Nuclear Explosion, July 16, 1945* (Albuquerque: University of New Mexico Press, 1984), 63.

25. Hempelmann, interview by Hacker. In this interview, Hempelmann asserted that Warren took too much credit both for raising concerns about radiation fallout

and for the planning and preparation of the health and safety dimensions of the Trinity test more generally. Rather than being in charge of the operation, according to Hempelmann, Warren served only in an advisory role. As a consultant, according to Hempelmann, "his role in the planning or whatever was really quite minimal."

26. J. O. Hirschfelder to J. R. Oppenheimer, "Strategic Possibilities Arising If a Thunderstorm Is Induced by Gadget Explosion," April 25, 1945, LANL.

27. Ibid.

28. Hubbard records in his journal that he arrived at Los Alamos on April 17, 1945. John M. Hubbard, "Journal of J. Hubbard, Meteorologist," 13, LANL. Copies of Hubbard's journal are at the LANL and in the Caltech library archives. Parts of the journal are also in Ferenc Szasz's papers at the University of New Mexico, Albuquerque.

29. Hubbard, "Journal," 19.

30. Ibid.

31. Szasz, *Day the Sun Rose Twice,* 77; Hubbard, "Journal," 110.

32. Hubbard, "Journal," 81.

33. Ibid., 90.

34. James F. Nolan, interview by Lansing Lamont, 1965, Harry S. Truman Library, Independence, MO; Warren, *Exceptional Man,* 785–790.

35. Hubbard, "Journal," 65.

36. J. O. Hirschfelder and John Magee to K. T. Bainbridge, "Danger from Active Material Falling from Cloud—Desirability of Bonding Soil near Zero with Concrete and Oil," June 16, 1945, LANL.

37. Joseph O. Hirschfelder, "The Scientific and Technological Miracle at Los Alamos," in *Reminiscences of Los Alamos, 1943–1945,* ed. Lawrence Badash, Joseph O. Hirschfelder, and Herbert P. Boida (London: D. Reidel, 1980), 75.

38. Hempelmann, interview by Hacker.

39. Ibid.

40. Nolan's military travel itinerary for June 17–21, 1945, "Itemized Schedule of Travel and Other Expenses," JFN papers.

41. Calutron is a name derived from California University Cyclotron.

42. Nolan, interview by Lamont.

43. James F. Nolan, "Medical Hazards of TR #2," June 20, 1945, LANL. There are a number of accounts, sometimes conflicting, of Nolan's famous encounter with Groves. For example, Hempelmann places the event on June 20, 1945, though has Nolan traveling with Paul Aebersold (a Berkeley-trained physicist and a new member of the Health Group) not alone, to Oak Ridge. Barton Hacker marks June 23, 1945, as the date of the encounter. Szasz has Nolan flying to Oak Ridge on June 20, carrying a report written by "McGee [*sic*], Hoffman, and Hempelmann." Szasz, *Day the Sun Rose Twice,* 65. Hempelmann, however, in his written history of the medical group's role in the Trinity test, stated that it was Nolan who prepared a "detailed plan of operation," which he took to Groves in Oak Ridge for his approval. Likewise, in a July 11, 1945, supplement

to the June 20, 1945, document, Aebersold included the following subtitle to the document: "Supplement to Medical Hazards of TR #2 by Capt. Nolan." P. C. Aebersold to L. H. Hempelmann, "TR Site Monitoring as of July 11, 1945 (Supplement to Medical Hazards of TR #2 by Capt. Nolan)," July 11, 1945, LANL. Also, Lamont, in his interview with Nolan, writes, "Nolan had to take *his* calculations and evacuation plans to Oak Ridge for approval by Gen. Groves in late June" (emphasis added). In Szasz's handwritten notes from the 1983 interview with Nolan, he documented Nolan saying, "We talked w / Staff Warren—wrote up report. Flew to Oak Ridge to talk w / Groves." Only later does he refer to the other ostensible authors, though he doesn't say they wrote the report, only that it was made up by them. It's likely that rather than "McGee [*sic*], Hoffman, and Hempelmann," Szasz was referring to Magee, Hirschfelder, and Hempelmann (James F. Nolan, interview by Ferenc Szasz, May 24, 1983, Ferenc M. Szasz Papers, Center for Southwest Research, University of New Mexico Library, Albuquerque). The interview took place nearly forty years after the historical moments being recollected. Concerning the timing, Nolan's official military itinerary indicates that he left Santa Fe at one o'clock on the morning of June 17 and arrived in Oak Ridge on June 18, and then departed from Oak Ridge at five thirty on the morning of June 20. It is likely, therefore, that Nolan actually spoke with Groves on June 19. Apart from Hempelmann's passing mention, there is no other record indicating that Aebersold was part of this journey. It's possible that Hempelmann recollected Aebersold as being in the mix because he was the author of the July 11, 1945, supplementary memo.

44. Nolan, "Medical Hazards of TR #2."

45. Hempelmann, interview by Hacker.

46. There are several variations to this quote. In *Day of Trinity*, Lamont cites Groves's words as "What are you, a Hearst propagandist?" (Lansing Lamont, *Day of Trinity* [New York: Atheneum, 1965], 127. Though in his interview notes, he records the question, in quotation marks, as "What's the matter with you, are you a Hearst propagandist?" (Nolan, interview by Lamont). Ferenc Szasz, in *Day the Sun Rose Twice,* offers the quote as "What are you . . . some kind of Hearst propagandist?" which is the same wording as in his interview notes (Szasz, *The Day the Sun Rose Twice,* 65; Nolan, interview by Szasz). In *Doctor Atomic,* John Adams quotes Groves asking, "What are you, a Hearst propagandist?" which is the wording from *Day of Trinity.* Lansing Lamont, *Day of Trinity* (New York: Atheneum, 1965), 127; Szasz, *Day the Sun Rose Twice,* 65; Adams, *Doctor Atomic.*

47. Nolan, interview by Lamont.

48. Louis Jacot, interview by Lansing Lamont, Lansing Lamont Papers, Harry S. Truman Library, Independence, MO.

49. Ibid.

50. It recently came to light that a fourth spy, Oscar Seborer, with the Russian code name of Godsend, was also working at Los Alamos between 1944 and 1946. Williams J.

Broad, "4th Spy Unearthed in U.S. Atomic Bomb Project," *New York Times,* November 24, 2019, A1, 17.

51. Nolan, interview by Lamont.

52. Nolan, interview by Szasz.

53. Warren, *Exceptional Man,* 799.

54. Hirschfelder, for example, remembered that, on the day before the test, because "we had such low priority . . . the best transportation we could get was an old automobile which we borrowed from Jim Tuck." Hirschfelder, "Scientific and Technological Miracle," 75.

55. L. H. Hempelmann and James F. Nolan to Kenneth Bainbridge, "Danger to Personnel in Nearby Towns Exposed to Active Material Falling from Cloud," memo, June 22, 1945, LANL.

56. Ibid.

57. Ibid.

58. Malloy, "'Pleasant Way to Die,'" 536–537.

59. Szasz, *Day the Sun Rose Twice,* 143.

60. J. O. Hirschfelder and John Magee to K. T. Bainbridge, "Improbability of Danger from Active Material Falling from Cloud," memo, July 6, 1945, LANL.

61. Hempelmann, interview by Hacker.

62. Louis Hempelmann, interview by Paul Henriksen and Lillian Hoddeson, January 31, 1986, LANL.

63. Hempelmann, interview by Hacker.

64. Ibid.

65. Ibid. Hempelmann also stated during a 1979 deposition, "We were very concerned of some of the workers during June and July of 1945. If it had not been that we had to get the bomb made as soon as possible all work would have stopped." Deposition of Louis H. Hempelmann, MD, December 20, 1979, *Bernice Lasovick v. United States of America,* 38–39, LANL. For a discussion of Hempelmann's concerns during this time, see also William S. Loring, *Birthplace of the Atomic Bomb: A Complete History of the Trinity Test Site* (Jefferson, NC: McFarland, 2019), 199.

66. Louis Hempelmann, interview by Paul Henriksen and Lillian Hoddeson, January 31, 1986, LANL; Louis Hempelmann, interview by Ferenc M. Szasz, January 29, 1982, Ferenc M. Szasz Papers, Center for Southwest Research, University of New Mexico Library, Albuquerque.

67. Hempelmann, interview by Henriksen and Hoddeson.

68. Szasz, *Day the Sun Rose Twice,* 143.

69. Louis Hempelmann, "History of the Preparation of the Medical Group for Trinity Test II," June 13, 1947, A1, LANL.

70. Louis Hempelmann, "Hazards of Trinity Experiment," April 12, 1945, LANL.

71. K. Bainbridge to Capt. T. O. Jones, "Legal Aspects of TR Tests," memo, May 2, 1945, NTA; Barton C. Hacker, *The Dragon's Tail: Radiation Safety in the Manhattan Project, 1942–1946* (Berkeley: University of California Press, 1987), 85.

72. Hempelmann, "Hazards of Trinity Experiment."

73. L. H. Hempelmann to J. G. Hoffman, "Procedure to Be Used by Town Monitors," July 10, 1945, LANL.

74. Ibid.

75. Joseph G. Hoffman to Lt. D. Daley, "Changes and Supplement to Town Monitoring," July 7, 1945, 2, LANL.

76. Hempelmann, interview by Hacker.

77. Ibid.

78. Hempelmann, interview by Henriksen and Hoddeson, 9.

79. Stafford Warren, interview by Lansing Lamont, April 20, 1964, Lansing Lamont Papers, Harry S. Truman Library, Independence, MO. Lamont stated, "Both men knew that the Army was not eager to pursue too diligently the possibilities of widespread fallout. The specter of endless lawsuits haunted the military, and most of the authorities simply wanted to put the whole test and its after effects out of sight and mind as quickly as possible." Lamont, *Day of Trinity,* 251.

80. Eileen Welsome, *The Plutonium Files: America's Secret Medical Experiment in the Cold War* (New York: Dial, 1999), 46.

81. Nolan, interview by Lamont. "It has been advised that no person should (of his own will) receive more than five (5) r. at one exposure." Nolan, "Medical Hazards of TR #2."

82. "Conference about Contamination of Countryside near Trinity with Radioactive Materials," present at conference: R. Oppenheimer, R. Tolman, L. H. Hempelmann, Col. Warren, Capt. Nolan, J. Hoffman, J. Hirschfelder, V. Weisskopf, Magee, Capt. T. Jones, and P. C. Aebersold, July 10, 1945, LANL. Regarding the acceptance of these high levels, Szasz writes, "The scientists put the evacuation levels at a high figure. This was done in part for reasons of secrecy, but the physicians also recognized that there would be no untoward biological effects from such a one-time exposure. They were not much concerned with remote effects. Awareness of the consequences of long-term, low-level exposure to radioactivity lay a generation in the future." Szasz, *Day the Sun Rose Twice,* 127.

83. Nolan, interview by Lamont.

84. Welsome, *Plutonium Files,* 47.

85. Hempelmann, interview by Hacker.

86. Nolan to Newcomb, August 12, 1957, JFN papers.

87. Conversation between Groves and Purnell, July 4, 1945, Groves Diary, Papers of Lt. Gen. Leslie R. Groves, National Archives, College Park, MD.

88. Deposition of Louis H. Hempelmann, 46–47.

89. Hempelmann, interview by Hacker.

90. Stafford Warren to James F. Nolan, July 22, 1945, JFN papers.

91. Ibid.

92. Warren highlighted this later in a document warning of the potential radiation dangers in the Marshall Islands. "Relatively low hazard after the New Mexico test was due to the fact that the column ascended to the great height that it did. Had it ascended to only 10,000 feet, the result might have been most disastrous." "Safety Predictions—Test Baker," Stafford Leak Warren Papers, UCLA Library Special Collections; also found in NTA.

93. Warren to Nolan, July 22, 1945, JFN papers.

94. Hempelmann, interview by Hacker.

95. Hempelmann, interview by Szasz.

96. Stafford Warren to Major Gen. Groves, "Report on Test II at Trinity," memo, July 21, 1945, RG 77, National Archives, College Park, MD.

97. William L. Laurence, *Dawn over Zero: The Story of the Atomic Bomb* (New York: Alfred A. Knopf, 1946), 10–12.

98. Jack Hubbard, "Return to Trinity," reflections from a return trip to Trinity on October 6, 1974, Stafford Leak Warren Papers, UCLA Library Special Collections.

99. Quoted in Szasz, *Day the Sun Rose Twice,* 89; and Lamont, *Day of Trinity,* 242.

100. Quoted in Szasz, *Day the Sun Rose Twice,* 91.

101. Szasz, *Day the Sun Rose Twice,* 124; Lamont, *Day of Trinity,* 244–245.

102. Szasz, *Day the Sun Rose Twice,* 126–127.

103. Entry for July 27, 1945, Groves Diary, Papers of Lt. Gen. Leslie R. Groves, National Archives, College Park, MD.

104. Szasz, *Day the Sun Rose Twice,* 132–133.

105. Hempelmann, interview by Henriksen and Hoddeson, 8.

106. Warren, interview by Lamont.

107. Barbara Kent, interview by author, July 11, 2019.

108. Quoted in Samuel Gilbert, "Inside America's Atomic State," Al Jazeera, February 16, 2016, https://www.aljazeera.com/indepth/features/2016/01/america-atomic-state-160107102647937.html.

109. Kent, interview by author; Robert Keller, interview by author, July 11, 2019.

110. Myrriah Gómez et al., *Unknowing, Unwilling, and Uncompensated: The Effects of the Trinity Test on New Mexicans and the Potential Benefits of Radiation Exposure Compensation Act (RECA) Amendments* (Albuquerque: Tularosa Basin Downwinders Consortium, February 2017).

111. Quoted in Gilbert, "Inside America's Atomic State."

112. Quoted in Lamont, *Day of Trinity,* 255.

113. Quoted in Szasz, *Day the Sun Rose Twice,* 145.

3. Delivering Little Boy

1. Lynn Vincent and Sara Vladic, *Indianapolis* (New York: Simon and Schuster, 2018), 67–68.

2. James F. Nolan to Richard F. Newcomb, August 12, 1957, James F. Nolan papers, in the author's possession (hereafter JFN papers).

3. Ibid.

4. Quoted in William Flynn, "The Day the Bomb Came to San Francisco," *San Francisco Chronicle,* August 2, 1970, A3.

5. Quoted in Vincent and Vladic, *Indianapolis,* 66.

6. Richard Newcomb, *Abandon Ship! The Saga of the U.S.S.* Indianapolis, *the Navy's Greatest Disaster* (New York: HarperCollins, 2001), 23.

7. Alice Blean to James F. Nolan, note accompanying clipping of Flynn, "Day the Bomb Came," JFN papers. The full note to Nolan reads, "Dear Jim—to hand down to your children! Does this make you a hero or a villain? We're fine. Hope you are. Love to Ann. Alice Blean."

8. Nolan was "authorized to carry a camera and to take photographs." Letter of order for: Captain James F. Nolan, 0522870, FA, July 9, 1945, JFN papers.

9. Vincent and Vladic observe that the repair work was not really finished. "There were projects that needed buttoning up, bulkheads to paint, and the slight but persistent list the ship had developed after workmen removed an aircraft catapult." Vincent and Vladic, *Indianapolis,* 73.

10. J. A. Flynn, Commander, US Navy, Executive Officer, "Memorandum to Officer Passengers," USS *Indianapolis,* July 12, 1945, JFN papers.

11. Flynn, "Day the Bomb Came." It's not entirely clear whether the crate contained material for the casing of Little Boy or for conventional bombs. According to Doug Stanton, the crate contained the integral components of the atom bomb known as Little Boy. Doug Stanton, *In Harm's Way: The Sinking of the USS* Indianapolis *and the Extraordinary Story of Its Survivors* (New York: Holt, 2001), 36. Vincent and Vladic write that the crate "contained miscellaneous unclassified materials that were to go with the officers to Tinian." Vincent and Vladic, *Indianapolis,* 69. Nolan recounted, "On the hanger deck there was a large crated piece of equipment which was, I think, a bomb casing which had nothing to do with the active material." Nolan to Newcomb, August 12, 1957, JFN papers. Furman recalled, "We made use of a large box of materials, which was to go with us to our Pacific base." An undated written account by Robert Furman of his mission transporting the bomb with Nolan aboard the USS *Indianapolis* (hereafter, Furman on the *Indy*), 9, Robert R. Furman Papers, Library of Congress.

12. Grover Carter to Colleen Mondor, August 14, 1996, Indianapolis Historical Society, Indianapolis.

13. Stanton, *In Harm's Way,* 30.

14. Nolan to Newcomb, August 12, 1957, JFN papers.

15. Ibid.

16. Newcomb, *Abandon Ship!,* 27; Stanton, *In Harm's Way,* 60.

17. Furman on the *Indy,* 12; draft of a speech, August 5, 1985, 3, Robert R. Furman Papers, Library of Congress.

18. Nolan to Newcomb, August 12, 1957, JFN papers.

19. Ibid.

20. Ibid.

21. Stanton, *In Harm's Way,* 20.

22. Fletcher Knebel and Charles W. Bailey II, *No High Ground* (New York: Harper and Brothers, 1960), 132.

23. Most accounts only refer to the presence of one canister. Vincent and Vladic, however, refer to the transportation of two canisters, one being a dummy canister and one actually containing the subcritical U-235. Furman described the two shipments as follows: "It was no bigger than two old-fashioned ice cream freezers, cylindrical and of shiny aluminum. . . . There were two such containers: varying from the other in form and actually not of the same interest, as far as replacement value was concerned, as the first. Consequently, we always used this second container when running trials or safety drills. Furman on the *Indy,* 5, Robert R. Furman Papers, Library of Congress. Richard Paroubek, who helped to carry the shipment off the *Indy* at Tinian, likewise remembers two canisters. "As we entered the cabin, three men were already there. We saw two lead canisters, about knee-high, with long steel pipes through rings on top." USS Indianapolis Survivors, *Only 317 Survived!* (Indianapolis: USS Indianapolis Survivors Organization, 2006), 396.

24. Nolan to Newcomb, August 12, 1957, JFN papers.

25. Ibid.

26. Ibid. On this particular scene, Newcomb adds, "Furman and Nolan were doubly amused, thinking back to their elaborate plans of lowering the canister into a raft or boat in case the ship had threatened to go down." Newcomb, *Abandon Ship!,* 34.

27. Charles B. McVay to James F. Nolan, "Change of Duty," memo, July 26, 1945, JFN papers.

28. For a full discussion of this, see Vincent and Vladic, *Indianapolis,* 429–430.

29. Stanton (*In Harm's Way,* 257) places Nolan, rather than Furman, at Guam talking to Haynes. Vincent and Vladic (*Indianapolis,* 307) have only Furman making this trip to Guam. Records from Nolan's file seem to confirm the latter, as Nolan reported, "After the sinking of the 'Indianapolis' Major Furman had the opportunity of visiting some of the survivors on Guam, and he talked to Dr. Haines [*sic*] about this at the time." Nolan to Newcomb, August 12, 1957, JFN papers.

30. See Stanton, *In Harm's Way,* 265–266. Before the proceedings, Hashimoto had been asked by lawyers on both sides whether it would have mattered whether the *Indianapolis* was zigzagging when he torpedoed the ship. Both times, he answered that it

would have made no difference. During the court proceedings, he again indicated that it would not have mattered, though the English translation was slightly more ambiguous in this instance. He was translated to have answered, "It would have involved no change in the method of firing the torpedoes, but some changes in the maneuvering." It's unclear why the defense lawyer did not seek clarification, because this was not exactly what Hashimoto intended to communicate. For a detailed discussion, see Vincent and Vladic, *Indianapolis,* 368.

31. Nolan to Newcomb, August 12, 1957, JFN papers.

32. Quoted in Stanton, *In Harm's Way,* 204.

33. Quoted in Vincent and Vladic, *Indianapolis,* 435–436.

34. Quoted in Stanton, *In Harm's Way,* 283.

35. Donald Blum to Colleen Mondor, February 27, 1996, Indianapolis Historical Society, Indianapolis.

36. Newcomb writes that at the time, with efforts to unify the armed forces being considered, "the Navy felt it was in a death struggle to prevent being swallowed up by the Army and Air Force." Newcomb, *Abandon Ship!,* 256.

37. Navy secretary James Forrestal and Fleet Admiral Ernest King, for example, rushed McVay's hearing after press began trickling out about some of these other matters. "We don't need that kind of publicity," Forrestal scolded his special assistant, Edward Hidalgo, before deciding with King to proceed "at once" with McVay's court-martial. Years later, navy lawyers resisted efforts to admit errors by the navy on the grounds that it would "open the Navy to litigation risks." Vincent and Vladic, *Indianapolis,* 338, 411.

38. Nolan to Newcomb, August 12, 1957, JFN papers.

39. Donald Leslie Collins, "Recollections of Nagasaki, 1945," chap. 7 in *Autobiography of Donald Leslie Collins,* 7.12, 13.

40. Harold Russ observes further that there were few survivors from these crashes because "the B-29 was a difficult plane to escape from." Harlow W. Russ, *Project Alberta: The Preparation of Atomic Bombs for Use in World War II* (Los Alamos: Exceptional Books, 1990), 48.

41. James F. Nolan in *The 509th Remembered: A History of the 509th Composite Group as Told by the Veterans That Dropped the Atomic Bombs on Japan,* ed. Robert Krauss and Amelia Krauss (Wichita: 509th Press, 2013), 153.

42. Jennet Conant, *109 East Palace: Robert Oppenheimer and the Secret City of Los Alamos* (New York: Simon and Schuster, 2005), 177.

43. Nolan to Newcomb, August 12, 1957, JFN papers.

44. Stephen Walker, *Shockwave: Countdown to Hiroshima* (New York: HarperCollins, 2005), 150–152; Robert S. Norris, *Racing for the Bomb: The True Story of General Leslie R. Groves, the Man behind the Birth of the Atomic Age* (New York: Skyhorse, 2002), 410–411; Leslie Groves, *Now It Can Be Told: The Story of the Manhattan Project* (New York: Harper and Brothers, 1962), 305–307.

45. James F. Nolan to Stafford Warren, "Monitoring Activities at Destination," July 28, 1945, JFN papers.

46. John Lansdale to Captain James F. Nolan, "Safeguarding Information," July 30, 1945, JFN papers.

47. Ibid.

48. Brendan McNally, "Burn after Reading," *The Rotarian,* March 2014, 49.

49. Ibid.

50. Quoted in Conant, *109 East Palace,* 140.

51. Nolan to Warren, "Monitoring Activities at Destination," July 28, 1945, JFN Papers.

52. "Dr. Nolan Tells B.H. Exchange Club of First Atom Bomb Delivery to Tinian," *Beverly Hills Citizen,* March 23, 1959.

53. Russ, *Project Alberta,* 64: "Prior to the start of the meeting the crew members were given a brief medical examination by Captain James F. Nolan, the Project A physician and radiologist"; Walker, *Shockwave,* 289–290.

54. Captain James F. Nolan, MC, to Col. S. L. Warren, MC, Oak Ridge, TN, "Additional Medical Activities at Destination," August 7, 1945, JFN papers.

55. Quoted in Knebel and Bailey, *No High Ground,* 213; Walker, *Shockwave,* 289–290.

56. Nolan to Warren, "Additional Medical Activities at Destination," August 7, 1945, JFN papers.

57. James F. Nolan, MD, to Robert J. Buettner, October 29, 1947, Stafford Leak Warren Papers, UCLA Library Special Collections.

58. Furman Diary, July 31, 1945, Robert R. Furman Papers, Library of Congress.

59. Furman Diary, August 28, 1945, Robert R. Furman Papers, Library of Congress.

60. Ibid.

61. Furman Diary, Robert R. Furman Papers, Library of Congress.

4. Hiroshima

1. Shields Warren, oral history interview by Peter D. Olch, October 10, 1972, 63, National Library of Medicine, National Institutes of Health, Bethesda, MD; H. W. Allen, memo establishing "Joint Commission for the Effects of the Atomic Bomb in Japan," October 12, 1945, Averill Liebow Papers, Medical History Library, Yale University.

2. See M. Susan Lindee, *Suffering Made Real: American Science and the Survivors at Hiroshima* (Chicago: University of Chicago Press, 1994), 23; and Shields Warren, interview by Olch, 62. However, in their 1956 report, Oughterson and Shields state that when Oughterson initiated efforts on behalf of the army in late August 1945, he "was not aware that other groups of American investigators were proceeding to Japan for a similar purpose." Ashley W. Oughterson and Shields Warren, eds., *Medical Ef-*

fects of the Atomic Bomb in Japan (New York: McGraw-Hill, 1956), 7. The latter appears the more accurate interpretation.

3. Leslie Groves to Thomas Farrell, August 12, 1945, Top Secret, Tinian Files, National Archives, College Park, MD.

4. Stafford Warren, *An Exceptional Man for Exceptional Challenges,* oral history interview by Adelaide Tusler (Los Angeles: UCLA Oral History, 1983), 615, 813.

5. Hymer L. Friedell, interview by Barton C. Hacker, June 12, 1979, Department of Energy, Nuclear Testing Archive, Las Vegas (hereafter NTA). Also, in a November 1, 1945, testimonial dinner, Warren recalled "having a great deal of difficulty in choosing the men who would go. . . . They had to be in uniform because of the military character of the operation. . . . Some of the men were bitterly disappointed because they couldn't go." Stafford Warren, "Odyssey in the Orient" (lecture at testimonial dinner sponsored by the Oak Ridge Medical Society, November 1, 1945), Stafford Leak Warren Papers, UCLA Library Special Collections (hereafter Stafford Warren Papers, UCLA). Eileen Welsome also notes that Hempelmann "no doubt felt disgruntled about being left behind." Eileen Welsome, *The Plutonium Files: America's Secret Medical Experiment in the Cold War* (New York: Dial, 1999), 109.

6. Louis Hempelmann, interview by Barton C. Hacker, June 3–4, 1980, NTA.

7. L. H. Hempelmann, "History of the Health Group (A-6), March 1943–November 1945," April 6, 1945, NTA.

8. "Investigation of the After Effects of the Bombing in Japan," chap. 6 in "Manhattan District History, Book 1, Vol. 4, Auxiliary Activities," 6.1–2, NTA.

9. Oughterson then presented the plan to Brigadier General Guy Denit for approval. In a letter to Denit dated August 28, 1945, he argued that a "study of the effects of the two atomic bombs used in Japan is of vital importance to our country." Among other reasons, he noted possible dangers of "residual radiation effects," which, though he viewed them as only a "remote" source of danger, "should be investigated at the earliest possible date." Denit approved Oughterson's plan and the recruitment of army personnel soon commenced. Oughterson would ultimately recruit a team of twelve medical officers and eleven enlisted. Quoted in Averill A. Liebow, "Hiroshima Medical Diary," *Yale Journal of Biology and Medicine* 38 (October 1965): 82.

10. Ibid., 85. The starting date of Liebow's diary is September 18, 1945, the day Liebow learned that he would be a part of the army delegation.

11. Like Oughterson, Shields Warren assumed "there wasn't anything being done" in terms of a postwar investigation of the medical effects of the bombs. Therefore, he approached the navy surgeon general Ross McIntyre and stressed the need to study the survivors of the bomb and "to get competent medical teams into the area." Persuaded as to the merits of this request, McIntyre ordered Shields Warren on September 8 to assemble a naval medical unit to go into Japan, which would ultimately be composed of fifteen officers and enlisted men. By this time, members of the Manhattan Project were already in Japan. Shields Warren, interview by Olch, 62.

12. H. W. Allen, memo establishing "Joint Commission for the Effects of the Atomic Bomb in Japan," October 12, 1945, Averill Liebow Papers, Medical History Library, Yale University.

13. See Lindee, *Suffering Made Real,* 117–142; and Welsome, *Plutonium Files,* 115.

14. Eisei Ishikawa and David L. Swain, trans., *Hiroshima and Nagasaki: The Physical, Medical, and Social Effects of the Atomic Bomb* (New York: Basic Books, 1981), 530.

15. Quoted in Gosuke Nagahisa, "RERF Chairman Expresses Words of Remorse and Appreciation to A-Bomb Survivors at 70th Anniversary Ceremony," *Chugoku Shimbun,* June 20, 2017, http://www.hiroshimapeacemedia.jp/?p=77599.

16. Daniel Lang, "A Fine Moral Point," *New Yorker,* June 8, 1946, 62. See also "Investigation of the After Effects," 6.39. This report states, "One of the major purposes that General Groves emphasized in directing the organization of the Manhattan District mission in August 1945 was that he wished to obtain a *quick* preliminary report on the after effects of the bombing of Hiroshima and Nagasaki. Therefore, as soon as the various groups had obtained the data available for such a quick report they returned to the United States, leaving further and lengthier investigation to other agencies who were on the ground" (emphasis in original).

17. Lang, "Fine Moral Point," 62.

18. Welsome, *Plutonium Files,* 110.

19. Memorandum of telephone conversation between General Groves and Lt. Col. Rea, Oak Ridge Hospital, 9:00 a.m., August 25, 1945, Correspondence ("Top Secret") of the Manhattan Engineer District, microfilm publication M1109, file 5G, National Archives, Washington, DC.

20. Ibid.

21. Louis Hempelmann, interview by Paul Henriksen and Lillian Hoddeson, January 31, 1986, 10, LANL.

22. Memorandum of telephone conversation between General Groves and Lt. Col. Rea, Oak Ridge Hospital, 9:00 a.m., August 25, 1945.

23. Entry for August 8, 1945, Groves Diary, Papers of Lt. Gen. Leslie R. Groves, National Archives, College Park, MD.

24. Robert S. Stone, MD, to Lieutenant Colonel H. L. Friedell, August 9, 1945, quoted in *Advisory Committee on Human Radiation Experiments: Final Report* (Washington, DC: US Government Printing Office, October 1995), 35.

25. Robert Oppenheimer to Brigadier General Thomas Farrell, memo, May 11, 1945, in *The Atomic Bomb and the End of World War II,* ed. William Burr, document 5, National Security Archive, https://nsarchive2.gwu.edu/nukevault/ebb525-The-Atomic-Bomb-and-the-End-of-World-War-II/documents/010.pdf.

26. Stafford Warren to Leslie Groves, "The Use of the Gadget as a Tactical Weapon Based on Observations Made during Test II," July 25, 1945, Stafford Warren Papers, UCLA.

27. See Sean L. Malloy, "'A Very Pleasant Way to Die': Radiation Effects and the Decision to Use the Atomic Bomb against Japan," *Diplomatic History* 36, no. 3 (June 2012): 542, where Malloy notes that "the Jacobson article turned out to be a boon for Groves." See also Robert J. Lifton and Greg Mitchell, *Hiroshima in America: Fifty Years of Denial* (New York: G. P. Putnam's Sons, 1995), 41–42, where Lifton and Mitchell also observe this outcome of the Jacobson incident. See also Paul Boyer, *By the Bomb's Early Light: American Thought and Culture at the Dawn of the Atomic Age* (Chapel Hill: University of North Carolina Press, 1994), 307.

28. Liebow writes that the mission of the Manhattan Project group was to "conduct a brief preliminary study of the effects for an immediate report to Washington. The major function was to determine whether there was residual radioactivity in order to safeguard our troops." Liebow, "Hiroshima Medical Diary," 84.

29. Donald L. Collins, "Pictures from the Past: Journeys into Health Physics in the Manhattan District and Other Diverse Places," in *Health Physics: A Backward Glance: Thirteen Original Papers on the History of Radiation Protection,* ed. Ronald L. Kathren and Paul L. Ziemer (New York: Pergamon, 1980), 41.

30. Ibid.

31. Ibid. In another account, Collins recalls asking Farrell, "Pardon me General, but it is my understanding that my mission is to measure the radioactivity in these areas." Donald Leslie Collins, "Recollections of Nagasaki, 1945," chap. 7 in *Autobiography of Donald Leslie Collins,* 7.13.

32. Collins, "Recollections of Nagasaki," 7.14.

33. Collins, "Pictures from the Past," 41; Donald Collins, oral history interview by Heather Wade, April 26, 2004, New York State Military Museum. In fact, Collins may well have read about their "findings" in *Stars and Stripes.* In an issue published on September 17, 1945, when Collins and his group were still in Okinawa awaiting transport into Nagasaki, the military newspaper reported on information given by Groves at a September 9 press conference held at the Trinity Site (to be discussed in this chapter). In the article, Groves is quoted as having stated, "11 days after the bomb fell Hiroshima apparently was safe from dangerous rays. . . . At any point beneath the impact of the explosion there was less than a tolerance dose of X-rays coming from the ground or air. That means, Groves said, that it is safe for anyone to live in that area permanently without risk." "Hiroshima Free of Death Rays, Report of Jap Experts Shows," *Stars and Stripes,* September 17, 1945.

34. "Our mission," as Collins understood it before the Tinian Island briefing, "was to survey the bombed cities of Hiroshima and Nagasaki, Japan and to assist the Japanese doctors in treating the injured." Collins, "Recollections of Nagasaki," 7.9–10.

35. "Investigation of the After Effects," 6.3.

36. James B. Newman Jr. to Leslie Groves, memo, October 1, 1945, states, "Furman's job completed Furman and his group will depart for mainland approximately 4 October [*sic*]." Tinian Files, National Archives, College Park, MD.

37. Account from Colonel R. C. Wilson in "Investigation of the After Effects," 6.45.

38. Entry for September 5, 1945, Furman's Diary, Robert R. Furman Papers, Library of Congress.

39. Marcel Junod, "The Hiroshima Disaster," *International Review of the Red Cross* 22 (September–October and November–December 1982): 6.

40. James F. Nolan to Robert J. Buettner, October 29, 1947, Stafford Warren Papers, UCLA; Stafford Warren, "Odyssey in the Orient"; "Investigation of the After Effects," 6.6.

41. Masao Tsuzuki, "Experimental Studies on the Biological Action of Hard Roentgen Rays," *American Journal of Roentgenology* 16 (August 1926): 134–150.

42. Quoted in Lang, "Fine Moral Point," 64. Marcel Junod also recalls a variation of this conversation while members of the Joint Commission stayed their first night on Miyajima Island. According to Junod, Tsuzuki said, "Tomorrow, when you go into Hiroshima, you will see the upshot of my experiment . . . 80,000 dead and 100,000 wounded. The effects of the atomic bomb are almost exactly the same. The magnitude of the experiment is greater, far greater, but that's all." Marcel Junod, *Warrior without Weapons* (New York: Macmillan, 1951), 266.

43. Leslie Groves to Thomas Farrell, September 5, 1945, Tinian Files, National Archives, College Park, MD.

44. James B. Newman to Leslie Groves, September 2, 1945, Tinian Files, National Archives, College Park, MD.

45. Wilfred Burchett, "The First Nuclear War," in *Hiroshima's Shadow,* ed. Kai Bird and Lawrence Lifschultz (Stony Creek, CT: Pamphleteer's, 1998), 68–69.

46. A September 11, 1945, issue of *Stars and Stripes* reported on this possibility: "The London Daily Express announced that one of its staff reporters, Peter Burchett, is under observation in Tokyo to establish whether white corpuscles in his blood had been affected by radioactivity during a recent visit to Hiroshima." "First Americans in Nagasaki See Atomic Havoc," *Stars and Stripes,* September 11, 1945.

47. Burchett, "First Nuclear War," 69.

48. Peter Wyden, *Day One: Before Hiroshima and After* (New York: Simon and Schuster, 1984), 326.

49. Stafford Warren, *Exceptional Man,* 644.

50. Wilson recalled, "Here we managed a successful landing despite bomb craters and the wreckage of many aircraft—one of which lay squarely on the runway." Account of General (formerly Colonel) R. C. Wilson in "Investigation of the After Effects," 6.48.

51. In Warren's recollections of this moment, he said, "We were met by a group of Japanese in uniform who had chairs drawn up and bottles of beer in baskets. . . . We couldn't wait for this so we all got in a bus and started off about noon." Stafford Warren, "Odyssey in the Orient."

52. Stafford Warren, "Odyssey in the Orient"; Morrison quoted in Lang, "Fine Moral Point," 66.

53. Stafford Warren, *Exceptional Man,* 590; Morrison quoted in Lang, "Fine Moral Point," 66.

54. Stafford Warren, *Exceptional Man,* 595–596; Stafford Warren, "Odyssey in the Orient"; Nolan to Buettner, October 29, 1947, Stafford Warren Papers, UCLA.

55. Junod, *Warrior without Weapons,* 295.

56. Ibid., 299.

57. John J. Flick, "Ocular Lesions following the Atomic Bombing of Hiroshima and Nagasaki," *American Journal of Ophthalmology* 31, no. 2 (February 1948): 137, 142.

58. Quoted in Junod, *Warrior without Weapons,* 270–271.

59. Junod, "Hiroshima Disaster," 13.

60. Ibid., 14–15.

61. Special Correspondent Iyo, "American Research Delegation Astonished: Pronounces in Hiroshima 'It Should Not Be Used,'" *Mainichi Shimbun,* September 11, 1945, 20.

62. Ibid. Outside the Hiroshima Memorial Peace Museum in Hiroshima is a small monument dedicated to the memory of Marcel Junod, which reads, in part, "On September 8, he entered the devastated city with no less than fifteen tons of prepared medicines. While occupied in surveying the actual extent of the appalling catastrophe, he himself treated many citizens who had fallen victim to the A-bomb. The medicines brought to the city through his endeavors were distributed to each aid station, saving thousands of A-bomb survivors. We erect this Monument to grateful remembrance of Dr. Junod for his humane acts and as a tribute to the International Red Cross for its continuing work of human compassion."

63. Stafford Warren, "Odyssey in the Orient."

64. Stafford Warren, *Exceptional Man,* 612.

65. A memo from Peer de Silva indicates that, at one point, the American officials wanted to bring Tsuzuki and Motohashi to the United States. In a memo dated October 29, 1945, de Silva writes, "It is intended that, upon return of the Atomic Bomb Mission to the United States, a request will be made to the War department to have two Japanese doctors sent to the United States to aid in compilation of medical data pertaining to the atomic bomb. These persons are: Dr. Masao Tsuzuki and Dr. Hitoshi Motohashi." Stafford Warren Papers, UCLA.

66. Stafford Warren, *Exceptional Man,* 611.

67. Thomas Farrell to Leslie Groves, September 10, 1945, Tinian Files, National Archives, College Park, MD.

68. Ibid.

69. Flick, "Ocular Lesions," 138, 141.

70. Quoted in W. H. Lawrence, "No Radioactivity in Hiroshima," *New York Times,* September 13, 1945, 4.

71. Quoted in Chad R. Diehl, *Resurrecting Nagasaki: Reconstruction and the Formation of Atomic Narratives* (Ithaca, NY: Cornell University Press, 2018), 121–122.

72. Stafford Warren, *Exceptional Man,* 813.

73. Stafford Warren to Gavin Hadden, June 17, 1948, Stafford Warren Papers, UCLA.

74. Stafford Warren to Leslie Groves, October 11, 1945, Tinian Files, National Archives, College Park, MD.

75. Warren to Hadden, June 17, 1948, Stafford Warren Papers, UCLA.

76. Stafford Warren, *Exceptional Man,* 668.

77. Howard W. Blakeslee, "Atom Bomb Turned Mile Ring of Desert into Jade-Like Glass," *Washington Post,* September 12, 1945, 1. Historian Janet Farrell Brodie accurately describes the event as a "carefully staged tour . . . providing false reassurance about the lack of radiation at the site and elsewhere in the area." Janet Farrell Brodie, "Radiation Secrecy and Censorship after Hiroshima and Nagasaki," *Journal of Social History* 48, no. 4 (2015): 847.

78. Charles B. Degges, "Crater of First A-Bomb Shown to U.S. Newsmen," *Los Angeles Times,* September 12, 1945, 4.

79. Even Farrell had conveyed to Groves in his secret September 10 memo that "summaries of Japanese reports previously sent are essentially correct, as to clinical effects of single radiation dose." Thomas Farrell to Leslie Groves, secret memo, September 10, 1945, Tinian Files, National Archives, College Park, MD.

80. Quoted in Blakeslee, "Atom Bomb," 1.

81. Malloy, "'Pleasant Way to Die,'" 538. See also the work of Barton Bernstein, who, in interviews with such Los Alamos luminaries as Luis Alvarez, Kenneth Bainbridge, Hans Bethe, Robert Brode, and Frank Oppenheimer, found that "not one believed that the high airburst had been conceived, even in part, in order to avoid radioactive ground contamination." Barton Bernstein, "Doing Nuclear History: Treating Scholarship Fairly and Interpreting Pre-Hiroshima Thinking about 'Radioactive Poisoning,'" *SHAFR Newsletter,* September 1996. While rummaging through the Ferenc M. Szasz Papers in the University of New Mexico Library archives in Albuquerque, I discovered an interesting and telling confirmation of Malloy's and Bernstein's position. In an early draft of his book on the Trinity test, Szasz had written that the Nagasaki and Hiroshima bombs were dropped as high as they were so that the explosion would not "spread radioactive particles through the region." Szasz gave a draft of the manuscript for review to meteorologist Jack Hubbard, who was deeply involved in the Trinity test. Hubbard wrote to Szasz in the margins, "I don't think this statement is true. I believe that the decision on detonation altitude for the Hiroshima and Nagasaki bombs was made on purely military grounds, actually to maximize blast damage. If there was any consideration of fallout I have never heard of it." Hubbard's handwritten comments in the margins of a draft of Szasz's manuscript, *The Day the Sun Rose Twice,* Ferenc M. Szasz Papers, Center for Southwest Research, University of New Mexico Library, Al-

buquerque. To provide just one example of the prevailing thinking before the Hiroshima and Nagasaki bombs, in a July 25, 1945, memo from Warren to Groves, Warren wrote, "If the detonation altitude is raised to approximately 2,000 ft. for more effective use of the blast . . ." Stafford Warren Papers, UCLA. No mention at all is made in the memo of the reduced levels of radiation that might be achieved by raising the explosion to this height.

82. Quoted in Blakeslee, "Atom Bomb," 1.

83. Telephone conversation between Hempelmann and Groves, August 25, 1945, Groves Diary, Papers of Lt. Gen. Leslie R. Groves, National Archives, College Park, MD.

84. Hempelmann, interview by Hacker.

85. Ibid.

86. Warren to Hadden, June 17, 1948, Stafford Warren Papers, UCLA.

87. Ibid.

88. Collins, "Recollections of Nagasaki," 7.26.

89. Warren, "Odyssey in the Orient."

90. Nolan to Buettner, October 29, 1947, Stafford Warren Papers, UCLA.

5. Tokyo and Nagasaki

1. James F. Nolan to Robert J. Buettner, October 29, 1947, Stafford Leak Warren Papers, UCLA Library Special Collections (hereafter Stafford Warren Papers, UCLA); "Investigation of the After Effects of the Bombing in Japan," chap. 6 in "Manhattan District History, Book 1, Vol. 4, Auxiliary Activities," 6.7, NTA.

2. Nolan to Buettner, October 29, 1947, Stafford Warren Papers, UCLA.

3. "A series of typhoons prevented Colonel Friedell's team from reaching Hiroshima until 26 September. His group had only about a week to carry out investigations designed to supplement the preliminary data collected by Farrell's party. Departing Hiroshima on 3 October, Friedell's team joined the Nagasaki group for the return trip to the United States." Vincent C. Jones, *Manhattan: The Army and the Atomic Bomb* (Washington, DC: Center of Military History, United States Army, 2007), 544–545.

4. Averill A. Liebow, "Hiroshima Medical Diary," *Yale Journal of Biology and Medicine* 38 (October 1965): 100.

5. James L. Nolan, "Los Alamos and the Atom Bomb through the Eyes of a Young Boy" (lecture at College of the Holy Cross, Worcester, MA, January 24, 2006).

6. For example, Major Kiyoshi Yamashina, of the Japanese Army Medical School, who did autopsy work in Hiroshima, complained when asked by the American doctors to "submit [his team's] autopsy findings and specimens." He said that doing so "made [them] keenly feel the wretchedness of a defeated nation." Kiyoshi Yamashina, "Recollections of the Time of the Atomic Bombing," 5, Averill Liebow Papers, Medical History Library, Yale University.

7. Nolan to Buettner, October 29, 1947, Stafford Warren Papers, UCLA.

8. Ibid.

9. Quoted in George Bishop, *Pedro Arrupe SJ* (Leominster, UK: Gracewing, 2007), 157.

10. In John Hersey's papers is a December 6, 1945, copy of Liebow's translation of Siemes's account, marked "Restricted." John Hersey Papers, Beinecke Library, Yale University.

11. John Hersey to Robert H. Donahugh, July 21, 1985, John Hersey Papers, Beinecke Library, Yale University.

12. Liebow, "Hiroshima Medical Diary," 121.

13. Ibid., 124.

14. John Hersey, *Hiroshima* (New York: Vintage Books, 1946), 75.

15. Liebow, "Hiroshima Medical Diary," 124.

16. Ibid., 128.

17. P. Siemes, "Atomic Bomb on Hiroshima, Eyewitness Account of P. Siemes," trans. Averill Liebow, 16, Averill Liebow Papers, Medical History Library, Yale University.

18. Ibid., 17–18.

19. Stafford Warren to Gavin Hadden, June 17, 1948, Stafford Warren Papers, UCLA. Of the Americans who were present during this conversation, Warren specifically names Nolan, Oughterson, and Kurt Kasznar.

20. Ibid.

21. Stafford Warren, *An Exceptional Man for Exceptional Challenges,* oral history interview by Adelaide Tusler (Los Angeles: UCLA Oral History, 1983), 947.

22. Robert J. Lifton and Greg Mitchell, *Hiroshima in America: Fifty Years of Denial* (New York: G. P. Putnam's Sons, 1995), 90; James Hershberg, *James B. Conant: Harvard to Hiroshima and the Making of the Nuclear Age* (New York: Alfred A. Knopf, 1993), 295, 761.

23. Norman Cousins, "The Literacy of Survival," in *Hiroshima's Shadow,* ed. Kai Bird and Lawrence Lifschultz (Stony Creek, CT: Pamphleteer's, 1998), 305.

24. Ibid.

25. Foreword to *Japan's Struggle to End the War,* by US Strategic Bombing Survey (Washington, DC: US Government Printing Office, July 1, 1946).

26. US Strategic Bombing Survey, *Japan's Struggle,* 45.

27. Sean L. Malloy, *Atomic Tragedy: Henry L. Stimson and the Decision to Use the Bomb against Japan* (Ithaca, NY: Cornell University Press, 2008), 162.

28. Warren to Hadden, June 17, 1948, Stafford Warren Papers, UCLA.

29. Nolan to Buettner, October 29, 1947, Stafford Warren Papers, UCLA.

30. Unusual about these photos is the presence of American military in them.

31. Donald Leslie Collins, "Recollections of Nagasaki, 1945," chap. 7 in *Autobiography of Donald Leslie Collins,* 7.24.

32. Ibid., 7.31.

33. Chad R. Diehl, *Resurrecting Nagasaki: Reconstruction and the Formation of Atomic Narratives* (Ithaca, NY: Cornell University Press, 2018), 145–167.

34. Raisuke Shirabe, *A Physician's Diary of the Atomic Bombing and Its Aftermath* (Nagasaki: Nagasaki Association for Hibakushas' Medical Care, 2002), 6–7. Also see Takashi Nagai, *Atomic Bomb Rescue and Relief Report* (Nagasaki: Nagasaki Association for Hibakushas' Medical Care, 2000), 16–17.

35. Warren to Hadden, June 17, 1948, Stafford Warren Papers, UCLA.

36. Shirabe, *Physician's Diary,* 5.

37. Nagai, *Atomic Bomb Rescue,* 4.

38. Shirabe, *Physician's Diary,* 47.

39. Margaret Nobuko Kosuge, "Prompt and Utter Destruction: The Nagasaki Disaster and the Initial Medical Relief," *International Review of the Red Cross* 89, no. 866 (June 2007): 300.

40. Ibid.

41. Quoted in ibid.

42. Ibid., 300–301.

43. Takashi Nagai, *The Bells of Nagasaki,* trans. William Johnston (Tokyo: Kodansha International, 1984), 56–59.

44. Ibid., 90.

45. Ibid., 90–93.

46. Ibid., 93.

47. Ibid., 92. See also Nagai, *Atomic Bomb Rescue,* 7. Here Nagai discusses what he calls "secondary radiation"—that is, radiation that "penetrated substances," causing what he termed a "secondary atomic explosion" or the creation of new radioactive isotopes. The effects of this secondary radiation were evident both among those who, like him and Shirabe, had received initial radiation and among those who "came to the site to clean up after the bombing." John Whittier Treat describes Nagai's work as "the most scientifically accurate first-hand document of the ground-level effects of nuclear weaponry" (John Whittier Treat, *Writing Ground Zero: Japanese Literature and the Atomic Bomb* [Chicago: Chicago University Press, 1995]), 311.

48. Charles B. Degges, "Crater of First A-Bomb Shown to U.S. Newsmen," *Los Angeles Times,* September 12, 1945, 4.

49. Takemae Eiji, *Inside GHQ: The Allied Occupation of Japan and Its Legacy,* trans. Robert Ricketts and Sebastian Swann (New York: Continuum, 2002), 428.

50. Thomas Farrell to Leslie Groves, September 14, 1945, Tinian Files, National Archives, College Park, MD. In this message, Farrell did try to provide something that might be of use to Groves. He observed that a naval doctor had taken some samples of dirt, wood, and metal in the blast area but that "no evidence was disclosed of any radioactivity in the materials collected." It's not clear whether he found no radioactivity or whether he did not disclose to Farrell whatever it was that he found. It's right after this line that he assures Groves of Warren's forthcoming detailed check.

51. Eisei Ishikawa and David L. Swain, trans., *Hiroshima and Nagasaki: The Physical, Medical, and Social Effects of the Atomic Bomb* (New York: Basic Books, 1981), 530.

52. Stafford Warren, *Exceptional Man,* 669.

53. Birchard Brundage to Stafford Warren, November 12, 1947, Warren Papers, UCLA.

54. Stafford Warren, *Exceptional Man,* 613–614.

55. Shirabe, *Physician's Diary,* 49.

56. Ibid., 47.

57. Donald L. Collins, "Pictures from the Past: Journeys into Health Physics in the Manhattan District and Other Diverse Places," in *Health Physics: A Backward Glance: Thirteen Original Papers on the History of Radiation Protection,* ed. Ronald L. Kathren and Paul L. Ziemer (New York: Pergamon, 1980), 41.

58. Collins, "Recollections of Nagasaki," 7.33.

59. In the final report of the Joint Commission, Shirabe and Kitamura are listed under the Nagasaki Medical College team, though it is also noted that "at one time or another all the surviving faculty members and medical students participated in the program of the Joint Commission," which would, of course, include Nagai. Ashley Oughterson et al., *Medical Effects of the Atomic Bombs: The Report of the Joint Commission for the Investigation of the Effects of the Atomic Bomb* (Washington, DC: US Department of Energy, April 19, 1951), 1:vii. Also, in Stafford Warren's files is an envelope of medical examination papers collected from Nagai's home.

60. Shields Warren, oral history interview by Peter D. Olch, October 10, 1972, 71, National Library of Medicine, National Institutes of Health, Bethesda, MD.

61. Quoted in John Dougill, *In Search of Japan's Hidden Christians: A Story of Suppression, Secrecy and Survival* (Tokyo: Tuttle, 2012), 195.

62. Paul Glynn, *A Song for Nagasaki* (San Francisco: Ignatius, 2009), 181–184.

63. Diehl, *Resurrecting Nagasaki,* 106.

64. Glynn, *Song for Nagasaki,* 181–184.

65. Tokusaburo Nagai, interview by author, September 11, 2018.

66. Lifton and Mitchell, *Hiroshima in America,* 13–22.

67. William Laurence, interview by Scott Bruns, March 28, 1964, 377–378, Columbia University Oral History Archives, Columbia University.

68. William L. Laurence, *Dawn over Zero: The Story of the Atomic Bomb* (New York: Alfred A. Knopf, 1946), 235–237.

69. Eileen Welsome, *The Plutonium Files: America's Secret Medical Experiment in the Cold War* (New York: Dial, 1999), 115.

70. As Takemae Eiji puts it, "The ABCC also was widely reviled for refusing to provide medical care. Its mission was to conduct 'pure' research for military, not humanitarian purposes, and scientists were under explicit orders not to render medical assistance to the people they examined. This was a political decision taken in

Washington, where officials feared that aiding victims of the bomb would imply an admission of US guilt, undermining America's moral leadership." Eiji, *Inside GHQ,* 430.

71. M. Susan Lindee, *Suffering Made Real: American Science and the Survivors at Hiroshima* (Chicago: University of Chicago Press, 1994), 128. See also Eiji, *Inside GHQ,* 430: "In fact, however, American and Japanese doctors often disobeyed orders and dispensed treatment, although this was done almost surreptitiously."

72. Shields Warren, interview by Olch, 67.

73. Liebow, "Hiroshima Medical Diary," 110.

74. Tomiko Morimoto West, interview by author, July 10, 2019.

75. Stafford Warren, *Exceptional Man,* 599.

76. Ibid., 608–609.

77. Ibid., 605.

78. David C. Milam, *The Last Bomb: A Marine's Memoirs of Nagasaki* (Austin: Eakin, 2001), 19.

79. Ibid., 605; Collins, "Recollections of Nagasaki," 7.39–40.

80. Collins, "Recollections of Nagasaki," 7.41.

81. Warren recalled the instructions that "had gone down in [his] ranks. 'We're not to have booty stripping. We'll have no assaults or rape. Be polite and don't cause any row.'" Stafford Warren, *Exceptional Man,* 593.

82. Collins, "Recollections of Nagasaki," 7.39.

83. "Part of Groves's ability to control the story lay in his use of secrecy and security classification." Robert S. Norris, *Racing for the Bomb: The True Story of General Leslie R. Groves, the Man behind the Birth of the Atomic Age* (New York: Skyhorse, 2002), 440.

84. Liebow, "Hiroshima Medical Diary," 123.

85. Ibid., 133.

86. James B. Newman Jr. to Leslie Groves, October 5, 1945, Tinian Files, National Archives, College Park, MD.

87. Ibid.

88. Shirabe, *Physician's Diary,* 53–54.

89. Stafford Warren, *Exceptional Man,* 662–663.

90. Michihiko Hachiya, *Hiroshima Diary: The Journal of a Japanese Physician, August 6–September 30, 1945,* trans. and ed. Warner Wells (Chapel Hill: University of North Carolina Press, 1955), 232.

91. Liebow, "Hiroshima Medical Diary," 121, 174.

92. Ibid., 237.

93. Ibid., 238–239.

94. Ibid., 239.

95. Nolan to Buettner, October 29, 1947, Stafford Warren Papers, UCLA.

6. Managing Radiation and the Radiation Narrative

1. Nolan was awarded the citation for Legion of Merit in October 1945 for his work "from June 1943 to July 1945," when he "devised and instituted plans for safeguarding the post against any possible disaster due to the handling of hazardous finished products. He organized and staffed the post medical facilities consisting of a seventy-five-bed hospital and a complete clinic serving five thousand persons. Through his inspiring devotion to duty, superior professional skill and executive ability he contributed in great measure to the elimination of health hazards for the personnel engaged in the vast research and production program necessary to the development of the Atomic Bomb. Captain Nolan's achievements reflect great credit upon himself and the military service." James F. Nolan papers, in the author's possession (hereafter JFN papers). Then in November 1945 he was given a Bronze Service Star for his role as part of the 509th Composite Group and his participation in the Eastern Mandates Campaign—that is, his role in the delivery of the bomb and his service on Tinian Island. JFN papers.

2. Lynne Handy, interview by author, March 23, 2015.

3. Stafford Warren to Major General L. R. Groves, cover letter to "Preliminary Report—Atomic Bomb Investigation," November 27, 1945, Stafford Leak Warren Papers, UCLA Library Special Collections (hereafter Stafford Warren Papers, UCLA).

4. Leslie Groves, testimony, in *Hearings before the Special Committee on Atomic Energy, United States Senate,* Seventy-Ninth Congress (Wednesday, November 28, 1945), 33.

5. Ibid., 31–37.

6. Eileen Welsome, *The Plutonium Files: America's Secret Medical Experiment in the Cold War* (New York: Dial, 1999), 113.

7. Stafford Warren to Leslie Groves, "Preliminary Report—Atomic Bomb Investigation," memo, November 27, 1945, 8, Stafford Warren Papers, UCLA.

8. Ibid., 4.

9. David Bradley, *No Place to Hide* (Boston: Little, Brown, 1948), 199.

10. Stafford Warren, interview by Barton C. Hacker, October 30, 1979, Department of Energy, Nuclear Testing Archive, Las Vegas (hereafter NTA).

11. James F. Nolan, interview by Lansing Lamont, 1965, Harry S. Truman Library, Independence, MO.

12. Groves, testimony, 34.

13. Warren to Groves, "Preliminary Report," memo, 1.

14. Groves, testimony, 36.

15. Ibid.

16. Louis Hempelmann, Clarence C. Lushbaugh, and George L. Voelz, "What Has Happened to the Survivors of the Early Los Alamos Nuclear Accidents?" (October 2, 1979, presented at the Conference for Radiation Accident Preparedness, Oak Ridge,

TN, October 19–20, 1979), 5, Los Alamos National Laboratory Archives (hereafter LANL).

17. Louis H. Hempelmann, Hermann Lisco, and Joseph G. Hoffman, "The Acute Radiation Syndrome: A Study of Nine Cases and a Review of the Problem," *Annals of Internal Medicine* 36, no. 2 (February 1952): 284.

18. Hempelmann, Lushbaugh, and Voelz, "What Has Happened?" 16.

19. L. H. Hempelmann to files, "Accident Report at Omega," July 6, 1945, LANL.

20. James F. Nolan to Stafford Warren, "Additional Medical Activities at Destination," secret memo, August 7, 1945, JFN papers.

21. Hempelmann, "Accident Report at Omega."

22. As Alex Wallerstein puts it, "The exigencies of the Second World War had privileged expediency over safety. . . . The Cold War, in spite of its many anxieties, could be taken at a more steady pace." Alex Wallerstein, "The Demon Core and the Strange Death of Louis Slotin," *New Yorker,* May 21, 2016.

23. J. F. Nolan, "History of Health Group during Interim Period, November 1945 to May 1946," April 16, 1945, LANL.

24. Ibid.

25. Ibid.

26. Quoted in Jonathan Weisgall, *Operation Crossroads: The Atomic Tests at Bikini Atoll* (Annapolis, MD: Naval Institute Press, 1994), 138.

27. Patrick Cleary, "Account of the Parajito Laboratory Accident of 21 May 1946," May 29, 1946, Production Materials for Louis Slotin Sonata, 1946–2006, Collected by Paul Mullin, New York Public Library (hereafter Slotin materials, NYPL).

28. Ibid.

29. Norris Bradbury to Marshall and Roger, memo, May 22–26, 1945, Slotin materials, NYPL.

30. Memo about "Meeting—May 23, 1946 2:30 p.m." to Louis Hempelmann, James F. Nolan, Paul Hageman, Harry O. Whipple, Darol Froman, Phil Morrison, Robinson, Newburger, C. W. Betts, Challis, Slotin materials, NYPL.

31. Norris Bradbury to Roger and Marshall, May 26, 1946, Slotin materials, NYPL.

32. A May 24, 1946, press release from Los Alamos stated, "In answer to inquiries, Dr. Bradbury stated the laboratory accident would not affect the projected Bikini tests." Slotin materials, NYPL.

33. Hempelmann, Lisco, and Hoffman, "Acute Radiation Syndrome," 284–285.

34. Nolan, interview by Lamont.

35. Hempelmann, Lushbaugh, and Voelz, "What Has Happened?," 2. The authors also observe later in the same follow-up study that "one might suspect that the myxedema of Case 4 [Graves], presumably radiation induced, may have promoted his coronary disease by elevating the blood cholesterol. This could well have precipitated the first heart attack." Ibid., 15.

36. C. W. Betts to Leslie Groves, "Radiation Accident at Site Y," May 27, 1946, Slotin materials, NYPL. "Dr. Slotin received a dose of 700 R and Dr. Graves received a dose of about 200 R. Doses of 100 R were received by Kline and Young."

37. N. E. Bradbury to Mrs. June Kline, May 25, 1946, Advisory Committee on Human Radiation Experiments, National Archives (hereafter ACHRE, National Archives), College Park, MD.

38. S. Allan Kline, "Estimated Damages to S. Allan Kline Resulting from Radiation Accident at Los Alamos, New Mexico in 1946," ACHRE, National Archives, College Park, MD.

39. S. Allan Kline to Caroll L. Tyler, March 13, 1951, ACHRE, National Archives.

40. C. L. Tyler to S. Allan Kline, response to March 13, 1951, letter, n.d., ACHRE, National Archives.

41. Clifford T. Honicker, "America's Radiation Victims: The Hidden Files," *New York Times Magazine,* November 19, 1989.

42. Betts to Groves, "Radiation Accident at Site Y," May 27, 1946, Slotin materials, NYPL.

43. "Relative Intensities," compiled 1:00 p.m., May 22, 1946, Slotin materials, NYPL. In another document, Joseph Hoffman provided an estimated dosage for all eight men. According to these estimates, Kline received a minimum of forty-five roentgens, a maximum of one hundred roentgens, and a probable sixty roentgens. "Estimates of Dosage Range," November 7, 1946, ACHRE, National Archives.

44. Louis H. Hempelmann to J. J. Nickson, December 10, 1946, ACHRE, National Archives.

45. Stafford Warren to Colonel K. D. Nichols, "Policy Matters," memo, December 28, 1946, ACHRE, National Archives.

46. Ibid.

47. Louis Hempelmann to Robert Kimball, December 7, 1949, ACHRE, National Archives.

48. Louis Hempelmann, interview by Barton C. Hacker, June 3–4, 1980, NTA.

49. Hempelmann, Lushbaugh, and Voelz, "What Has Happened?" 16.

50. Stafford Warren, testimony, in *Hearings before the Special Committee on Atomic Energy, United States Senate,* Seventy-Ninth Congress (February 15, 1946), 510.

51. James B. Newman Jr. to Leslie Groves, October 5, 1945, Tinian Files, National Archives, College Park, MD.

52. John J. Flick, "Ocular Lesions following the Atomic Bombing of Hiroshima and Nagasaki," *American Journal of Ophthalmology* 31, no. 2 (February 1948): 139.

53. US Strategic Bombing Survey, *The Effects of the Atomic Bombs on Hiroshima and Nagasaki* (Washington, DC: US Government Printing Office, June 30, 1946), 15.

54. Ashley W. Oughterson and Shields Warren, eds., *Medical Effects of the Atomic Bomb in Japan* (New York: McGraw-Hill, 1956), 88–89. See also Harry M. Cullings, in reference to the same report: "From Table 4.4 of that reference, it may be calculated

that -30,000 (42% of 72,000 injured survivors in Hiroshima and 13,000 (51%) of 25,000 injured survivors in Nagasaki were estimated to have sustained 'radiation injury' often in combination with other injuries." Harry M. Cullings, "Impact on the Japanese Atomic Bomb Survivors of Radiation Received from the Bombs," *Health Physics* 106, no. 2 (February 2014): 284.

55. Shields Warren and Rupert Draeger, "The Pattern of Injuries Produced by the Atomic Bombs at Hiroshima and Nagasaki," *U.S. Naval Medical Bulletin* 46, no. 9 (September 1946): 1350.

56. Ibid., 1352–1353.

57. Nello Pace and Robert Smith, "Measurement of the Residual Radiation Intensity at the Hiroshima and Nagasaki Atomic Bomb Sites," (April 16, 1946), Naval Medical Research Institute, 1–3, Stafford Warren Papers, UCLA. See also Averill A. Liebow, Shields Warren, and Elbert De Coursey, "Pathology of Atomic Bomb Casualties," *American Journal of Pathology* 25, no. 5 (1949): 853–1927. Regarding the bombs dropped in Japan, the authors observe, "Potentially of greater significance may be the neutrons, for they can be projected for considerable distance through the atmosphere. Their effectiveness in damaging tissue is several times greater than that of gamma rays, measured in roentgens equivalent physical (rep)." Ibid., 861.

58. Pace and Smith, "Measurement," 2.

59. Eisei Ishikawa and David L. Swain, trans., *Hiroshima and Nagasaki: The Physical, Medical, and Social Effects of the Atomic Bomb* (New York: Basic Books, 1981), 79, 151.

60. Greg Mitchell, *Atomic Cover-Up: Two U.S. Soldiers, Hiroshima and Nagasaki, and the Greatest Movie Never Made* (New York: Sinclair Books, 2012), 30–35; Welsome, *Plutonium Files,* 119.

61. Entry for September 10, 1945, in Diary of Kiyoshi Tanimoto, 101–102, John Hersey Papers, Beinecke Library, Yale University.

62. Welsome, *Plutonium Files,* 119.

63. Mitchell, *Atomic Cover-Up,* 30–31.

64. David C. Milam, *The Last Bomb: A Marine's Memoirs of Nagasaki* (Austin: Eakin, 2001), 23.

65. See Susan Southard, *Nagasaki: Life after Nuclear War* (New York: Penguin, 2015), 223–224; Welsome, *Plutonium Files,* 119; Tetsuji Imanaka et al., "Gamma-Ray Exposure from Neutron-Induced Radionuclides in Soil in Hiroshima and Nagasaki Based on DS02 Calculations," *Radiation and Environmental Biophysics* 47, no. 3 (2008): 331–336; and George D. Kerr et al., "Workshop Report on Atomic Bomb Dosimetry—Residual Radiation Exposure: Recent Research and Suggestions for Future Studies," *Health Physics* 105, no. 2 (2013): 140–149.

66. Stafford Warren to Leslie Groves, "The Use of the Gadget as a Tactical Weapon Based on Observations Made during Test II," July 25, 1945, Stafford Warren Papers, UCLA. Janet Farrell Brodie notes that Warren's memo may have been intentionally ambiguous. She describes it as "a masterful blend of reassurance and of realistically

honest assessment of radiological dangers." Janet Farrell Brodie, "Radiation Secrecy and Censorship after Hiroshima and Nagasaki," *Journal of Social History* 48, no. 4 (2015): 855. Thus, the memo supplied enough "reassurance" for Groves to focus on that which supported his preferred narrative about the effects of radiation.

67. Sean L. Malloy, "'A Very Pleasant Way to Die': Radiation Effects and the Decision to Use the Atomic Bomb against Japan," *Diplomatic History* 36, no. 3 (June 2012): 539; Leslie Groves to George C. Marshall, July 30, 1945, Top Secret, Manhattan Project File, Folder 4, Trinity Test, National Archives, Washington, DC, http://www.nuclearfiles.org/menu/library/correspondence/groves-leslie/corr_groves_1945-07-30.htm.

68. Malloy, "'Pleasant Way to Die,'" 540.

69. Quoted in "No Two-Headed Baby Salmon," *New York Daily News,* April 28, 1957.

70. Leslie Groves to Stafford Warren, May 8, 1958, Stafford Warren Papers, UCLA.

71. Brodie similarly observes that after Trinity, Warren wrote memos to Groves that were intentionally ambiguous and that minimized "the radiation dangers" in order to "placate Groves." Brodie, "Radiation Secrecy," 855.

72. Southard, *Nagasaki,* 224; Brodie, "Radiation Secrecy," 851. Lindee identifies 1962 as the year when the Japanese government began to include "early entrants" as deserving of assistance for medical treatment. Lindee, *Suffering Made Real,* 9.

73. Southard, *Nagasaki,* 177.

74. Radiation Effects Radiation Foundation, *A Brief Description* (Hiroshima: Radiation Effects Radiation Foundation, April 2016), 26–30.

75. Information from permanent exhibit at the Atomic Bomb Medical Museum, Atomic Bomb Disease Institute, Nagasaki University Graduate School of Biomedical Science.

76. Radiation Effects Radiation Foundation, *Brief Description,* 30.

77. Ibid., 31; information from permanent exhibit at the Atomic Bomb Medical Museum, Nagasaki University Graduate School of Biomedical Science.

78. Southard, *Nagasaki.* See also Cullings, "Impact on the Japanese," 281. Cullings writes, "Survivors experienced psychosocial effects such as uncertainty, social stigma, or rejection, and other social pressures." Hiroshima survivor Tomiko Morimoto West had a cousin who had been so injured by the bomb that he "had a hard time finding a wife because of his disfigurement." West also told me of a "very good friend" whose mother had been "a very good-looking lady" but had also been disfigured by the bombing. When her husband returned from overseas after the war, "he divorced her because she was so disfigured." Tomiko Morimoto West, interview by author, July 10, 2019.

79. Deposition of Louis H. Hempelmann, MD, December 20, 1979, 31, *Bernice Lasovick v. United States of America,* LANL.

80. Welsome, *Plutonium Files,* 15–19.

81. Louis Hempelmann to Robert Oppenheimer, "Health Hazards related to Plutonium," August 16, 1944, NTA. Hempelmann wrote, "A great deal of concern has

been expressed during the past two weeks by members of the Chemistry Division about the inability of the Medical Group to detect dangerous amounts of plutonium in the body. This concern was occasioned by the accidental explosion of 10 milligrams of Plutonium in Don Mastick's face."

82. Robert Oppenheimer to Louis Hempelmann, August 16, 1944, NTA.

83. Louis Hempelmann to Robert Oppenheimer, "Medical Research Program," August 29, 1944, NTA.

84. Louis Hempelmann to Robert Oppenheimer, "Meeting of Chemistry Division and Medical Group," March 26, 1945, NTA. It appears that Hempelmann, Warren, Friedell, Joseph W. Kennedy, Arthur Wahl, and Wright Langham attended this meeting.

85. *Advisory Committee on Human Radiation Experiments: Final Report* (Washington, DC: US Government Printing Office, October 1995), 241.

86. Hymer L. Friedell to Commanding Officer, Santa Fe Area, Santa Fe, New Mexico, Attention: Capt. James Nolan, "Shipping of Specimens," April 16, 1945, NTA.

87. Welsome, *Plutonium Files,* 121.

88. *Advisory Committee,* 244.

89. Quoted in Welsome, *Plutonium Files,* 321.

90. Quoted in ibid., 324.

91. *Advisory Committee,* 267.

92. Remarks by President William J. Clinton in acceptance of human radiation final report, October 3, 1995, Old Executive Office Building, Washington, DC.

93. Welsome, *Plutonium Files,* 470.

94. Lynne Handy, interview by author, March 23, 2015.

95. James L. Nolan, "Los Alamos and the Atom Bomb through the Eyes of a Young Boy" (lecture at College of the Holy Cross, Worcester, MA, January 24, 2006).

96. *Advisory Committee,* 267.

97. Quoted in Welsome, *Plutonium Files,* 5.

98. "Osaka University Probe the Atomic Bomb in Depth," *Mainichi Shimbun,* September 14, 1945.

99. Quoted in Samuel Gilbert, "Inside America's Atomic State," Al Jazeera, February 16, 2016, https://www.aljazeera.com/indepth/features/2016/01/america-atomic-state-160107102647937.html

100. *Advisory Committee,* 37.

101. Ibid., 269.

7. Bikini and Enewetak

1. Quoted in Jonathan M. Weisgall, *Operation Crossroads: The Atomic Tests at Bikini Atoll* (Annapolis, MD: Naval Institute Press, 1994), 107.

2. Quoted in Robert C. Kiste, *The Bikinians: A Study of Forced Migration* (Menlo Park, CA: Cummings, 1974), 28.

3. Kisti, *Bikinians,* 22–26; Weisgall, *Operation Crossroads,* 105.

4. Robert Oppenheimer to President Harry S. Truman, "Concerns about Atomic Testing—Cover Letter Attached," May 3, 1946, Digital National Security Archive, President's Secretary File, Harry S. Truman Library.

5. President Harry S. Truman to Dean Acheson, "Concerns about Atomic Testing—Cover Letter Attached," May 7, 1946, Digital National Security Archive, President's Secretary File, Harry S. Truman Library.

6. Quoted in Weisgall, *Operation Crossroads,* 13.

7. Quoted in ibid., 14.

8. Quoted in ibid., 87.

9. James P. Delgado, *Nuclear Dawn: The Atomic Bomb from the Manhattan Project to the Cold War* (Oxford: Osprey, 2009), 151.

10. Stafford Warren, *An Exceptional Man for Exceptional Challenges,* oral history interview by Adelaide Tusler (Los Angeles: UCLA Oral History, 1983), 858.

11. Stafford Warren to James F. Nolan, April 19, 1946, Department of Energy, Nuclear Testing Archive, Las Vegas (hereafter NTA).

12. L. Berkhouse et al., *Operation Crossroads 1946,* United States Atmospheric Nuclear Weapons Tests, Nuclear Test Personnel Review (Washington, DC: Defense Nuclear Agency, Department of Defense, May 1, 1984), 56–57.

13. Stafford Warren, *Exceptional Man,* 855–856.

14. Ibid., 867.

15. Quoted in John Crosby, *Out of the Blue: A Book about Radio and Television* (New York: Simon and Schuster, 1952), 7.

16. Weisgall, *Operation Crossroads,* 199.

17. Ibid., 9.

18. Ibid., 9, 223.

19. "Safety Predictions—Test Baker," 5, Stafford Leak Warren Papers, UCLA Library Special Collections. The document can also be found in NTA.

20. Ibid., 14–16.

21. Weisgall, *Operation Crossroads,* 228; Keith M. Parsons and Robert A. Zaballa, *Bombing the Marshall Islands: A Cold War Tragedy* (New York: Cambridge University Press, 2017), 26.

22. "Forrestal and Blandy Get Close-Up of Sakawa Sinking and Other Ruins," *New York Times,* July 3, 1946.

23. Ibid.

24. Quoted in Weisgall, *Operation Crossroads,* 196.

25. Quoted in "Forrestal and Blandy"; and "Bikini Atom Bomb Not So Powerful as One at Nagasaki, Blandy Says," *New York Times,* July 3, 1946.

26. David Bradley, *No Place to Hide* (Boston: Little, Brown, 1948), 109–110.

27. Quoted in Weisgall, *Operation Crossroads,* 236.

28. Louis Hempelmann, interview by Barton C. Hacker, June 3–4, 1980, NTA.

29. Ibid.

30. Stafford Warren, *Exceptional Man,* 903–904.

31. Ibid., 911.

32. Ibid., 124–126.

33. Quoted in Weisgall, *Operation Crossroads,* 242.

34. Anthony Guarisco, testimony, in *Hearings before the Committee on Veterans' Affairs, United States Senate,* Ninety-Ninth Congress (December 11, 1985), 589. I was told by another researcher that, in an interview with Warren's wife, she confirmed that he had nightmares for years about Crossroads.

35. Quoted in Bradley, *No Place to Hide,* 138.

36. Quoted in ibid., 162–163.

37. Anne Chambers, "A Study of the Relocation of Two Marshallese Atoll Communities," *Kroeber Anthropological Society Papers* 44 (1971): 38.

38. Kiste, *Bikinians,* 112–113.

39. Weisgall, *Operation Crossroads,* 270.

40. R. R. Newell, "Report of Medico-legal Board," August 19, 1946, NTA.

41. Ibid.

42. Weisgall, *Operation Crossroads,* 275–278; Eileen Welsome, *The Plutonium Files: America's Secret Medical Experiment in the Cold War* (New York: Dial, 1999), 174–175. Fred C. Thompson, Operation Crossroads participant and central-east vice president of the National Association of Radiation Survivors, provided evidence during his testimony before the Senate Veterans' Affairs Committee on December 11, 1985. Thompson stated that of 1,054 replies from Operation Crossroads participants, 75 percent had some kind of problem, including "195 cases of cancer, 124 of cardiovascular, 104 deforming arthritis, 90 bone-to-muscle syndrome, 107 genetic effects in offspring, 81 sterile, and 81 dead." Concerning his own medical issues, Thompson stated that about sixteen years after Crossroads, "I began to have a lot of trouble with my joints, especially in my wrist forearms, and shoulders. The joint problems and pain have intensified until I am now in constant pain and walking with difficulty using a cane. I have had both hands operated on and my teeth removed. I have a heart condition, and have just learned I have diabetes. I blame all this on the radiation I received at Operation Crossroads." Fred C. Thompson, testimony, in *Hearings before the Committee on Veterans' Affairs, United States Senate,* Ninety-Ninth Congress (December 11, 1985), 512–513.

43. Weisgall, *Operation Crossroads,* 276; Tom Wicker, "Serving His Country," *New York Times,* August 29, 1983, A19.

44. Jack Adair Tobin, "The Resettlement of the Enewetak People: A Study of a Displaced Community in the Marshall Islands" (PhD diss., University of California, Berkeley, 1967), microfilm, 27.

45. L. H. Berkhouse et al., *Operation Sandstone 1948,* United States Atmospheric Nuclear Weapons Tests, Nuclear Test Personnel Review, DNA 6033F (Washington,

DC: prepared by the Defense Nuclear Agency as executive agency for the Department of Defense, December 19, 1983), 18.

46. Chambers, "Study of the Relocation," 34.

47. "Marshall Islands: A Chronology: 1944–1983" (July 1983), A Publication of the Micronesia Support Committee, Honolulu, Hawaii, 9, David J. Bradley Papers, Rauner Special Collections Library, Dartmouth College.

48. Tobin, "Resettlement of the Enewetak People," 30.

49. Berkhouse et al., *Operation Sandstone 1948,* 2.

50. Barton C. Hacker, *Elements of Controversy: The Atomic Energy Commission and Radiation Safety in Nuclear Weapons Testing, 1947–1974* (Berkeley: University of California Press, 1994), 20.

51. Ibid.

52. Chapter 5 of a military report on Operation Sandstone indicates that the "7.6.8 Advisory Unit," was "commanded or directed by" "J. F. Nolan, AEC." Chapter 8 of the same report notes that "at this time Dr. Nolan, Dr. Whipple, and Captain Knowlton came aboard the BAIROKO to act as advisors on matters of radiological safety." In a February 29, 1948, memo included in an appendix of this report, US Navy Commander Frank Winant lists "Dr. James F. Nolan, Dr. Harry Whipple, and Dr. Norman P. Knowlton, Jr." under the following heading: "Upon reporting to Task Group 7.6 the following civilians are to be further assigned to Task Unit 7.6.8 (ADVISORY UNIT) for primary duty." "Operation Sandstone, Nuclear Explosions, 1948," (March 20, 1948), 37, 58, 162–163, NTA.

53. "Operation Sandstone, Nuclear Explosions, 1948," (March 20, 1948), 6, NTA.

54. J. E. Hull, "Atomic Weapons Tests, Eniwetok Atoll, Operation Sandstone, 1948, Report to the Joint Chiefs of Staff," vol. 1, annex 1, pt. 3, p. 246, NTA.

55. Ibid., 246–247.

56. "Operation Sandstone, Nuclear Explosions, 1948" (March 20, 1948), 27.

57. Ibid.

58. Frank I. Winant Jr., Commander, USN, to Dr. James F. Nolan, Task Group 7.6, May 28, 1948, James F. Nolan papers, in the author's possession.

59. C. Thomas et al., *Analysis of Radiation Exposure for Naval Personnel at Operation Sandstone,* (McLean, VA: prepared by the Science Applications International Corporation for the Defense Nuclear Agency, August 15, 1983), 3, https://www.dtra.mil/Portals/61/Documents/NTPR/4-Rad_Exp_Rpts/5_DNA-TR-83-13_Analysis_of_Rad_Exposure_for_Naval_Personnel_at_Op_SANDSTONE.pdf.

60. Hacker, *Elements of Controversy,* 33.

61. "Operation Sandstone Radiation Injuries," July 27, 1948, 2, Los Alamos National Laboratory Archives.

62. Louis Hempelmann to Robert Stone, June 28, 1948, 2, Los Alamos National Laboratory Archives.

63. Ibid.

64. Hacker, *Elements of Controversy*, 34.

65. Parsons and Zaballa, *Bombing the Marshall Islands*, 65.

66. Ibid., 73–82. In his testimony before the Senate Veterans' Affairs Committee, Robert Conrad acknowledged that three-quarters of the Rongelapese experienced beta burns and that some, years later, developed thyroid tumors. Robert Conrad, testimony, in *Hearings before the Committee on Veterans' Affairs, United States Senate*, Ninety-Ninth Congress (December 11, 1985), 499–500.

67. Susanne Rust, "How the US Betrayed the Marshall Islands, Kindling the Next Nuclear Disaster," *Los Angeles Times*, November 10, 2019; Trevor Nace, "Fears Grow That 'Nuclear Coffin' Is Leaking Waste into the Pacific," *Forbes*, May 27, 2019. Nace places the amount in the Runit Dome at "73,000 cubic meters of radioactive soil," or 2.58 million cubic feet, as does Kyle Swenson in "The U.S. Put Nuclear Waste under a Dome on a Pacific Island. Now It Is Cracking Open," *Washington Post* blogs, May 20, 2019, https://www.washingtonpost.com/nation/2019/05/20/us-put-nuclear-waste-under-dome-pacific-island-now-its-cracking-open/.

68. Rust, "How the US Betrayed."

69. Walter J. Hickel, *Who Owns America* (Englewood Cliffs, NJ: Prentice-Hall, 1971), 208.

70. David Bradley, testimony, in *Hearings before the Committee on Veterans' Affairs, United States Senate*, Ninety-Ninth Congress (December 11, 1985), 490.

71. Ibid, 491–492.

72. Ibid., 487.

73. Ibid., 487, 492.

8. Dr. Nolan and the Quandary of Technique

1. Robert Futoran, interview by author, April 10, 2019. See also James F. Nolan, Juan Araujo Vidal, and John H. Anson, "Early Experiences in the Treatment of Carcinoma of the Uterine Cervix with Cobalt-60 Teletherapy and Intracavitary Radium," *American Journal of Obstetrics and Gynecology* 72, no. 4 (October 1956): 789–803. In this article, Nolan, Vidal, and Anson note that on July 1, 1948, they began to treat patients using a "450 kv.; 5 mm. Cu H.V.L. x-ray apparatus" for the purposes of external radiation therapy (789). This is likely the device provided to Nolan by the military.

2. Lynne Handy, interview by author, September 4, 2015.

3. James L. Nolan, "Los Alamos and the Atom Bomb through the Eyes of a Young Boy" (lecture at College of the Holy Cross, Worcester, MA, January 24, 2006).

4. Carl Maag et al., *Shot Hood: A Test of the Plumbbob Series*, United States Atmospheric Nuclear Weapons Tests, Nuclear Test Personnel Review (Washington, DC: Defense Nuclear Agency, Department of Defense, May 13, 1983), 18.

5. According to the Atomic Heritage Foundation, as of April 2018, the government had received 34,372 claims and paid out over $2 billion in settlements for

Nevada downwinders and others affected by radiation from nuclear testing. "Nevada Test Site Downwinders," Atomic Heritage Foundation, July 31, 2018, https://www.atomicheritage.org/history/nevada-test-site-downwinders.

6. Albert Borgmann, "Technology as a Cultural Force: For Alena and Griffin," *Canadian Journal of Sociology* 31, no. 2 (2006): 353.

7. Ibid., 353–354.

8. A diagram of the "Nolan applicator" is included in the 1963 publication of *Cancer of the Female Reproductive Organs.* As described in figure 49 of the book, "Diagrammatic illustration of the Nolan applicator. Angle of the tandem is adjustable, and removable ovoids of different sizes are available. Filtration is included within the ovoids to decrease radiation of the rectum and bladder." Alfred I. Sherman, *Cancer of the Female Reproductive Organs* (St. Louis: C. V. Mosby, 1963), 111.

9. James F. Nolan and Edith Quimby, "Dosage Calculations for Various Combinations of Parametrial Needles and Intracervical Tandems," *Radiology* 40, no. 4 (April 1943): 391–402; James F. Nolan and William Stambo, "Dosage Calculations for Various Plans of Intravaginal X-Ray Therapy," *Radiology* 49, no. 4 (1947): 462–475; James F. Nolan and James P. Steele, "Carinoma of the Endometrium: Measurements of the Radiation Distribution around Various Multiple Capsule Applications of Radium in Irregular Uteri," *Radiology* 51, no. 2 (1948): 166–176; Alfred Sherman, James F. Nolan, and Willard M. Allen, "The Experimental Application of Radioactive Colloidal Gold in the Treatment of Pelvic Cancer," *American Journal of Roentgenology and Radium Therapy* 64, no. 1 (1950): 75–85; James F. Nolan, "Cancer of the Cervix, Vulva, and Vagina," *California Medicine* 99, no. 3 (September 1963): 189–196; James F. Nolan, C. Paul Morrow, and John Anson, "Factors Influencing Prognosis," *Gynecologic Oncology* 2 (1974): 300–307; Wilfredo Hernandez-Linares et al., "Carcinoma In Situ of the Vagina: Past and Present Management," *Obstetrics and Gynecology* 56, no. 3 (September 1980): 356–360; Neville F. Hacker et al., "Superficially Invasive Vulvar Cancer with Noda Metastases," *Gynecologic Oncology* 15 (1983): 65–77.

10. James F. Nolan, "The Risks and Hazards Thereof" (presidential address at the Fifty-Third Annual Meeting of the American Radium Society, Mexico City, March 15–18, 1971), published in *American Journal of Roentgenology* 114, no. 1 (January 1972): 3.

11. Ibid., 4.

12. Ibid.

13. Nolan's colleague Robert Futoran remembers that he and Nolan would wear film badges for detecting radiation once every thirty days and would record the level of exposure as though it were for the full thirty days, thus significantly underrepresenting how much radiation they were actually getting. Futoran, interview by author.

14. Nolan, "Risks and Hazards Thereof," 4.

15. Ibid.

16. Ibid., 5.

17. "From Alamogordo to Los Angeles Tumor Unit," *Medical Tribune,* May 4, 1970, 4; Lynne Handy, interview by author, September 4, 2015.

18. Lynne Handy, interview by author, March 23, 2015.

19. Nolan, "Risks and Hazards Thereof," 5.

20. Ibid.

21. Ibid. Nolan is referring to the story of the ten lepers in the Gospel of Luke 17:11–19.

22. Nolan, "Risks and Hazards Thereof," 5.

23. Ibid., 6.

24. Futoran, interview by author.

25. Nolan, "Risks and Hazards Thereof," 6.

26. Borgmann, "Technology as a Cultural Force," 353.

27. William Laurence, interview by Scott Bruns, March 28, 1964, 374, Oral History Archives, Columbia University.

28. Ibid., 378.

29. Ray Kurzweil, *The Singularity Is Near: When Humans Transcend Biology* (London: Penguin Books, 2005), 28.

30. Quoted in Christianna Reedy, "Kurzweil Claims That the Singularity Will Happen by 2045," Futurism, October 5, 2017, https://futurism.com/kurzweil-claims-that-the-singularity-will-happen-by-2045. See also Kelly McSweeney, "Ray Kurzweil Predictions Persist: Is Technological Singularity Next?," *Now,* January 31, 2019, https://now.northropgrumman.com/ray-kurzweil-predictions-persist-turns-70/.

31. Kurzweil, *Singularity Is Near,* 29.

32. Neil Postman, *Building a Bridge to the 18th Century* (New York: Alfred A. Knopf, 1999), 42.

33. Borgmann, "Technology as a Cultural Force," 353.

34. Jon Else, *The Day after Trinity: Robert Oppenheimer and the Atomic Bomb* (New York: Voyager, 1995), CD-ROM.

35. Quoted in Else, *The Day after Trinity,* supplemental files, 50.

36. Chevalier quoting Oppenheimer in Else, *The Day after Trinity,* supplemental files, 51.

37. Jacques Ellul, "The Technological Order," *Technology and Culture* 3, no. 4, Proceedings of the Encyclopedia Britannica Conference on the Technological Order (Autumn 1962): 394.

38. Jeffrey P. Greenman, Read Mercer Schuchardt, and Noah J. Toly, *Understanding Jacques Ellul* (Eugene, OR: Cascade Books, 2012), 23.

39. Greenman, Schuchardt, and Toly summarize this point: "Technique can become the all-embracing consciousness of the mechanical world." Ibid. *Technique,* according to Ellul, refers to "the totality of methods rationally arrived at and having absolute efficiency (for a given stage of development) in every field of human activity." Jacques Ellul, *The Technological Society* (New York: Alfred A. Knopf, 1964), xxv.

40. Ellul, "Technological Order," 410. On this point, see also Robert Wuthnow, *Restructuring of American Religion* (Princeton, NJ: Princeton University Press, 1988).

41. Ellul, *Technological Society,* 96.

42. Ellul writes, "Scholars now generally agree that the watershed between the older society and the typical society dominated by technique came around 1945." Jacques Ellul, *Perspectives of Our Age,* ed. Willem H. Vanderburg (Berkeley: Anansi, 1981), 28.

43. Ellul, *Technological Society,* 95. See also Sonya D. Schmid, "Data, Discourse, and Disruption: Radiation Effects and Nuclear Orders," in *The Age of Hiroshima*, ed. Michael D. Gordin and G. John Ikenberry (Princeton, NJ: Princeton University Press, 2020), 243–258. Schmid observes that "the Chernobyl catastrophe exposed the artificiality of the distinction between military and peaceful applications that had taken decades to set up and had come to appear as natural." Schmid, "Data, Discourse, and Distruption," 254.

44. Kenneth Glazier, "The Decision to Use Atomic Weapons against Hiroshima and Nagasaki," *Public Policy* 18 (Winter 1969): 515.

45. Quoted in Samuel A. Goudsmit, *Alsos* (Los Angeles: Tomash, 1947), 76.

46. Ellul, *Technological Society,* 99.

47. Nolan, "Risks and Hazards Thereof," 6.

48. Thomas Hughes, *American Genesis: A Century of Invention and Technological Enthusiasm, 1870–1970* (Chicago: University of Chicago Press, 2004).

49. Quoted in Else, *Day after Trinity,* supplemental files, 108.

50. Ibid.

51. US Atomic Energy Commission, *In the Matter of J. Robert Oppenheimer: Transcript of Hearing before the Personnel Security Board, April 13, 1954* (Washington, DC: US Government Printing Office, 1954), 2:266.

52. Bill Joy, "Why the Future Doesn't Need Us," *Wired,* April 2000, 243.

53. Ellul, *Technological Society,* 87.

54. Joy, "Why the Future," 243.

55. Ibid., 250.

56. Ibid., 256.

57. See Joseph Masco, *The Nuclear Borderlands: The Manhattan Project in Post–Cold War New Mexico* (Princeton, NJ: Princeton University Press, 2006), 24–25.

58. Ibid., 25.

59. Ellul, "Technological Order," 412.

60. Ibid.

61. Nicholas Carr, *The Shallows: What the Internet Is Doing to Our Brains* (New York: W. W. Norton, 2010); David Rothenberg, "How the Web Destroys the Quality of Students' Research Papers," *Chronicle of Higher Education,* August 15, 1997, A44; Mark Bauerlein, *The Dumbest Generation: How the Digital Age Stupifies Young Americans and Jeopardizes Our Future* (New York: Penguin, 2008); David Shenck, *The End of Patience* (Bloomington: Indiana University Press, 1999); Sherry Turkle, *Alone Together:*

Why We Expect More from Technology and Less from Each Other (New York: Basic Books, 2011); Nicholas Carr, "Is Google Making Us Stupid?," *Atlantic,* July / August 2008.

62. See Robert Putman, *Bowling Alone: The Collapse and Revival of American Community* (New York: Simon and Schuster, 2000). Putnam sees "cyberbalkanization," the phenomenon by which the "Internet enables us to confine our communication to people who share precisely our interests," as a threat to "bridging social capital." Ibid., 177–178. It seems the term *cyberbalkanization* was coined by Marshall Van Alstyne and Erik Brynjolfsson in a related discussion in their paper "Electronic Communities: Global Village or Cyberbalkans," March 1996, http://web.mit.edu/marshall/www/papers/CyberBalkans.pdf.

63. Katrina Brooker, "'I Was Devastated': Tim Berners-Lee, the Man Who Created the World Wide Web, Has Some Regrets," *Vanity Fair,* August 2018, https://www.vanityfair.com/news/2018/07/the-man-who-created-the-world-wide-web-has-some-regrets; "30 Years On, What's Next #ForTheWeb?," Web Foundation, March 12, 2019, https://webfoundation.org/2019/03/web-birthday-30/.

64. "30 Years On."

65. Ibid. See also Tim Berners-Lee, "I Invented the Web. We Can Fix It," *New York Times,* November 29, 2019, A29. Here Berners-Lee writes, "I had hoped that 30 years from its creation we would be using the web foremost for the purposes of serving humanity. . . . However, the reality is much more complex. Communities are being ripped apart as prejudice, hate, and disinformation are peddled online. Scammers use the web to steal identities, stalkers use it to harass and intimidate their victims, and bad actors subvert democracy using clever digital tactics. The use of targeted political ads in the United States' 2020 presidential campaign and in elections elsewhere threatens once again to undermine voters' understanding and choices."

66. Brooker, "'I Was Devastated.'"

67. Ibid.

68. Greg Milner, *Pinpoint: How GPS Is Changing Technology, Culture, and Our Minds* (New York: Norton, 2016), 111–137.

69. Ibid., xviii–xix.

70. Michael Sandel, *The Case against Perfection* (Cambridge, MA: Harvard University Press, 2007). On this point, see especially chapter 3 of Sandel's book.

71. D. T. Max, "Beyond Human," *National Geographic,* April 2017, 40–63; "Brave New Dialogue," editorial, *Nature Genetics* 51, no. 365 (2019), https://www.nature.com/articles/s41588-019-0374-2.

72. Joy, "Why the Future," 248.

73. Ferenc Morton Szasz, *The Day the Sun Rose Twice: The Story of the Trinity Site Nuclear Explosion, July 16, 1945* (Albuquerque: University of New Mexico Press, 1984), 152.

74. Quoted in ibid., 157.

75. Ibid.

76. Peter Berger, *Invitation to Sociology: A Humanistic Perspective* (New York: Anchor Books, 1963), 121, 176.

77. Ellul, "Technological Order," 410.

78. Borgmann, "Technology as a Cultural Force," 359.

79. Wuthnow, *Restructuring of American Religion,* 268–296.

80. Borgmann, "Technology as a Cultural Force," 360.

81. Ellul, *Technological Society,* xxvii.

82. Ibid., xxxi.

83. Ibid., xxxiii.

84. Peter Berger, *Invitation to Sociology,* 176.

85. Ellul, *Technological Society,* xxix, xxxi.

86. Ibid., xxxii.

87. Sean L. Malloy, "'A Very Pleasant Way to Die': Radiation Effects and the Decision to Use the Atomic Bomb against Japan," *Diplomatic History* 36, no. 3 (June 2012): 526–528.

88. Ellul, *Technological Society,* xxxiii.

89. Ibid., xxxi.

90. Nolan, "Risks and Hazards Thereof," 6.

9. 1983

1. Robert S. Norris and Hans M. Kristensen, "Global Nuclear Weapons Inventories, 1945–2010," *Bulletin of the Atomic Scientists* 66, no. 4 (2010): 81.

2. Matt Novak, "Reagan Thought This 1983 Nuclear Apocalypse Movie Validated His Nuclear Policy," *Paleofuture* (blog), Gizmodo, April 17, 2017, quoting Reagan's diary entry of October 10, 1983, https://paleofuture.gizmodo.com/reagan-thought-this-1983-nuclear-apocalypse-movie-valid-1794377982.

3. Quoted in Dawn Stover, "Facing Nuclear Reality: 35 Years after *The Day After,*" *Bulletin of the Atomic Scientists,* December 13, 2018, https://thebulletin.org/facing-nuclear-reality-35-years-after-the-day-after/.

4. National Conference of Catholic Bishops, *The Challenge of Peace: God's Promise and Our Response: A Pastoral Letter on War and Peace* (Washington, DC: US Conference of Catholic Bishops, May 3, 1983), 2, http://www.usccb.org/issues-and-action/human-life-and-dignity/war-and-peace/nuclear-weapons/upload/statement-the-challenge-of-peace-1983-05-03.pdf.

5. Greg Mitchell, *Atomic Cover-Up: Two Soldiers, Hiroshima and Nagasaki, and the Greatest Movie Never Made* (New York: Sinclair Books, 2012).

6. "Los Alamos," *Our Times with Bill Moyers,* June 26, 1983, CBS News Archives.

7. Ibid.

8. Hans Bethe, "The Technological Imperative," *Bulletin of the Atomic Scientists* 41, no. 7 (August 1985): 34–36.

9. Victor Weisskopf, "Los Alamos Anniversary: 'We Meant So Well,'" *Bulletin of the Atomic Scientists* 39, no. 7 (August / September 1983): 24–26.

10. Ibid., 25.

11. Ibid., 26.

12. Ferenc Morton Szasz, *The Day the Sun Rose Twice: The Story of the Trinity Site Nuclear Explosion, July 16, 1945* (Albuquerque: University of New Mexico Press, 1984), 176.

13. Paul Olum, "Hiroshima: Memoir of a Bomb Maker . . . 'the Gadget,'" History News Network, Columbian College of Arts and Sciences, George Washington University, July 5, 2002, http://hnn.us/articles/171.html. Olum's previously unpublished memoir was supplied to the History News Network by George Beres.

14. Ibid.

15. "Frightened for the Future of Humanity," *New York Times*, April 24, 1983, E21. The reprinted version of Olum's petition letter is introduced in the *New York Times* with the following: "The following statement was signed by 70 scientists who contributed to the development of the first atomic bomb, in 1943."

16. Ibid.

17. Most of the signatures on the Szilard petition were of scientists at the Met Lab in Chicago. Copies of Szilard's petition made it to Los Alamos, but Oppenheimer shut down support of the document. See Peter Wyden, *Day One: Before Hiroshima and After* (New York: Simon and Schuster, 1984), 177–179.

18. Gregg Herken, "Mad about the Bomb," *Harper's*, December 1983, 55.

19. Ann Nolan to James F. Nolan, September 21, 1945, James F. Nolan papers, in the author's possession.

20. Ibid.

21. James F. Nolan, interview by Ferenc Szasz, May 24, 1983, Ferenc M. Szasz Papers, Center for Southwest Research, University of New Mexico Library, Albuquerque.

22. Bill Reynolds, interview by author, December 10, 2018.

23. Ibid.

24. Lynne Handy, interview by author, March 23, 2015.

25. "From Alamogordo to Los Angeles Tumor Institute," *Medical Tribune Report*, May 4, 1970.

26. P. Siemes, "Atomic Bomb on Hiroshima, Eyewitness Account of P. Siemes," trans. Averill Liebow, 18, Medical History Library, Yale University.

27. Noah Bierman, "Trump Warns North Korea of 'Fire and Fury,'" *Los Angeles Times*, August 8, 2017.

28. Quoted in "Dad's Images of Death," *Las Vegas Review-Journal*, August 6, 2007, https://www.reviewjournal.com/news/dads-images-of-death/.

29. Lynne Handy, interview by author, March 23, 2015.

30. Quoted in "Dad's Images of Death," *Las Vegas Review-Journal,* August 6, 2007, https://www.reviewjournal.com/news/dads-images-of-death/.

31. "10 Year Old Boy Carries Dead Baby Bro to Cremation," *Editor's Journal* (blog), August 8, 2014, https://theeditorsjournal.wordpress.com/2014/08/05/10-year-old-boy-carries-dead-baby-bro-to-cremation/.

32. Quoted in Douglas Martin, "Joe O'Donnell, 85, Dies; Long a Leading Photographer," *New York Times,* August 14, 2007.

33. Quoted in Joe O'Donnell, *Japan 1945: A U.S. Marine's Photographs from Ground Zero* (Nashville: Vanderbilt University Press, 2005), 84; and Szasz, *Day the Sun Rose Twice,* 157.

34. Wyden, *Day One,* 363–364.

35. "Medical Center Opens," *New Mexican* (Santa Fe), January 27, 1952, clipping of article, with handwritten note, in JFN papers.

Acknowledgments

Researching this book was a great adventure, and I was aided by many people and institutions along the way. In the early stages of the project, I enjoyed a semester of leave at the Oakley Center for the Humanities and Social Sciences. While at the Oakley Center, I presented material from what eventually became Chapter 7 and benefited from the comments of the other Oakley fellows. I also twice presented material from the project in our department's colloquium series and received welcome feedback from my colleagues in the Anthropology and Sociology Department at Williams College. Several student research assistants, including Ashley Arnold, Erin Curley, Marianna Garcia, Joyce Tseng, and Ashley Villareal, assisted me on various parts of the book project. In 2019, I spent a semester as a fellow at the Institute for Human Ecology and visiting professor in sociology at the Catholic University of America. I thank both Brandon Vaidyanathan and Joseph Capizzi for providing me with the time and space to research and write during this phase. While in Washington, DC, I presented material from the book in a variety of venues and had engaging conversations about the project with, among others, Vincent Kiernan and William Saunders.

I visited and / or collected material from a number of archives and was assisted by the courteous and resourceful staff at these institutions: the Los Alamos National Lab; the Nuclear Testing Archive in Las Vegas; the Los Alamos Historical Society; the Center for Southwest Research at the University of New Mexico, Albuquerque; the National Archives in College Park, Maryland; the Library of Congress; the Yale University Medical Historical Library; the Beinecke Library at Yale University; the New York Public

Library; Rauner Special Collections Library at Dartmouth College; the Indianapolis Historical Society; the US Naval Institute Research Library; Bernard Becker Medical Library at the Washington University School of Medicine; the Howard Gotlieb Archival Research Center at Boston University; the Harry S. Truman Library; Special Collections of the Charles E. Young Research Library at the University of California, Los Angeles; the San Ildefonso Pueblo Museum; the CBS News Archives; the Hiroshima Memorial Peace Museum; the Atomic Bomb Medical Museum at Nagasaki University; the Nagasaki Atomic Bomb Museum; the Museum of Medical History at the Hiroshima University School of Medicine; and the library at the Radiation Effects Research Foundation in Hiroshima.

A 1945 World Fellowship funded my research in Japan. In Nagasaki, Hiroshima, and Tokyo, I gained much from conversations with (and was given useful material by) several people, including Masako Fukushima, Eric J. Grant, Akiko Kubota, Michael Milward, Kazuo Miyata, Tokusaburo Nagai, Rie Nakanishi, Ohtsura Niwa, Mayumi Oda, Mari Shimomura, Stanislaus Keisaka Shionoya, Tasaki Toru, Robert Ullrich, and Kenichi Yokota.

I received invaluable input from family and friends who generously shared their memories of my grandfather, including Robert Futoran, Karen Nolan, Eric Thorson, John Reynolds, Marta Reynolds, Kate Campion, Chris Nolan, Annie Games, Alice Judd, and Clare Nolan. Especially helpful was the input I received from Lynne Handy and Bill Reynolds, both of whom kindly read a draft of the manuscript. I also owe thanks to my late and beloved father, who saved and protected the small secret archive that served as the inspiration for this book.

I'm grateful to Michael Aronson and Nicholas Carr, who read and thoughtfully commented on early drafts of the manuscript, and to Jonathan Imber, who did the same with a later version. Renee Fox, David C. Schindler, and Will Nolan read and offered useful input on sections of the book. Yumi Farwell aided me with translation work. John Forbes was the first to draw my attention to the life and work of the Nagasaki radiologist Takashi Nagai, while Pia Joliffe, at a later stage, offered additional input on Nagai. Tina Cordova was a valuable resource for information on the Trinity downwinders, as were Barbara Kent and Bob Keller. Joyce Landsverk shared important papers and photos from her father, Donald Collins, on his time in Japan after the end of World War II. Gregg Herken and Ken Olum aided me with information on the fortieth-anniversary reunion in

Los Alamos, and Sasha Davis provided a template for an updated map of the Marshall Islands.

Input from Sara Vladic, Lynn Vincent, and Atsuko Iida deepened my understanding of the story of the USS *Indianapolis*. Discussions with Jack Niedenthal and Jonathan Weisgall were instructive regarding US involvement in the Marshall Islands. I also benefited from conversations with Chad Diehl on the postwar history of Nagasaki; Tomiko Morimoto West on her experience in Hiroshima during and after the August 6 bombing; David Furman on his father's travels with my grandfather; Rose Frisch, Henry Frisch, and Andrew Hanson on James F. Nolan's work at the Los Alamos Hospital; Mary Kirby on some of the developments discussed in Chapter 8; and Cindy Kelly on the Manhattan Project in general. I had many helpful discussions with the historian Jessica Chapman, with whom I cotaught a course on the early nuclear age at Williams College.

I owe a great deal to Ian Malcolm, my editor at Harvard University Press. To work with so supportive, intelligent, and competent an editor as Ian has been a much-appreciated gift. Finally, I thank Cathy, whose wisdom, patience, and direct advice have deeply influenced this work, as well as the thinking and perspective of the one who wrote it.

Illustration Credits

Page 10: Human Radiation Experiments / Atomic Heritage Foundation
Pages 16, 18, 54 (top and bottom), 66, 67, 72, 73, 78, 88, 92, 93, 94 (top and bottom), 108, 114, 115, 143, 173, 177, 199, 227, 230: James F. Nolan papers, in the author's possession
Pages 20, 23: Los Alamos Historical Society
Pages 39, 43, 46, 147: Los Alamos National Laboratory Archives
Pages 95, 97, 98: Mainishi Shimbun
Page 99: Averill A. Liebow Collection / Yale University Archives
Page 102: US Army White Sands Missile Range Public Affairs Office
Page 103: AP Photo
Pages 109, 116: © James L. Nolan, Jr.
Page 120: Tokusaburo Nagai
Page 124: Surveys of Hiroshima and Nagasaki / Atomic Heritage Foundation
Page 126 (top): Stafford Leak Warren Papers, UCLA Library Special Collections
Page 126 (bottom): David and Joyce Landsverk
Pages 168, 181, 183: David J. Bradley Papers, Rauner Special Collections Library, Dartmouth College Library
Page 175, 176, 178: US Navy
Page 186: Sasha Davis
Page 193: Wikimedia Commons
Page 223: Gregg Herken
Page 232: Joe O'Donnell

Index

Index

Index

Index

Index

Index

Index